CLINICAL ONCOLOGY

CLINICAL ONCOLOGY

Basic principles and practice

Third Edition

ANTHONY J NEAL MD MRCP FRCR

Consultant in Clinical Oncology at St. Luke's Cancer Centre, Guildford, Surrey, UK

PETER J HOSKIN MD MR FRCP FRCR

Consultant in Clinical Oncology at Mount Vernon Hospital, Northwood, Middlesex and Reader in Oncology at Royal Free and University College London Medical Schools, UK

A member of the Hodder Headline Group
LONDON

First published in Great Britain in 1997
This impression reprinted in 2003 by
Arnold, a member of the Hodder Headline Group,
338 Euston Road, London NW1 3BH
Second impression 1998

Co-published in the United States of America by
Oxford University Press Inc.,
198 Madison Avenue, New York, NY 10016
Oxford is a registered trademark of Oxford University Press

Whilst the advice and information in this book are believed to be true and
accurate at the date of going to press, neither the authors nor the publisher
can accept any legal responsibility or liability for any errors or omissions
that may be made. In particular (but without limiting the generality of the
preceding disclaimer) every effort has been made to check drug dosages;
however, it is still possible that errors have been missed. Furthermore,
dosage schedules are constantly being revised and new side-effects
recognized. For these reasons the reader is strongly urged to consult the
drug companies' printed instructions before administering any of the drugs
recommended in this book.

British Library Cataloguing in Publication Data
A catalogue record for this book is available from the British Library

Library of Congress Cataloging-in-Publication Data
A catalog record for this book is available from the Library of Congress

ISBN 0 340 76409 0   2401561x.

2 3 4 5 6 7 8 9 10

Commissioning Editor: Joanna Koster
Production Editor: James Rabson
Production Controller: Deborah Smith
Cover Design: Terry Griffiths

Papers used in this book are natural, renewable and recyclable products.
They are made from wood grown in sustainable forests. The logging and
manufacturing processes conform to the environmental regulations of the
country of origin.

Typeset in 9/11 Palatino by Charon Tec Pvt. Ltd, Chennai, India
Printed and bound in Spain

What do you think about this book? Or any other Arnold title?
Please send your comments to **feedback.arnold@hodder.co.uk**

CONTENTS

PREFACE

Approximately 1 million people in the European Union die from malignant disease each year, representing approximately one in four of all deaths. Many more will develop cancer but will be successfully treated for it. The management of cancer patients will therefore form a significant part of the daily practice of most doctors in clinical specialities and general practice.

This concise textbook has been written to provide an insight into the basic principles and practice of clinical oncology. With both general and site-specific chapters, it provides a readily available source of information on the epidemiology, aetiology, pathology, presentation, staging, management and prognosis of malignant disease. Recent advances and topical issues are covered. Whilst written primarily for undergraduates in medicine, the content is also highly relevant to junior doctors, nurses with an interest in oncology and other healthcare professionals who wish to acquire a core of basic knowledge in this field. The text of this third edition has been fully revised, the statistics updated and many new figures added to illustrate key points.

A. J. Neal and P. J. Hoskin
2002

1 PATHOGENESIS OF CANCER

Pathogenesis is defined as 'the manner of development of a disease'. An understanding of the causes of a given cancer is an integral part of formulating strategies for successful treatment, screening and prevention. We owe much of our current understanding to epidemiologists who have discovered associations between different cancers and a number of genetic and environmental factors. In many cases, these lead directly to malignancy (e.g. smoking and lung cancer). It is becoming increasingly clear that changes in the host genome are the final common pathway in the process of carcinogenesis whatever the initial aetiology. However, in most patients with cancer it is still not possible to identify why that particular person developed cancer.

GENETIC FACTORS

The 23 pairs of human chromosomes contain the genetic material of the cell made up of unique sequences of deoxyribonucleic acid (DNA) base pairs which code for the amino acid building blocks of proteins responsible for all the basic metabolic processes that enable the individual cells to survive, reproduce and express properties characteristic of their tissue of origin. Subtle changes in the genes comprising the chromosome may lead to a malignant tumour characterized by loss of the normal cellular mechanisms responsible for control of proliferation, cell differentiation, programmed cell death (apoptosis), cellular organization and cellular adhesion. The uncoupling of the usual balance between cell loss and multiplication leads to growth of the tumour and its subsequent invasion both locally and at distant sites.

Over the last few decades, the field of molecular biology has made great progress in elucidating the likely mechanisms of carcinogenesis. Much of this is due to the development of techniques for the isolation and identification of genetic material such as the polymerase chain reaction and gel electrophoresis. It is becoming apparent that genetic aberrations can be found in the majority of human cancers. The site of the genes responsible can be inferred by 'linkage studies' on individual members of families in which there is an inherited pattern of cancer incidence. The known positions of marker genes are used to deduce where the cancer gene lies along a given chromosome. The gene can then be sequenced, cloned and used to test patients thought to harbour the gene.

Factors suggesting a genetic predisposition to cancer include:

- family clustering of a specific type(s) of cancer
- cases occurring in very young individuals relative to the age distribution of that cancer within the rest of the population
- associations noted between different tumour types
- multiplicity of cancers, e.g. bilaterality

The genetic aberrations associated with cancer can be classified according to whether they are associated with activated oncogenes or tumour suppressor genes.

ACTIVATED ONCOGENES

These are genes which, when expressed, code for a protein that is related in some way to the proliferative cycle of cells or cell differentiation. These products may be growth factors, growth factor receptors on the cell surface or the chemicals that transmit the receptor signals from the cytoplasm to the nucleus. These oncogenes are well preserved throughout the evolutionary scale, remaining very similar right down to primitive organisms such as yeasts. Their overexpression or amplification leads to uncoupling of the usual cell loss/gain equilibrium in favour of cell multiplication, resulting in an increase in cell numbers and ultimately a clinically apparent tumour. They are activated during the intense cell proliferation and differentiation of embryogenesis, but in the mature cells are suppressed by regulating genes at other points along the chromosome. DNA strand breaks (e.g. due to ionizing radiation or chemical carcinogens) with aberrant repair or translocations of genetic material may lead to loss of the genes responsible for regulation of a given oncogene. This may in turn lead to its activation.

The best-characterized example is that of the Philadelphia chromosome of chronic myeloid leukaemia, which is confined to the malignant clone and can be identified in 95 per cent of patients with the disease. There is a translocation of part of chromosome 9 to chromosome 22 and vice versa, placing the *abl* oncogene from chromosome 9 adjacent to the breakpoint cluster region (*bcr*) on chromosome 22. The fusion of these genes leads to the transcription of a protein with tyrosine kinase activity, which leads to leukaemic transformation by increasing myelocyte proliferation.

TUMOUR SUPPRESSOR GENES

Each cell has one of a pair of tumour suppressor genes on each homologous chromosome, and both must be inactivated for the cancer to develop. This means that individuals from a 'cancer family' with only a single gene inherited owing to a 'germ line' mutation have a normal phenotype, act as carriers, but will develop cancer if the second gene is lost because of a somatic mutation or other form of genetic miscoding. Normal individuals must lose both genes by a somatic mutation for a sporadic cancer to develop. Thus, tumour suppressor genes cause cancer not by amplification or overexpression (as with oncogenes) but by loss of their function.

The best known example of a tumour suppressor gene is the *P53* gene which has been called 'the guardian of the genome' and is found to be mutated in the majority of sporadic cancers. It is also mutated

TABLE 1.1   Inherited diseases associated with the development of cancer

Disease	Type of cancer
Autosomal dominant	
Familial polyposis coli	Adenoma/carcinoma of the colon/rectum
Gardener's syndrome	Adenoma/carcinoma of the colon/rectum
Multiple endocrine neoplasia	Endocrinologically active adenomata types I and II (see Chapter 14)
von Recklinghausen's disease	Neurofibromas, schwannoma, phaeochromocytoma
Palmar/plantar tylosis	Carcinoma of the oesophagus
Gorlin's syndrome	Basal cell carcinoma of skin, medulloblastoma
von Hippel–Lindau disease	Cerebellar haemangioblastoma, hypernephroma
Autosomal recessive	
Albinism	Melanoma, basal cell and squamous cell carcinomas of the skin
Xeroderma pigmentosum	Melanoma, basal cell and squamous cell carcinomas of the skin
Ataxia telangiectasia	Acute leukaemia
Fanconi anaemia	Acute leukaemia
Wiskott–Aldrich syndrome	Acute leukaemia
Bloom's syndrome	Acute leukaemia
Chromosomal disorders	
Down's syndrome (trisomy 21)	Acute leukaemia
Turner's syndrome (XO)	Dysgerminoma

in Li Fraumeni syndrome, characterized by cancers of the breast, adrenal glands, leukaemia, gliomas and soft-tissue sarcomas. This gene is involved in inducing cell cycle arrest which allows cells with DNA damage to repair these mutations before entering mitosis. Mutation of *P53* therefore makes the cell susceptible to carcinogenic mutations. Other examples include the retinoblastoma gene, which is located on chromosome 13, breast cancer susceptibility genes *BRCA1* (chromosome 17) and *BRCA2* (chromosome 13), the Wilms' tumour gene on chromosome 11 and the familial polyposis coli gene on chromosome 5.

Some examples of inherited diseases associated with the development of cancer are listed in Table 1.1.

CHEMICAL FACTORS

Cigarette smoking

Polycyclic aromatic hydrocarbons in the tar (e.g. benzpyrene) rather than the nicotine are carcinogenic. Smoking is strongly associated with carcinomas of the lung (squamous and small cell variants), oral cavity, larynx, bladder and pancreas.

Asbestos

A history of asbestos exposure is usually elicited from dockers, plumbers, builders and engineers and is associated with carcinomas of the lung, and mesotheliomas of the pleura and peritoneum. The blue variant is particularly carcinogenic.

Products of the rubber and aniline dye industry

Both β-naphthylamine and azo dyes are carcinogenic. These substances and their products are excreted in the urine, and cause cancers of the renal pelvis, ureter and bladder.

Wood dust

Inhalation of hardwood dusts has been associated with adenocarcinoma of the nasal sinuses, first described in workers in the furniture factories of High Wycombe, UK.

Soot

Before the advent of vacuum machines for cleaning chimneys, there was an increased risk of carcinoma of the scrotum in chimney sweeps owing to trapping of soot in the rugosity of the scrotal skin and poor personal hygiene.

Tar/bitumen

As with cigarette smoke, polycyclic aromatic hydrocarbons may lead to cancer of exposed skin.

Mineral oils

An increased risk of skin cancer was noted in workers using spinning mules owing to exposure to lubricating oils.

Chromates, nickel

These substances are associated with the development of lung cancer.

Arsenic

Its use as a 'tonic' during the early twentieth century led to multiple basal and squamous cell carcinomas of the skin. It has also been associated with lung cancer.

Aflatoxin

This is a product of the fungus *Aspergillus flavus*, which is a contaminant of poorly stored cereals and nuts, and causes hepatocellular carcinoma.

Nitrosamines

These are products of the action of intestinal bacteria on nitrogenous compounds in ingested food and have been implicated in stomach cancer.

Vinyl chloride monomer

Industrial exposure has led to angiosarcomas of the liver and cerebral gliomas.

Alkylating chemotherapy agents

The addition of alkyl groups to the DNA double-helix drastically changes its configuration and leads to difficulty when the cell undergoes mitosis or meiosis, ultimately leading to loss and distortion of the genome. Use of these agents in the chemotherapy of lymphoma has led to an increased risk of acute myeloid leukaemia in long-term survivors.

PHYSICAL FACTORS

Physical factors may cause direct damage to the genome, such as DNA strand breaks or point mutations, both of which may lead to an aberration either of the gene sequence or of the genes themselves. This is a phenomenon of everyday life and the changes are either repaired by cellular protection mechanisms or are so severe that the cell perishes and does not multiply. However, if the effects are such that these mechanisms for repair are overloaded, the cell may divide and the genetic error expresses itself, possibly leading to a cell with a malignant phenotype. Since the skin and mucosal surfaces are exposed to the external environment, it is these that are most prone to physical carcinogenic influences.

SOLAR RADIATION

Excessive ultraviolet exposure in normal individuals or minimal amounts in susceptible individuals (e.g. albinos, xeroderma pigmentosum) may lead to melanoma, basal cell carcinoma and squamous carcinoma (Fig. 1.1).

IONIZING RADIATION

Several categories of exposure can be identified and implicated in carcinogenesis.

- *Excessive background radiation* Radon gas is colourless and odourless, being a daughter product from the radioactive decay of uranium in the Earth's crust, particularly in granite-rich areas. It seeps into homes and reaches its highest level during winter, when ventilation of dwellings is at its minimum. When inhaled, solid (α-particle emitting) daughter products may be deposited on the bronchial epithelium, leading eventually to lung cancer. Uranium miners are at particular risk, and many have died of lung cancer in Eastern Europe and Germany. Japanese atomic bomb survivors have an increased incidence of a number of solid tumours, particularly breast cancer, and radioiodine exposure from atomic bomb test fallout has caused thyroid cancer. Radium ingested by watch dial painters has led to bone sarcomas caused by concentration of the element in the skeleton.

- *Excessive diagnostic radiology exposure* There was an increased risk of carcinoma of the breast in a cohort of women that had many chest fluoroscopies to monitor iatrogenic pneumothoraces. The use of Thorotrast (containing thorium, which has similar properties to radium) as a contrast agent led to tumours of the hepatobiliary tract and nasal sinuses.

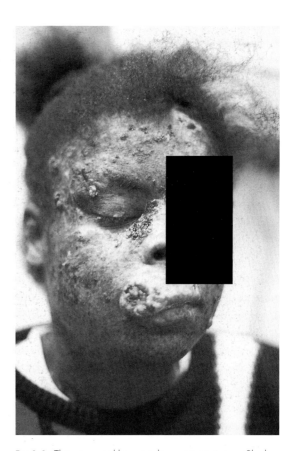

FIG 1.1 This young girl has xeroderma pigmentosum. She has developed multiple facial solar keratoses and skin cancers due to exposure to ultraviolet radiation.

- *Therapeutic radiation* Breast irradiation for postpartum mastitis has caused breast cancer and there is an increased incidence of papillary carcinoma of the thyroid after thyroid irradiation for benign disease. Soft tissue sarcomas may arise at the edge of a previously irradiated area and skin carcinomas may arise in previously irradiated skin.

HEAT

Carcinomas of the skin have been described in chronic burn scars and the skin of Indians who wear heating lamps against their skin for warmth. Claypipe smokers are at risk of carcinoma of the lip.

CHRONIC TRAUMA/INFLAMMATION

Carcinomas may arise at sites of chronic skin/mucosal damage (e.g. the tongue adjacent to sharp

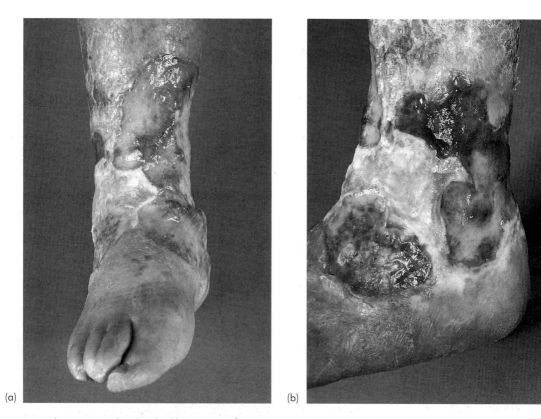

(a)   (b)

FIG 1.2 A large venous skin ulcer had been present for many years on the medial malleolus of the ankle. More recently, it had enlarged and become irregular in shape with everted margins. Biopsy confirmed the clinical diagnosis of squamous carcinoma. (a) Frontal view; (b) lateral view.

teeth or a syphilitic lesion), at the site of a sinus from chronic osteomyelitis or inflammatory bowel disease, chronic venous (Marjolin's) ulcer on the lower limb (Fig. 1.2), or colonic carcinoma after chronic ulcerative colitis. Calculi and the associated infection may predispose to carcinomas of the urinary and hepatobiliary tracts. Skin cancers may arise in scarring from a previous burn (Fig. 1.3) and lung scars from previous tuberculosis may lead to adenocarcinoma.

VIRAL FACTORS

Viruses reproduce by integrating their own genes with those of the infected host, and in doing so the gene sequence of host chromosomes is adjusted. This may in turn lead to deregulation of oncogenes or inactivation of tumour suppressor genes, ultimately resulting in malignant transformation.

Evidence suggesting that a viral infection may have led to a tumour includes:

- geographical and community case clustering;
- serological evidence of infection;
- visualization of viral particles in the tumour cells; or
- identification of viral genome in the tumour DNA.

General observations include the following:

- the prevalence of infection is always much higher than the incidence of the associated tumour;
- additional factors (e.g. genetic, immune) must be operative for malignant transformation;
- there is usually a long latent period between infection and presentation with cancer.

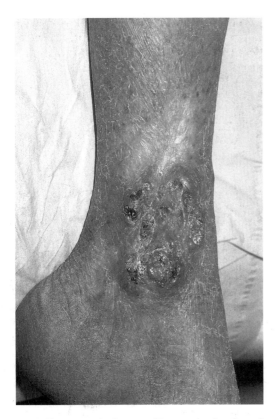

FIG 1.3 This woman had sustained burns to the skin above the lateral malleolus of the ankle 10 years earlier. She then developed nodularity and ulceration within the scar. Biopsy confirmed squamous carcinoma.

Some specific viruses related to cancer include the following.

HEPATITIS B VIRUS

There is a high lifetime incidence (up to 100 times) of hepatoma in parts of Africa where hepatitis B is endemic and there are many chronic carriers of the virus.

EPSTEIN–BARR VIRUS (EBV)

There is very strong evidence that this is the causative agent of undifferentiated nasopharyngeal carcinoma in South-East Asia, B-cell lymphomas in the immunosuppressed and Burkitt's lymphoma in Africa; there is also evidence linking it with Hodgkin's disease.

HUMAN PAPILLOMA VIRUS (HPV)

Types 16 and 18 are responsible for warts in humans and are associated with cervical intra-epithelial neoplasia (CIN) and cancers of the anal canal and vulva.

HUMAN T-CELL LYMPHOTROPIC VIRUS TYPE 1 (HTLV-1)

This is a retrovirus related to the human immunodeficiency virus (HIV, HTLV-3) and causes adult T-cell lymphoma leukaemia in the endemic regions of Japan and the Caribbean, where more than 95 per cent of cases have positive viral serology.

HUMAN HERPES VIRUS TYPE 8

This is the causative agent in acquired immune deficiency syndrome (AIDS)-associated Kaposi's sarcoma and primary effusion lymphoma.

IMMUNE FACTORS

There is evidence that the body's immunosurveillance system mediated by T cells is capable of mounting an immune response to tumour cells. This manifests as a lymphocytic infiltrate in tumours such as seminoma and melanoma, which correlates with a favourable prognosis, the phenomenon of spontaneous regression in hypernephroma and melanoma, and the objective responses seen when the T-cell population is boosted by cytokines, such as interleukin 2 and interferon. There is evidence that immunosuppression leads to development of some forms of cancer, some of which are mediated by viruses.

ACQUIRED IMMUNE DEFICIENCY SYNDROME

Up to 40 per cent of patients with AIDS will ultimately develop some form of malignant disease (see Chapter 20).

DRUG-INDUCED MYELOSUPPRESSION

Transplant recipients receiving steroids and azathioprine or cyclosporin have an increased incidence of Kaposi's sarcoma, non-Hodgkin's lymphoma and skin cancer.

ENDOCRINE FACTORS

Many cells have receptors for hormones on their surface, within their cytoplasm and nucleus. Overstimulation of these receptors by endogenous or exogenous hormones may lead to excessive cell proliferation, usually resulting in an adenomatous change but sometimes malignancy.

Excessive endogenous steroids (e.g. from a granulosa cell tumour of the ovary) or long-term exogenous oestrogens (e.g. high-dose oestrogen-only oral contraceptive or hormone replacement therapy) may predispose to hyperplasia of the endometrium which may progress to a well-differentiated adenocarcinoma. Similarly, excess physiological secretion of hormones may lead to hyperplasia, adenomatous change and eventually malignant transformation. For example, chronic severe iodine deficiency leads to a rise in thyroid-stimulating hormone (TSH), leading to goitre and, in some cases, follicular carcinoma.

UNDERSTANDING THE CAUSE OF CANCER – THE CONTRIBUTION TO PATIENT CARE

Identification of the aetiological agents responsible for cancers is vital for identifying individuals at high risk. Avoiding exposure of employees to industrial carcinogens either by the issue of protective clothing or restricted access is a vital part of health and safety practice to prevent cancers. Similarly, screening of high-risk asymptomatic individuals may be indicated, e.g. regular urine cytology in rubber workers at risk of bladder cancer. Identification of cancer patients in whom industrial exposure to a carcinogen is implicated will entitle the patient to industrial injuries compensation.

Understanding the cause of cancer also forms the backbone of more general health education programmes aimed at reducing tobacco consumption and exposure to excessive ultraviolet irradiation.

Molecular biology has already given us a particularly valuable insight into the mechanisms of carcinogenesis. Specific applications include:

- risk factor determination;
- genetic counselling;
- therapy;
- screening;
- prevention.

The ultimate goal of such research must be to give a greater understanding of cancer and ultimately facilitate more effective cancer therapies. The identification of precise genetic abnormalities may in turn make it possible to insert the appropriate genetic code into the genome (e.g. to replace a missing tumour suppressor gene) or inactivate/downregulate an overexpressed oncogene, thereby reversing the cellular processes underlying the malignant phenotype.

Examples of such translational research include the development of the monoclonal antibody trastuzumab (Herceptin: see chapter 8) which is a very active treatment in women with breast cancers that overexpress a receptor of the epidermal growth factor family, *HER2*.

The antibody imatinib (Glivec) is another example of rational drug design. It is highly active for blast-phase chronic myeloid leukaemia, as the tyrosine kinase protein it targets is BCR-ABL, produced by the Philadelphia chromosome (see above). Similarly, the recognition of gastro-intestinal stromal tumours (GISTs) and their overexpression of *c-kit* has led to an effective therapeutic option with imatinib in a tumour that was previously unresponsive to conventional treatments (see Chapter 9).

2 PRINCIPLES OF CANCER DIAGNOSIS AND STAGING

Diagnosis and staging are vital for determining the optimum management of a patient with cancer.

SECURING A TISSUE DIAGNOSIS

Cancer treatment usually involves major procedures with significant toxicity and the diagnosis of cancer has profound psychological, social and physical consequences for the patient. It is therefore mandatory to be certain of the diagnosis before informing the patient or starting therapy. This may entail a simple biopsy or a more invasive procedure such as a laparotomy or craniotomy. As a rule of thumb, the least invasive means of obtaining tissue should be employed. However, occasionally, several attempts at obtaining tissue from an ill-defined and poorly accessible tumour prove unsuccessful or the patient may be unfit to undergo an essential procedure by virtue of age or general condition. Under these circumstances, clinical judgement and common sense must prevail. Clearly, it would be inappropriate to investigate exhaustively an elderly and infirm person with an extensive asymptomatic brain tumour or widespread metastatic disease if no treatment or change in management would be considered. Specific methods of obtaining tumour tissue include the following techniques.

CYTOLOGY OF BODY FLUIDS

A small specimen of body fluid (e.g. sputum, ascitic fluid, pleural fluid, urine or cerebrospinal fluid) may be spun down and the cells in it stained and examined under the microscope within minutes of its collection. An experienced cytologist can then give an immediate and accurate diagnosis. The false-positive rate is very low although false-negatives occur due to errors in interpretation or sampling. This analysis has the advantage that the specimen can often be collected as an outpatient procedure with minimal discomfort and it gives a result quickly so that treatment can start as soon as possible.

CYTOLOGY OF TISSUE SCRAPINGS

Superficial cells are removed from a body surface (e.g. skin, vagina, cervix, bronchial mucosa or oesophageal mucosa) by scraping or brushing, before being stained and examined under the microscope. The advantages and limitations are the same as for fluid cytology.

FINE NEEDLE ASPIRATION

Fine needle aspiration (FNA) entails the passage of a fine-gauge hypodermic needle into a suspected tumour. Ultrasound or computed tomography (CT) guidance may be necessary for deep-seated tumours that cannot be palpated, such as those at the lung apex or retroperitoneum. Cells are aspirated, smeared onto a microscope slide and sent to a cytologist. This method is particularly useful for discriminating between reactive and malignant lymphadenopathy and for assessing breast lumps.

NEEDLE BIOPSY

This is more invasive than FNA. A core of tissue is taken with a biopsy needle (e.g. Trucut) under local anaesthetic and the specimen is sectioned after fixing and mounting in wax, which means that the result will not be available for several days after collection. The larger specimen makes a false-negative result less likely.

INCISION BIOPSY

A small ellipse of tissue is taken from the edge of the tumour using a small scalpel under local anaesthetic. A punch biopsy instrument can be used instead of a scalpel to obtain a core of tissue.

EXCISION BIOPSY

The tumour is excised *in toto* with a narrow margin of normal tissue. Unlike the other investigations, this has the advantage of removing the lesion, which may be curative for benign tumours and certain skin malignancies if the microscopic margins are clear. It can, however, make further management difficult if the original boundaries of the tumour are not apparent after excision.

PRINCIPLES OF CANCER STAGING

Once the diagnosis has been confirmed, the stage of the cancer, which defines the size and extent of the tumour, must be ascertained. Staging has several purposes:

- it defines the locoregional and distant extent of disease;
- it helps to determine the optimum treatment;
- it permits a baseline against which response to treatment can be assessed;
- it provides prognostic information.

Staging entails a detailed assessment as to the local extent of the tumour and whether there is evidence of spread elsewhere (e.g. regional lymphatics, distant metastases). This will in turn help the referring specialist and oncologist to decide on the most appropriate therapy. For example, a patient with distant metastases is unlikely to be a candidate for aggressive surgery to remove the primary tumour but may be a candidate for systemic treatment such as chemotherapy. Alternatively, the detection of lymph node metastases alone may indicate to the surgeon that excision of the primary tumour should be combined with a lymph node dissection and/or systemic adjuvant therapy. Detailed surgical staging is also valuable to the radiotherapist in deciding the volume of tissue to be irradiated.

Staging permits assessment of the response to treatment. A thorough assessment of the tumour dimensions prior to therapy will permit a critical evaluation of the response to treatment at a later date. Accurate measurements in two planes perpendicular to each other can be used as a crude measure of tumour size before, during and after therapy.

Staging provides a guide to the likely prognosis. In most cancers, the ultimate outcome and therefore life expectancy is related to the stage. Patients with metastatic disease at presentation will clearly fare worse than patients with disease localized to the site of origin. The only tumours that are potentially curable when distant metastases are present are seminoma, teratoma, choriocarcinoma, lymphoma and leukaemia.

Staging may be *clinical*, based on the clinician's history and examination, *non-clinical*, comprising blood tests and radiological studies, or *pathological*, based on the surgical specimen.

History

A thorough and systematic history can reveal symptoms that may suggest the need for specific staging investigations or a certain disease stage. For example, systemic symptoms such as weight loss, anorexia, malaise and fever raise the suspicion of metastatic disease. Specific symptoms at a site distant from the primary tumour may also be suspicious of distant metastases, e.g. skeletal pain, early morning headache, haemoptysis, hepatic pain.

Examination

A full physical examination should be performed in all cases. The primary tumour's size, shape, position and mobility should be recorded, preferably with a diagram. The regional lymph nodes should be carefully palpated: nodes involved are enlarged, usually non-tender, hard and may be fixed to each other, the overlying skin or underlying tissues. The sclerae should be examined for jaundice and the abdomen palpated for hepatomegaly in which the liver is typically hard and knobbly. The chest should be examined for signs of collapse, consolidation or effusion. The skin should be surveyed for any abnormal appearances, which may be biopsied if suspicious. A detailed neurological examination should be performed to exclude focal or global

TABLE 2.1 Interpretation of abnormal screening blood tests

Test result	Interpretation
Normochromic normocytic anaemia	Suggests possibility of advanced cancer
Leucoerythroblastic anaemia	Suggests heavy bone marrow infiltration
Elevated alkaline phosphatase with normal gammaglutamyltransferase ± elevated calcium	Suggests possible bone metastases
Elevated alkaline phosphatase ± gammaglutamyltransferase ± bilirubin	Suggests possible liver metastases

neurological deficit, and the fundi examined to exclude papilloedema. Tenderness over sites of bone pain is suspicious and should be followed by appropriate radiographs.

Investigations

A knowledge of the patterns of spread of tumours will aid the selection of staging investigations. All patients should have a full blood count, liver function tests, calcium and alkaline phosphatase tests. The interpretation of deranged values is outlined in Table 2.1. Measurement of the erythrocyte sedimentation rate (ESR) is useful in lymphoma and myeloma. A chest X-ray should be performed in all cases to exclude obvious pulmonary metastases, with equivocal cases proceeding to a CT scan of the thorax. In the case of bone/soft tissue sarcomas, a CT scan of the thorax is justified at the outset as this will be more sensitive and if positive may spare the patient major surgery. Other investigations may be indicated, depending on site and nature of the malignant disease:

- plain radiographs;
- liver ultrasound;
- isotope bone scan;
- computed tomography/magnetic resonance imaging;
- other specialized investigations (e.g. bone marrow trephine, lumbar puncture lymphangiography);
- tumour marker assays.

PLAIN RADIOGRAPHS

Plain radiographs of the skeleton should be taken at sites of any unexplained bone pain, particularly if affecting a long bone, as these are prone to pathological fracture (Fig. 2.1) which may be prevented if the metastasis is detected early. A skeletal survey comprising views of the skull, thoracic spine, lumbar spine and pelvis is indicated in suspected myeloma.

LIVER ULTRASOUND

This forms part of the routine staging of gastrointestinal malignancies as these metastasize to the liver via the portal circulation. It is sensitive, specific, non-invasive and more readily available than CT or magnetic resonance imaging (MRI). It is, to some extent, operator dependent and the final hard-copies can be difficult for the non-radiologist to interpret.

ISOTOPE BONE SCAN

This is a useful way of imaging the whole skeleton. It is routinely performed as part of the staging of prostate cancer, which has a propensity for early dissemination to the skeleton, but is otherwise reserved for patients with widespread skeletal symptoms or when plain radiographs are equivocal for metastatic disease. A metastasis leads to an osteoblastic response, which in turn leads to increased accumulation of the bone-seeking radioisotope and therefore a hot spot (Fig. 2.2). Myeloma bone lesions are not particularly well visualized as they do not evoke a significant osteoblastic response. A very diffuse involvement of the skeleton may produce an intense uptake of isotope producing a 'superscan'. Bone scans can be unreliable in assessing response to therapy in the short term, an activity may be increased at the sites of metastatic disease with regression of the metastasis and subsequent bone healing.

COMPUTED TOMOGRAPHY

Computed tomography gives good soft tissue and bone contrast. A CT scan of the thorax, abdomen

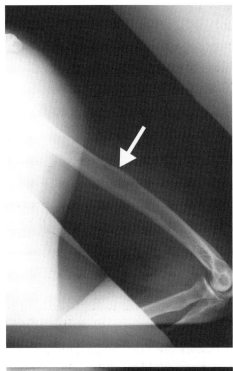

(a)

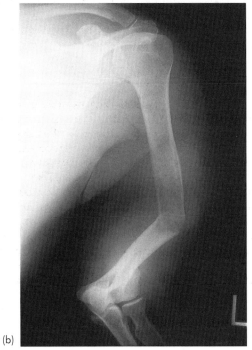

(b)

FIG 2.1 Plain radiographs of the humerus in a patient with lung cancer and a painful arm. (a) Lytic metastasis in the mid-shaft; this was noted by the radiologist but no prophylactic treatment was undertaken. (b) Subsequent pathological fracture at the same site.

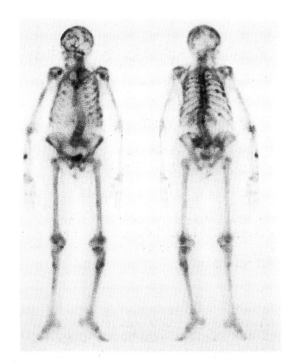

FIG 2.2 Isotope bone scan (anterior and posterior views) showing multiple skeletal metastases from breast cancer. Radioactive technetium has been injected and taken up by the skeleton, particularly in regions of increased bone metabolism. Note the uptake in the kidneys and bladder due to urinary excretion of isotope. Metastases are seen in the skull, ribs, spine, pelvis and femora.

and pelvis is indicated for potentially curable tumours with a propensity for widespread multiple metastases and is performed in all cases, e.g. lymphoma, germ-cell tumours of the testis. It has superseded lymphangiography in the staging of these patients, and is able to demonstrate enlarged lymph nodes that would otherwise not be visualized by lymphangiography, e.g. retrocrural lymph nodes (Fig. 2.3). A CT scan of the chest is valuable for excluding pulmonary metastases when the chest X-ray appearances are equivocal or in the case of tumours with a propensity for pulmonary metastases, such as testicular tumours and soft tissue/bone sarcomas. A CT scan of the pelvis is valuable in tumours of the urogenital tract to delineate the extent of the primary and exclude enlarged lymph nodes. Abnormal lymph nodes on CT are defined as >1 cm in diameter, although CT cannot detect abnormal lymph node architecture and therefore cannot distinguish between benign and malignant enlargement. Localized CT imaging may be used to position a needle for biopsy of a mass.

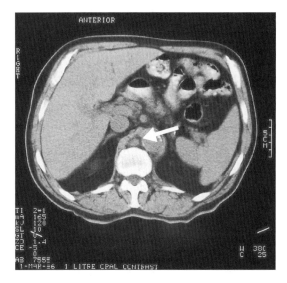

FIG 2.3 Computed tomography scan of the upper abdomen in a patient with a testicular tumour. A significantly enlarged retrocrural lymph node is seen. This would not have been visualized using the now obsolete staging technique of lymphangiography.

MAGNETIC RESONANCE IMAGING

Magnetic resonance imaging gives soft tissue contrast superior to that of CT and superb anatomical definition in transverse, sagittal and coronal views (Fig. 2.4). No ionizing irradiation is involved and it is therefore better for investigating young children and pregnant women. Contraindications include cardiac pacemakers, metallic intracranial vessel ligation clips, previous metallic intraocular foreign bodies and claustrophobia. It is particularly sensitive for imaging the brain and spinal cord (where it is replacing myelography). Magnetic resonance imaging is useful for patients with apparently solitary cerebral metastases on CT as a means of excluding multiplicity which may be important in determining optimal management, and is the investigation of choice for patients with primary central nervous system (CNS) tumours. It has a role in the delineation of the local extent of soft tissue sarcomas and primary liver tumours prior to definitive surgery where the tumour can be related to adjacent major blood vessels, and is the staging method of choice for pelvic tumours (e.g. carcinomas of the prostate, cervix, rectum). It may be useful in determining the nature of persistent skeletal symptoms when plain radiographs and isotope bone scans are both normal (Fig. 2.5).

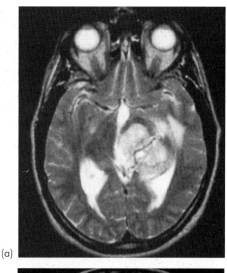

(a)

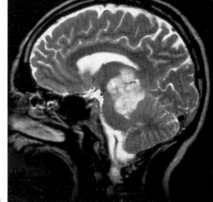

(b)

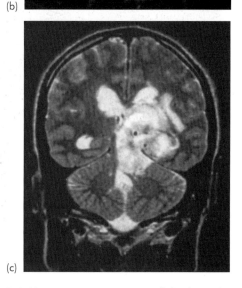

(c)

FIG 2.4 Magnetic resonance image of the brain showing (a) transverse, (b) sagittal and (c) coronal views. The images show a large glioma impinging on the brainstem.

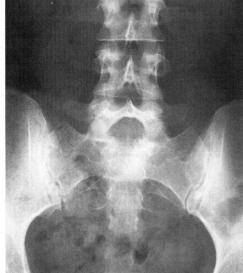

(a)

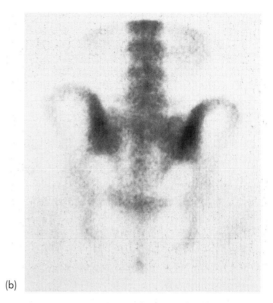

(b)

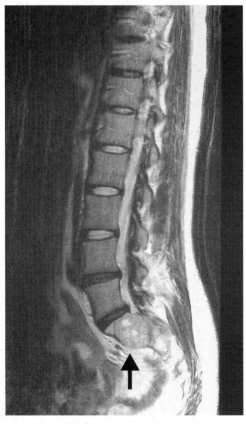

(c)

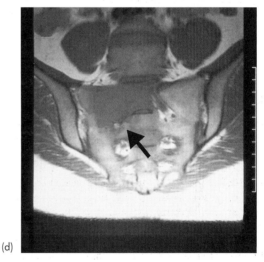

(d)

FIG 2.5 This woman with previously treated breast cancer presented with sciatica. (a) Normal plain radiograph of lower lumbar spine and adjacent pelvis. (b) Isotope bone scan of the same region showing normal, symmetrical uptake. (c) Sagittal magnetic resonance image of the lumbar spine and sacrum showing a soft tissue mass at S1. (d) Transverse magnetic resonance image showing a large metastasis in the superior aspect of the sacrum impinging on the ipsilateral S1 nerve root.

POSITRON EMISSION TOMOGRAPHY (PET)

This entails the systemic administration of positron-emitting molecules, such as fluorodeoxyglucose (FDG) and ^{11}C methionine. These tracers are preferentially taken up by fast-metabolizing tissues (e.g. tumours) and can then be detected and their uptake spatially localized. These studies provide entirely different functional information from the structural information obtained from CT and MRI, and can provide a whole-body snapshot of the likely sites of disease activity. This can be of particular value in the assessment of residual soft tissue masses after chemotherapy (e.g. lymph node masses in lymphoma and testicular tumours), where the presence of viable tumour may be distinguished from fibrosis and/or necrosis.

OTHER SPECIALIZED INVESTIGATIONS

Bone marrow aspirate and trephine

This is a relatively non-invasive method for obtaining a sample of bone and bone marrow for microscopic examination. It is particularly useful in the diagnosis and staging of haematological malignancies (lymphoma, myeloma, leukaemia) and some solid tumours (small cell carcinoma of the lung, Ewing's tumour of bone).

Lumbar puncture

Some tumours have a particular propensity to spread to the CNS, particularly the meninges, and the CNS may act as a sanctuary allowing malignant cells to survive systemically administered chemotherapy. It is relatively easy to obtain a specimen of cerebrospinal fluid from the lumbar subarachnoid space, which can then be submitted for cytological examination. Lumbar puncture forms part of the routine staging of high-risk non-Hodgkin lymphomas (e.g. primary testicular lymphomas, those with bone marrow involvement and lymphomas affecting the paranasal sinuses).

Lymphangiography

This entails the injection of a blue vital dye into the first web space of the foot (the dye is taken up by lymphatics, permitting visualization) and cannulation of a small subcutaneous lymph vessel into which radiographic contrast can be injected. Although superseded by CT and MRI, it does outline the architecture of pelvic and lower para-aortic nodes and identifies nodes of normal size with metastatic deposits. It also opacifies the nodes for many months, allowing monitoring of nodal disease status by serial plain radiographs.

Tumour marker assays

Tumour markers are usually proteins associated with the malignant process. Common methods of detection include:

- immunohistochemistry;
- fluorescence *in situ* hybridization (FISH).

Tumour markers in the serum are useful in many aspects of cancer management, and testicular tumours provide a number of examples (Table 2.2). The following are examples of tumour markers used for other tumour types:

- oestrogen receptor and CA15-3 in breast cancer;
- carcinoembryonic antigen (CEA) in colorectal cancer;
- prostate-specific antigen (PSA) in prostate cancer;
- CA125 in ovarian cancer;
- CA19-9 in pancreatic cancer;
- α-fetoprotein (AFP), β-human chorionic gonadotrophin (HCG) and lactate dehydrogenase (LDH) in testicular teratoma/seminoma;
- thyroglobulin in follicular carcinoma of the thyroid;
- calcitonin in medullary carcinoma of the thyroid;
- S100 in melanoma and other neuroendocrine tumours;
- 24-hour urinary vanillylmandelic acid (VMA) in phaeochromocytoma;
- 24-hour 5-hydroxyindoleacetic acid (5-HIAA) in carcinoid tumours;
- urinary Bence-Jones protein, serum paraprotein and immunoglobulin electrophoresis in myeloma.

THE TNM STAGING SYSTEM

The origins of this staging system go back to the 1940s. Since then it has evolved into a comprehensive

TABLE 2.2 Role of serum tumour markers in the management of patients with testicular tumours

Role	Example
Diagnosis	Elevation of AFP suggests teratomatous elements, elevated HCG suggests trophoblastic elements while elevated LDH is associated with seminomatous elements
Staging	Failure of AFP/HCG/LDH to return to normal after orchidectomy suggests residual disease elsewhere
Prognosis	Very high levels of AFP/HCG are associated with poor prognosis in testicular teratoma
Indicator of response	Failure of AFP/HCG/LDH to fall with chemotherapy suggests resistant disease
Detection of relapse	Sudden elevation of AFP/HCG/ LDH while in clinical remission suggests subclinical relapse

AFP, α-fetoprotein; HCG, β-human chorionic gonadotrophin; LDH, lactate dehydrogenase.

system covering all types and stages of cancer. It is accepted and contributed to by the most eminent cancer research groups such as the World Health Organization, International Union Against Cancer and International Society of Paediatric Oncology. A formalized, universally applied staging scheme has several advantages. First, it aids the clinician in their appreciation of the extent of the cancer and gives a meaningful guide to likely prognosis. Second, it gives a consistency in the reporting of clinical trials and facilitates an exchange of meaningful information between clinicians without ambiguity, even if they do not speak the same language.

The system describes the anatomical extent of the disease by using three components:

- 'T' for the primary tumour;
- 'N' for regional lymph nodes;
- 'M' for distant metastases.

Each of these categories is assigned a number according to the extent of disease, which will vary according to anatomical site and type of malignancy.

Other categories include:

- Tis – carcinoma *in situ*;
- T0 – no evidence of primary;
- Tx – primary cannot be assessed;
- Nx – nodes cannot be assessed;
- Mx – metastases cannot be assessed;
- Gl – well differentiated;
- G2 – moderately differentiated;
- G3 – poorly differentiated;
- G4 – undifferentiated;
- pT/N/M – pathological staging.

The reader is referred to the site-specific chapters in this book for more detailed staging descriptions.

USE OF PATHOLOGICAL INFORMATION

The pathologist plays a vital role in tumour diagnosis. The information on a pathology report is an integral part of the decision-making process for the clinician. Essential details include:

- tumour size and macroscopic appearance;
- tissue of origin;
- benign versus malignant;
- if malignant, primary versus secondary;
- tumour differentiation (i.e. grade);
- degree of local invasion (blood vessels, lymphatic vessels, nerve fibres, organ capsule);
- number of regional lymph nodes retrieved and number involved;
- host immune response;
- tumour excised with an adequate margin of normal tissue;
- immunocytochemical markers (e.g. HER2 in breast cancer).

Much of this information is of prognostic value and may assist in determining the optimal treatment of the patient. The recent advances in immunocytochemistry have allowed pathologists to identify the tissue of origin in very poorly differentiated tumours (see Chapter 21), which has improved the management of this small group of patients. It is not only courteous but essential that as much relevant clinical information as possible is put onto any form submitted to the pathologist.

3 DECISION MAKING AND COMMUNICATION

The following chapters describe clear treatment policies for different types of malignant disease. These policies are based upon a knowledge of the natural history of the disease and, as detailed in the previous chapter, details of its extent (i.e. the clinical or pathological stage of the tumour).

However, the practice of clinical oncology demands more than simple application of these instructions in an uncritical fashion. The individualization of treatment for any given patient will be influenced by sociological, economic and psychological factors as well as oncological principles. The three levels of decision making used when formulating a treatment policy for an individual are:

- the decision to treat or not to treat;
- treatment intent, whether radical or palliative; and
- specific aspects of treatment policy regarding local, systemic and supportive therapy. Figure 3.1 illustrates the various options for treatment.

TO TREAT OR NOT TO TREAT

Not every patient in whom a diagnosis of cancer is made will benefit from active treatment of their disease. There is, for example, good evidence to show that active local treatment in the form of radiotherapy for inoperable carcinoma of the bronchus will have no impact whatsoever on the survival of a patient. It follows, therefore, that in asymptomatic patients diagnosed with this condition treatment will only be meddlesome and indeed may detract from that patient's quality of life by invoking side effects for no positive outcome. However, it is equally important that those patients that develop symptoms from

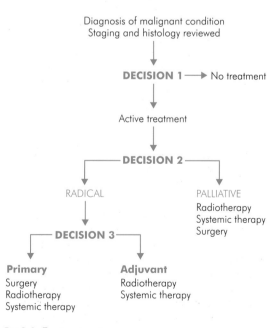

Fig 3.1 Treatment options.

a bronchial carcinoma are not denied treatment by operating a blanket policy of no treatment for these patients. The decision to treat a patient will be based not only on their clinical state but also on the availability of treatment facilities and the emotional response of the patient and their relatives. It is often very difficult for a patient to accept that, having been told they have cancer, no treatment is proposed beyond occasional visits to their doctor, even though the treatment may have no proven benefit.

A more comfortable scenario in which a no-treatment decision may be taken is when the prognosis is so good and the risk of relapse so small that treatment for all patients will result in overtreatment with consequent side-effects for the majority. An example of this situation is the management of stage 1 testicular teratoma following orchidectomy, where the probability of relapse is around 20 per cent and the use of tumour markers and scans enables early diagnosis of relapse in a tumour that is readily cured on exposure to appropriate chemotherapy. This is a much easier scenario for the patient, who will readily accept that they are almost certainly cured and require no further treatment other than close follow-up for a year or two.

Treatment should always have a positive benefit for the patient but treatment outcome is not entirely predictable. The decision to treat or not then becomes a matter of balancing the probability of improving a patient's condition, whether by symptom control with palliative treatment or by cure with radical treatment, against the toxicity and disturbance to lifestyle that treatment will entail. Thus, it is possible to justify an intensive course of chemotherapy with major side-effects when there is a high probability of cure but more difficult to do so in a patient with limited life expectancy in whom only minor symptom improvement can be anticipated.

RADICAL OR PALLIATIVE TREATMENT

Radical treatment is that which is given with the intent of long-term control or cure for the patient, whereas palliative treatment is that which is given to improve the quality of life for a patient with no implied impact upon their survival.

While this may seem to be a clear distinction, in practice it may be difficult to define treatment aims in these terms. For example, a patient presenting with small cell lung cancer may be offered a course of

radical treatment comprising intensive chemotherapy and perhaps also chest radiotherapy. However, it is recognized that while this treatment may prolong survival, the likelihood of cure is less than 15 per cent. Thus, the treatment intent, although radical, will result for most patients in only very limited benefit. Conversely a patient with breast cancer relapsing with a single site of painful bone metastases may receive a low palliative dose of radiation for pain relief only, yet live for several years.

In most cases, however, the decision of treatment intent if not outcome will be clear. Those patients that present with localized tumours accessible to local therapy and those with metastatic disease from chemosensitive tumours such as germ cell tumour or lymphoma will be offered radical treatment. Those that present with metastatic disease from other tumours and those that relapse after primary treatment will, with few exceptions, fall into the palliative group.

It should be noted that palliative treatment has the aim of improving a patient's well-being, usually through treatment for specific local symptoms such as pain, obstruction or haemorrhage. It should follow therefore that patients who have cancer for which radical treatment is not appropriate and that have no symptoms do not require palliative treatment. The concept of prophylactic palliative treatment, in other words treatment to prevent symptoms emerging, is, for most patients, inappropriate and in the asymptomatic patient introduces treatment toxicity with little likelihood of benefit. There may be occasional exceptions to this concept, for example the prophylactic fixation of a bone with extensive osteolytic disease and impending pathological fracture. As always, the probability of treatment benefit must be weighed against the natural history of the condition and probability of disease-related and treatment-related symptoms.

LOCAL, REGIONAL OR SYSTEMIC TREATMENT

As a general principle, a primary malignant tumour will require ablation with local treatment, which may be surgical excision and/or radiation treatment. Similarly, metastatic disease requires systemic treatment which may be chemotherapy or hormone therapy.

Local treatment may involve simple excision of a tumour, removal of the entire organ or removal of the involved organ and regional tissues at risk of tumour involvement. In the past there have been advocates of extensive local surgery in the hope of improving cure; however, such approaches are only rational where a tumour is known to develop locally and then spread in a predictable fashion. In practice, most common tumours are thought to spread at an early stage in their evolution through blood and lymphatic dissemination of tumour cells. For this reason the use of radical regional surgery is usually inappropriate. This is well illustrated in the case of breast cancer where it is now clear that survival is largely independent of local treatment for a given stage of disease. Thus, radical mastectomy is no better at curing breast cancer than simple removal of the lump from the breast.

Although local control of a tumour is an important goal, most patients die from cancer because of metastatic disease. Where a cancer has been detected prior to the establishment of metastases then radical local treatment can result in cure. However, the natural history of many cancers is such that even relatively early tumours will already be associated with distant micrometastases. In these cases, improvements in survival are likely to come only from the use of systemic treatment.

ADJUVANT TREATMENT

Adjuvant treatment is the prophylactic use of local or systemic treatment following primary treatment of a malignant tumour to prevent recurrence.

The most common form of adjuvant treatment given today is probably the use of postoperative radiotherapy following excision of a malignant tumour, for example irradiation of the breast following local excision of an early carcinoma. Such adjuvant treatment may add significantly to patient morbidity and it is important, therefore, to consider the relative merits of treatment or no treatment in these situations. For example, the risk of local relapse in the breast following simple excision with no radiotherapy is around 30–50 per cent, depending upon tumour size. On this basis, if all patients are treated following lumpectomy, half may never have required treatment; the difficulty lies in predicting accurately those that will relapse. A further consideration is the fact that local relapse following lumpectomy may be treated successfully in many women and will still occur in 5–10 per cent even with radiotherapy. It has also been shown that adding

radiotherapy to the breast alone after simple excision does not improve survival. The decision to offer a woman breast radiotherapy following excision of a malignant breast lump has therefore to balance the potential benefits with the likely side-effects for each individual patient and, in this case, the substantial reduction in likelihood of local relapse in the breast from 50% to 5% will be seen in most cases to justify a relatively simple, low morbidity treatment.

The use of adjuvant systemic therapy is also one in which decisions to offer a particular treatment may be questioned and where the acute morbidity is often considerable. There are, in fact, few sites of cancer where the use of adjuvant systemic therapy is of proven value. The area where there has been the greatest endeavour and the most reliable information is once again breast cancer. There is now little doubt that an overall survival benefit is achieved by offering women with early operable breast cancer some form of adjuvant systemic therapy. In postmenopausal women tamoxifen is recommended. This reduces the likelihood of dying from breast cancer by one-third and is a simple treatment involving the administration of a single tablet daily for a number of years with few, if any, associated side effects. Therefore the decision in this case is reasonably straightforward. In contrast, there is a less reliable effect of tamoxifen in premenopausal women with an oestrogen receptor-negative tumour, and at present chemotherapy is recommended. However, this treatment involves 6 months of intravenous chemotherapy with attendant side-effects. Furthermore, its greatest efficacy lies in those patients with positive axillary lymph nodes, but even so the difference in survival at 10 years between women that receive chemotherapy and those that do not in prospective randomized trials is only 6 per cent. Therefore, the treatment decision for adjuvant chemotherapy in a premenopausal patient with negative lymph nodes in whom there may be only a small probability of advantage for the individual becomes more difficult.

It can be difficult to translate clinical trial and population-based data to the individual patient. Breast cancer is a common cancer and so even a very small treatment effect of, say, an improvement in survival of 5 per cent over 10 years will result in many thousands of women world-wide living for longer after breast cancer. However, for the individual woman the odds that she will benefit from adjuvant treatment in that setting are small and it is possible that she will undergo a toxic treatment with no effect on her ultimate survival.

It is also difficult for those around the patient, be they family, friends or physicians, to evaluate and balance the risks of having a toxic treatment against the risk of relapse, particularly when there can never be the certainty of cure. There is evidence to suggest that patients have a much lower threshold for accepting treatment, even where there is significant associated toxicity, than would the nurses or doctors who look after them.

QUALITY OF LIFE

While survival will always be the most important end-point of cancer treatment there is increasing concern and interest in the quality of life that a patient with cancer may enjoy and the impact of different treatment regimes upon this. Measurement of quality of life has become an increasingly sophisticated exercise. Early attempts relied heavily upon assessments by a physician on a broad scale measuring physical performance status as illustrated in Chapter 6 (see Table 6.2). A true measure of the quality of life for an individual can, however, only be acquired from that individual, and a number of formal patient questionnaire-based scales have now been developed. These include the Rotterdam symptom checklist, the Hospital Anxiety Depression (HAD) score and the European Organization for Research and Treatment of Cancer (EORTC) standardized quality of life questionnaire (EORTC QLQ-C30), consisting of a core questionnaire to which can be added disease site-specific modules. The place for quality of life assessments in clinical trials will be discussed later in this chapter.

COMMUNICATION

Communication in oncology is no different from that of any other branch of medicine. There are, however, specific features in this area of practice which require consideration. In Western society the term 'cancer' remains one which is surrounded by fear and dread for most of the population. In other cultures it may not even be considered in open discussion. Many patients passing through an oncology unit will have incurable and ultimately fatal disease requiring special skills in communication and support. These issues may span the entire range of oncological treatment from radical treatment, which may

require lengthy consideration and discussion with the patient regarding choices between different treatment options, and at the other extreme imparting news that cancer may be incurable for a particular patient and that death is imminent.

Patients are increasingly well informed and wish to discuss the details of their disease and options for treatment rather than be faced with instructions. The diagnosis of cancer is often associated with many emotional responses which will colour the interview with a patient, including anger, frustration, guilt and despair. These may present considerable barriers to open discussion particularly where there is a perception that earlier medical care has been inadequate or delayed the diagnosis of their cancer.

Communication with a patient is affected by many factors relating to both the patient and the healthcare professional attempting to impart information. These include environment, culture and content.

Environment

Wherever possible, important discussions imparting news of a diagnosis of cancer, discussions relating to treatment options and the 'bad news interview' informing that the condition may be incurable and terminal should be carried out in an environment that is comfortable for the patient. Privacy is an important issue often difficult to achieve in a busy ward and wherever possible a dedicated side-room or communication room should be available. Where possible, the patient should be adequately clothed and not given important information during the process of physical examination or while still undressed.

If possible and provided that this is desired by the patient they should have a relative or friend accompanying them or, alternatively, a health professional with whom they have empathy, for example their ward nurse. Despite inevitable pressures on the time available for such interviews the patient should not be aware of time pressures which may hinder their willingness to interact and ask questions.

Culture

There will be cultural differences in the way in which a diagnosis of cancer, a potentially fatal illness and death are approached. Increasingly, however, in Western civilization a direct approach is recognized as preferable. The word 'cancer' should not be avoided or hidden behind euphemisms. A clear and simple explanation of the disease relevant to that particular patient and the treatment options should be given. Patients may be unfamiliar with surgical procedures, and the processes of radiotherapy and chemotherapy which should always be qualified by additional explanation. It is always unwise to assume that a patient has any background information unless confirmed. It is often helpful early in a consultation to ask the patient to give their understanding of their illness or the treatments being offered against which background further discussion can proceed. A particular pitfall to avoid relates to fellow health-professionals who may be disadvantaged by the assumption that they already are familiar with their condition and will have decided on the treatment they wish to receive; this is usually far from the case and they will welcome putting aside any background knowledge they may have acquired for a full and simple explanation of their position.

Content

Three common consultations can be identified in oncology which present specific challenges in communication; these are the choice between different radical or palliative treatments, the discussion of likely prognosis and discussion of matters related to the process of dying.

TREATMENT CHOICES

Where there is a choice of treatment this should be laid out for the patient and, in each case, the possible advantages and disadvantages discussed. It may be difficult for practitioners to give a balanced view of treatment options outside their own area of interest and it may be useful for such discussions to include more than one specialist. Realistic estimates of success should be given with clear explanation of the expected end point, whether 'cure', by which the patient will interpret a complete return to normal life and normal life expectancy, 'control' of the disease, which may be only temporary or simply control of symptoms without any impact perhaps on survival.

There is a recognized need to clearly highlight possible side-effects of treatment, in particular those that may result in a long-term alteration in lifestyle for the patient. Again, realistic estimates of the likelihood of this occurring and the balance between side-effect incidence and likelihood of positive benefit should be discussed.

It is well recognized that most patients do not retain information from their initial interview for long and that a significant amount of the information will be forgotten or misinterpreted. It is therefore important that written information is given to the patient to support the facts imparted in the interview and that this is followed up by an opportunity for the patient to return for further discussion. A readily available point of contact should be given to the patient and often it is helpful for another health-care professional such as a specialist nurse to be available to them to discuss matters further.

PROGNOSIS

Prediction of life expectancy is notoriously difficult and there is considerable evidence that estimates by health-care professionals are often widely inaccurate. It is often difficult for patients and their relatives to accept that their medical advisers cannot give an accurate picture of the future. In general, precise figures are likely to be inaccurate, misleading and disturbing for the patient. However, it is usually possible to estimate survival in terms of days, weeks, months or years and where lengthy survival is to be expected a percentage likelihood of surviving say 5 years can be given. This should, however, be carefully interpreted since it is often difficult for patients to relate life table curves giving a probability of survival at any point to their own individual survival.

The point at which patients wish to discuss such matters in detail will vary, with some wishing to consider this in detail from the outset but many preferring to leave the matter unspoken for some time or on occasions throughout their illness until their final days. This should be respected and the issue dealt with sensitively giving patients the opportunity to ask specific details of their outlook but not necessarily giving bald and alarming statements of a short prognosis. Open questions such as 'Is there anything else you would like to ask?' may give them the lead to pursue specific areas of concern when they wish to do so.

DYING

The mention of death and dying is often avoided by both carers and patients, perhaps in an attempt to avoid facing the inevitability of this event. However, meaningful discussions with a patient that has advanced incurable cancer can only progress once the notion of dying has been accepted, even if only to subsequently agree not to mention it further. Patients and their relatives will often hide behind euphemisms such as 'the end' or 'when it's all over', while health-care professionals may use terms such as 'very serious' or 'incurable' to introduce the idea that an illness is fatal. Realistic expectations are important for practical issues to be faced such as where and by whom the patient wishes to be cared for in their last days, clarification of their wishes in the form of a will and where dependent children are involved arrangements for their future care. Patients and their relatives are often concerned over the process of dying rather than the event itself and it is important to explore these fears with appropriate reassurance as to the availability and efficacy of symptom control and nursing care. Above all it is important not to avoid the issue when faced with direct questions from the patient but to reply honestly and with sensitivity.

Difficulties in communication

EXPECTATIONS VERSUS REALITY

For many patients the reality of a serious illness and the possibility of death is dealt with by unrealistic expectations from their treatment and their carers. This can be projected as anger and dissatisfaction when treatment failure is encountered. It is important that unrealistic expectations are not fuelled by unrealistic predictions of outcome from treatment and that such responses are met sympathetically but with clear and accurate information of realistic outcomes.

LACK OF KNOWLEDGE

Many patients may find it difficult to accept that their advisers do not understand the details of their disease process or can attribute any cause to it. Patients often focus on events in their life and seek confirmation that this was the possible cause or not for their cancer. This is usually impossible in practice to confirm or refute. Similarly, events may occur in their disease course which are unexpected and cannot necessarily be explained by previous experience. Health-care professionals should not be reluctant to admit that they do not know or understand events and this is far better than fabrication of possible mechanisms that have no real basis.

IDENTIFICATION

Patients that may be contemporaries of their carers and children are particularly likely to provoke strong emotional responses. This is a normal reaction to events and should be recognized as such but not be allowed to cloud objectivity. If this is found to be an overwhelming difficulty health-care professionals should have access to an alternative colleague who can take their place or support them through difficult patient events.

CONFLICT WITHIN FAMILIES

The diagnosis of a life-threatening illness or impending death may unveil underlying conflicts between a patient and other family members. There is often guilt that the patient has not been given sufficient attention, symptoms have been missed and that more should have been done. This may be transferred to those looking after the patient as complaints relating to their diagnosis and care. Other more complex tensions may emerge with unmasking of relationship difficulties between partners or parents and children. There may be attempts to 'protect' the patient by asking professionals to withhold information which relatives may see as distressing. Throughout, the important principle to keep sight of is that it is the patient who is pre-eminent and while dealing with relatives sympathetically, the patient's wishes should at all times be respected first.

CONCLUSION

Decision-making in oncology is not as straightforward as a simple knowledge of the disease process may imply. Relating the large body of knowledge regarding disease outcome, treatment outcome and treatment-related morbidity to an individual patient can be difficult. The probability of benefit from any treatment may be interpreted differently by each patient so that while one might accept a 90 per cent probability of cure as very favourable, another will find a 10 per cent probability of relapse unacceptable. Treatment decisions rely on an accurate and realistic presentation of the facts but individual interpretations may come to very different conclusions from the same facts.

CLINICAL EVIDENCE AND CLINICAL TRIALS

Ultimately treatment decisions rely upon interpretation of the available data for a given clinical situation. Different sources of data, however, have different levels of reliability when applying them to a patient population. Perhaps the least reliable, but often most memorable, is that of the anecdote recalling the course of a similar patient treated in the past. The most reliable data will come from the results of a large randomized trial addressing a specific question. A grading of the levels of clinical evidence has recently been introduced as follows.

- Level Ia – meta-analysis of randomized controlled trials.
- Level Ib – evidence from one or more randomized trial.
- Level IIa – evidence from a non-randomized trial.
- Level III – evidence from descriptive studies.
- Level IV – evidence from expert committee reports or clinical experience.

Types of clinical trial

A particular clinical question, whether in cancer treatment or any other speciality, can be addressed in a number of ways as categorized above. Types of trial include:

- randomized controlled trials;
- case-control studies;
- cohort studies.

DEVELOPMENT OF NEW TREATMENTS

A clearly defined path for new treatment development in the clinical setting is defined as shown in Fig. 3.2.

RANDOMIZED CONTROLLED TRIALS

These are statistically the most reliable way of comparing two or more different treatments in a population of patients. The characteristics of the population are defined and patients fulfilling these criteria are allocated to one of the treatment options by a random process akin to tossing a coin, but more usually derived from a computer-generated list of random numbers. In this way, fluctuations in the population

which may affect the outcome of treatment are distributed evenly across the treatment groups, allowing a true comparison of the treatment to be made.

Endpoints

It is important at the outset of a trial to define the endpoints by which the results will be judged. This will also guide the assessments which will be required during the trial to have the appropriate information to address the main questions posed by the trial. Endpoints are often defined as *primary* reflecting the main question addressed by the trial and *secondary* which will include other important outcomes such as side effects. Common endpoints will include:

- survival;
- disease-free survival;
- response;
- toxicity;
- quality of life.

Survival is the commonest endpoint for a large trial comparing two or more treatments for cancer. While apparently straightforward in its definition in large trials, times of death may be difficult to trace, particularly when it lasts over several years or the condition has a relatively long natural history, for example patients in trials of initial treatment for breast cancer. It is also important to have documented the cause of death. This will allow a comparison of not only overall survival but also disease-specific survival (i.e. counting only those patients dying from the disease under investigation). It is always important, however, to analyse all causes of death since this may on occasions reveal an excess of deaths from complications of the treatment. A typical example of this related to long-term analysis of the results of radiotherapy for breast cancer, where a reduction in breast cancer death rate is seen in patients receiving radiotherapy, but overall survival between those receiving radiotherapy and those that did not is no different. The explanation for this apparent anomaly was explained by an excess of non-cancer deaths, predominantly cardiovascular disease in the radiotherapy group which negated their reduction in breast cancer deaths.

Disease-free survival is defined by the period during which a patient remains in remission, without detectable disease, following treatment. It may be further subdefined as 'local disease-free survival', taking into account only relapse within a specified site which would typically be the primary site of the cancer after a local treatment, such as surgery or radiotherapy, which would not be expected to

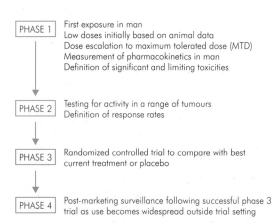

PHASE 1   First exposure in man
           Low doses initially based on animal data
           Dose escalation to maximum tolerated dose (MTD)
           Measurement of pharmacokinetics in man
           Definition of significant and limiting toxicities

PHASE 2   Testing for activity in a range of tumours
           Definition of response rates

PHASE 3   Randomized controlled trial to compare with best
           current treatment or placebo

PHASE 4   Post-marketing surveillance following successful phase 3
           trial as use becomes widespread outside trial setting

FIG 3.2 Path for new treatment development.

directly influence more distant sites. 'Distant disease-free survival' may also be used to assess a treatment for metastatic disease. It is important in the design of a trial to take into account where this is used as an endpoint that relapse may only be defined by specific tests which will have to be performed at specific time-points. For example if a patient is most likely to relapse with lung metastases detected on a chest X-ray, where the trial design defines a chest X-ray to be performed once a year, relapse can only be defined once a year, assuming that the patient did not become symptomatic and obtain a chest X-ray for their clinical management in the meantime. This would obviously then only give a very crude picture of the pattern of relapse, and if the treatment being tested delayed appearance of metastases by less than 12 months this would not be detected. A design that called for a chest X-ray every 2–3 months during the period of risk might be more suitable in such a scenario. It is also important to realize that patients can only be compared by disease-free interval if they are likely to become disease free; for example, it is a very common endpoint for trials after local treatment of early breast cancer where virtually all patients are 'disease free' at last on routine investigations, but of little value in trials of treatment for metastatic disease where only modest response rates might be anticipated.

In these patients a similar concept may however be applied using symptom response rather than tumour response and measuring 'symptom-free survival'.

Response may be an important endpoint when testing new treatments to see whether they are effective. There are recognized formal definitions of response as follows.

- Complete response (CR) – complete disappearance of all detectable disease for a period of at least 1 month.
- Partial response (PR) – a 50% reduction in measurable disease for at least 1 month.
- Stable disease (SD) – a reducing of <50% in measurable disease or no increase in size for at least 1 month.
- Progressive disease (PD) – any increase in size of measurable disease during the assessment period.

Response may be quoted as overall response rates (OR or RR) which will usually include CR + PR but it is important to check on precise definitions as some investigators will include stable disease in this category.

Toxicity is a vital component in assessing the outcome of any clinical trial since, ultimately, any benefit will be judged alongside the side-effects invoked to achieve it. Toxicity will include the immediate effects observed during the trial and may take the form of laboratory measures such as full blood count or renal function and symptom scores for expected side-effects of treatment. It is also important to consider later effects after treatment has been completed, and specific issues that may arise from cancer trials include the effects of treatment on fertility and the induction of second malignancies.

Quality of life measures will give a global view of the impact of the intervention to be tested, taking into account the response of the disease, side-effects of treatment and also the more complex issues of the psychological and sociological consequences of the disease and its treatment.

Measurement of endpoints

This is a very important component of the design of any trial and requires a knowledge of the natural history of the disease being studied, as illustrated in the example above, together with a knowledge of the effects of the treatment interventions to be tested which will usually be available from preceding use of the agents in phase 1 and 2 trials (see below). There are two important considerations in deciding how measurement should be included in a trial:

- timing;
- measurement.

Timing must be defined to give useful information but without burdening the patient or investigators with unnecessary measurements. In the early part of a trial more measures are likely than later on, the most intensive being during treatment. However, as illustrated by the example of annual chest X-rays in a disease which may relapse in a few months, appropriate time-points for assessment after treatment must also be incorporated. The nature of most cancer is for these to be most intensive over the first 2–3 years after treatment and then to become less intrusive as the high risk period for relapse passes.

Measurement may require a range of methods to be applied.

- *Death* is a clear endpoint but tracing patients after treatment to different centres and defining cause of death may be more troublesome. In some countries, cancer registries may be able to supply the information independently.
- *Clinical measurement* of a tumour mass may appear straightforward but clear parameters will need to be defined, for example whether maximum diameter, minimum diameter or a calculated area

or volume is to be used. Ideally, measurements are made by observers independent from those treating the patients or, if by the investigators then they should be blinded to the treatment received. Trials which do not include these safeguards may be open to bias.

- *Radiological measurements* should similarly be carefully defined and ideally judged by an independent radiologist or preferably a central panel convened for the trial. This allows any variation between observers to be ironed out and greater uniformity in the observations will be achieved.
- *Laboratory measures* are, in general, more objective but validation of the laboratory methods used is important, or again it is preferable to use a single reference laboratory distant from the treating centre with mechanisms in place to notify investigators of clinically relevant abnormal results.
- *Measurement of symptoms* is much more difficult. There are a number of accepted and validated measuring tools for common problems such as pain or vomiting and wherever possible these should be employed rather than individualized scales from a single trial or centre. These will typically take the form of categorical scales based on a none, mild, moderate, severe format or visual analogue scales using measured lines for patients to mark the extent of a symptom on. Critical to achieving good data is careful explanation and continued support during the data collection. It is, however, important wherever possible to have data completed by the patient themselves rather than a surrogate.
- *Quality of life instruments* are detailed questionnaires relating to the patient's emotional and physical well-being. They can be general or may have additional 'disease-specific modules' addressing issues which may be pertinent to a particular tumour site, for example urinary and sexual function in carcinoma of the prostate. Common examples used in cancer trials are the FACT (Functional Assessment of Cancer Treatment) and EORTC QLQ-C30 quality of life questionnaires.
- *Health economic assessments* are increasingly an integral component of randomized trials assessing new treatments as it becomes apparent that the resources allocated to health care in the developed world can no longer match the availability and demand for increasingly complex and expensive treatments. Demonstration of cost-effectiveness is therefore an important component of any clinical trial evaluating new cancer treatments. The tools for evaluating this are also becoming more complex as it becomes clear that a simple balance sheet approach cannot address the issues that may arise. Attempts are made to relate the treatment effect with the length of time over which benefit may occur, resulting in concepts such as the Quality Adjusted Life Year (QALY) to measure treatment outcome.

Important examples include the introduction of adjuvant chemotherapy for common cancers such as breast cancer or colorectal cancer where for many patients the actual benefit may be small, and the adoption of expensive procedures such as bone marrow transplantation on an increasingly wide basis. The need for considerable expertise and supportive therapies also means that cancer treatment increasingly has become concentrated in large specialized cancer centres, often many miles from the patient's home and district general hospital.

Placebo-controlled trials

These trials will be appropriate where a new treatment is being tested in a situation where there is no recognized standard treatment with which to compare it. While it may be possible to compare the new treatment with no treatment, there is always the possibility that simply the process of delivering a treatment, whether a drug or other intervention will have an unexpected beneficial or harmful effect. The use of a placebo which will be made to resemble the active treatment as closely as possible reduces this possibility. Placebos are most effective in trials which are 'blinded'. This refers to a situation in which either the investigator or subject do not know the difference between the placebo and active drug (single-blind design). The optimum design is a double-blind trial in which neither the investigator nor the subject are aware whether a placebo or active drug is being used. Where there is already a recognized treatment against which the new treatment is to be tested then placebo-controlled trials are inappropriate as the control arm will be the standard best available treatment. A further alternative approach, particularly in testing a new treatment in advanced cancer is to use as a control arm best supportive care. This is a concept referring to optimized symptom control as distinct from the use of 'anticancer' treatment, addressing the important issue of maintaining a high level of care for the patients in a trial not receiving the new treatment while allowing a test of the new treatment in the setting of active, advanced malignancy.

Randomization

This describes the method by which subjects in a trial are distributed into different groups. In oncology this will usually be comparing different treatments. Most trials have two 'arms': the standard arm, which should be the recognized best available treatment or where there is none then this will be a 'no treatment' or placebo arm, and the experimental arm in which the new treatment will be tested. In most trials there will be balanced randomization, that is, the trial will comprise equal numbers in each of the arms of the trial. Occasionally, however, a design may be used in which there is a weighted randomization, for example a 2:1 distribution of subjects, usually in favour of the experimental arm (i.e. twice as many subjects in the experimental arm as the control). Randomization should take place through an independent trials office totally separate from the facilities in which the trial will be undertaken; usually, this will involve computer-generated blocks of random numbers which will then allocate subjects to their arm of the trial. This may be accessed by researchers through a telephone call, fax or increasingly a voice-activated computer programme.

Stratification

Stratification may be built into the design of a trial. This is to ensure that subgroups within the trial population which may have different prognoses are equally distributed. In oncology this may mean that trials are stratified by tumour stage or performance status. This means that, at randomization, each tumour stage or performance status group will be independently randomized, ensuring an equal distribution of stages or performance status across the arms of the trial. This precaution also aids later analysis using the stage or performance status subgroups without prejudice. Multicentre trials often also stratify by treatment centre.

Trial statistics

The major drawback of a randomized trial is that in order to achieve a result that is statistically sound, large numbers of patients are required. The total number required will be defined beforehand by the trial statistician who will be able to predict the number needed to give a defined level of statistical certainty for a given change in response rate from a known baseline. For example, if a standard treatment has a known response rate of 70% and a 5-year survival of 45%, the trial investigators must decide what improvement upon this they would expect, or wish to detect, in their trial. They will then need to define the power of the trial (i.e. how certain they wish to be of their result at the end). The precise number of patients will be affected by

the degree of error in the trial results that will be accepted by those designing the trial. There are two types of error recognized:

- type I (α) error in which a difference may be observed which does not really exist; and
- type II (β) error in which a true difference may be missed.

These will commonly be set at an α error of 0.05 and a β error of 0.2 (often referred to as 80% power). This means that it will be accepted that there is a 5 per cent chance of the result observed being false. As a general principle, the stricter the statistical constraints (i.e. the smaller the α and β errors accepted and the smaller the difference between the arms of the trials to be detected) the larger the numbers required. As an example, for a trial in a condition where with standard treatment the 5-year survival is 50%, to detect a 10% increase in survival with a new treatment in a two-arm randomized trial accepting an α error of 0.5 and a β of 0.2, a total of 760 patients will be required. Trials designed to show equivalence (i.e. no difference between the treatment arms) require the highest numbers.

The 'p' value is often quoted alongside results of a clinical trial. This essentially relates to the α error accepted in the result. The conventional value required before a result is considered statistically significant is $p = 0.05$ which can be seen to relate to an α error of 0.05 and means that there is a 5 per cent chance of the results not being a true reflection of the comparison in the trial, or in other words there can be a 95 per cent certainty that the result is a true result.

Trial infrastructure

Such trials demand an extensive infrastructure within a dedicated central clinical trials unit which will coordinate the trial and provide a central point for randomization, data collection and analysis. It should be separate from the investigators entering and treating patients in the trial, who are usually based in many different centres all accruing relatively small numbers of patients. A randomized clinical trial may take several years before it is completed and can be analysed to give reliable results that will be translated into clinical practice. It is important during the running of such a trial that any new information from other trials which may affect the relevance of the outcome are considered and that any unexpected toxicity or difference in response is evaluated within the trial. For this reason most large trials will have associated with them a data monitoring committee (DMC) usually comprising a statistician and two or three clinicians or scientists that are not involved in that particular trial. They will review the results of the trial at defined times, perhaps annually or after accrual of a defined number of subjects (e.g. after every 100 patients entered). They may recommend early closure of a trial if a large number of unexpected toxicities are found in one arm, or if a sufficiently large difference emerges between the arms of the trial early on which was unexpected and unlikely to be reversed by larger numbers. The data seen by the DMC must at all times remain confidential from the investigators involved in running the trial. In practice, early closure is rare in a well designed clinical trial but the DMC is an important component to ensure that patients are not given inappropriate treatment.

Ethics of clinical trials

It is a fundamental principle in designing and partaking in a clinical trial comparing two treatments that the patient should not be disadvantaged compared with other patients not taking part in the trial. For this to be satisfied the investigators must be confident that there is no proven advantage for the new treatment over the existing management and, equally, that there is no evidence of any greater toxicity which would disadvantage the patient. This will be based on information gained from earlier phase I and phase II trials. However, it has been shown that patients taking part in clinical trials have a better outcome than those who do not, possibly because of adherence to a rigid protocol and the greater clinical input that inevitably accompanies trial participation.

Meta-analysis

A meta-analysis is a means of overcoming the problem of patient numbers. This arises because most innovations in treatment have only a modest impact upon outcome; an improvement in survival of more than 10 per cent from any new intervention is very unusual. Other new treatments may not even be expected to improve survival but may be aimed at reducing toxicity or improving quality of life. Any clinical observation is inherently unreliable in statistical terms and will carry a range around which a repeat observation may be expected to fall – this is often quoted as the 95 per cent confidence interval (CI) within which 95 per cent of repeated observations might be expected to fall. The smaller the

number of observations the wider will be the confidence interval. To be certain that the observations in two groups of patients are truly different, there must be no overlap of the confidence intervals. Where there is a big difference, even relatively wide confidence limits will not overlap, but for a small, true difference the confidence interval needs to be as small as possible to demonstrate the difference and this will only be achieved with a large number of patients.

A meta-analysis therefore attempts to include as many patients as possible who have been reported to have entered trials addressing a particular question. This approach has been used for several tumour sites of which breast cancer provides an excellent example. For a number of years a series of individual clinical trials across the world have addressed the question as to whether adding hormone therapy or chemotherapy to the primary treatment can prolong survival. The results of individual trials failed to give a clear answer, with some showing benefit and others no benefit. A meta-analysis has therefore been performed combining the results of all known trials in this area and demonstrating in 30 000 women that adjuvant tamoxifen conveys a 6.2 per cent survival advantage after 10 years and in 10 000 women that polychemotherapy carries a 6.3 per cent survival advantage after 10 years. These figures illustrate the very small overall survival effect seen and explain why series of small trials gave conflicting results. With such large numbers, as in the overview, however, small differences can be found with a high level of statistical reliability as demonstrated by the very low p-value associated with this data; the tamoxifen result above has a p-value of <0.00001, (i.e. only a 1 in 10 000 chance that the observation is not real).

CASE-CONTROL STUDIES

In many situations, particularly in rare tumours, where it is not possible to study large numbers of patients, randomized trials are not practical. The next best type of trial is the case-control trial in which a new treatment is given to a series of patients and then compared with previous patients, or patients treated differently in another centre. It is important in such a comparison to attempt to exclude any factors that might affect the result other than the treatment being tested. This is achieved by selecting matched controls (i.e. patients with otherwise identical characteristics to one of the new treatment group with whom they are matched). Parameters which it is important to match for include age, sex, tumour stage and histological type, together with any other known prognostic factors. The comparison may be refined by selecting two matched controls for each patient receiving the new treatment.

The difference between the two groups is often quoted as an odds ratio (OR) comparing the probability of an event (e.g. death or tumour recurrence) occurring in the control group with that in the new treatment group.

COHORT STUDIES

Cohort studies are not usually of value in comparing two different treatments but are used in particular to investigate aetiological factors. As their name suggests, they are observational studies in which a group of patients (a cohort) is monitored over a period of time for a particular outcome (e.g. development of or death from cancer). This type of study is usually reported in terms of relative risk, comparing the incidence in the cohort with that of a control cohort. The value of this type of study is in defining the natural history of a particular tumour type and evaluating the impact of potential aetiological agents.

CONCLUSION

Subsequent chapters will describe for different tumour types their aetiology, natural history and various treatment options. The accuracy of this depends critically upon the data from which this information is derived. It can be seen that there are many pitfalls in obtaining and interpreting the results of clinical data sets. Any advances in cancer management depend critically upon rigorous evaluation with close attention to the design and interpretation of clinical trials to ensure that reliable outcome data is acquired to further advance knowledge. It also demands that clinicians and patients of the future are sufficiently informed to understand and partake in clinical trials.

4 PRINCIPLES OF SURGICAL ONCOLOGY

The local treatment of malignant disease involves the use of surgery, radiotherapy or a combination of the two. Surgery is essentially a local treatment while radiotherapy offers locoregional treatment covering a wider area and is less constrained by anatomical boundaries and surgical technique. Optimum initial management of the primary tumour and regional metastases is vital if later relapse is to be avoided, and close liaison between surgeon and oncologist is required to enable the best use of each modality.

MANAGEMENT OF THE PRIMARY TUMOUR

Surgery for a malignant tumour may have several components:

- tissue biopsy to establish the diagnosis;
- removal of malignant disease with a clear margin of normal tissue;
- repair, reconstruction and restoration of function.

The last item may vary according to the extent of resection and anatomical site, from simple primary wound closure to major reconstruction of bone and soft tissue with vascularized grafts and prostheses.

The type of surgery required will be determined by the type of tumour and the anatomical site, and may include:

- wide local excision of the tumour mass (e.g. local excision of a breast lump);
- removal of part of an organ and surrounding tissue (e.g. partial glossectomy and neck dissection for a carcinoma of the tongue);
- Removal of an entire organ (e.g. laryngectomy, cystectomy or hysterectomy).

En bloc removal of the immediate lymphatic drainage areas is usually an integral part of any cancer surgery (e.g. hysterectomy for cervical cancer includes pelvic lymphadenectomy).

Radiotherapy will give equivalent local control rates to surgery for small tumours (<5 cm) in many sites and has the potential advantage in certain sites of being able to preserve anatomical structure and function. For example, in the treatment of cancer of the larynx radical radiotherapy can result in tumour eradication with voice preservation, in contrast to the surgical alternative which is total laryngectomy. However, against this must be balanced the need for close postradiotherapy surveillance and that a significant proportion (around 20 per cent) of patients will still come to surgery. Furthermore, surgery following radiotherapy may be technically more difficult and have a higher complication rate. As with surgical management, irradiation of a local tumour must include areas of potential spread. A common approach to enable high radiation doses to be concentrated at the site of the tumour mass is to use a shrinking field technique. This involves:

- initial treatment of a wide area to cover all potential routes of microscopic spread, together with the primary tumour and regional lymphatics;
- a boost to the primary tumour site alone with a margin of 1–2 cm.

COMBINED SURGERY AND RADIOTHERAPY

The combination of surgery with radiotherapy has two potential advantages and applications:

- it enables the extent of surgery to be limited by treating sites of microscopic disease immediately adjacent to the primary site with radiotherapy (e.g. the use of local excision and radiotherapy in place of mastectomy for breast cancer);
- for large tumours (>5 cm), local control rates are, in general, better for combined therapy than either modality alone.

Combined treatment may involve the use of preoperative or postoperative radiotherapy. The relative merits of each approach are shown in Table 4.1. There is no evidence that preoperative

TABLE 4.1 Relative merits of pre- and postoperative radiotherapy

Preoperative radiotherapy	Postoperative radiotherapy
Early radiotherapy	No delay to surgery
Enables preoperative preparation for planned surgery	True pathological staging may be masked by preoperative radiotherapy
Surgery may be easier if tumour shrinks preoperatively	Pathology of surgical specimen may guide later radiotherapy
	Lower dose of radiotherapy needed for microscopic disease

or postoperative radiotherapy is more effective in ultimate tumour control.

MANAGEMENT OF REGIONAL LYMPH NODES

The common epithelial tumours such as those of the lung, breast, head and neck region and pelvis metastasize through two routes: the lymphatic system and the blood circulation. Clinically involved lymph nodes and those at high risk of microscopic involvement require active treatment.

Surgery

Surgery is indicated for the immediate draining nodes around a primary tumour. Radical dissection of the involved node chain should be considered, and may involve:

- axillary dissection for breast cancer;
- radical neck dissection for head and neck sites;
- inguinal node dissection for vulval, anal or penile cancers treated with primary surgery.

A more conservative approach, sentinel lymph node mapping, is increasingly being used for breast cancer and melanoma. This entails identification of the 'sentinel' lymph node. This is the node which is first to receive lymph from the tumour-bearing tissue. Methylene blue dye and/or radiolabelled colloid microspheres are injected preoperatively to allow peroperative removal of this lymph node(s). If involved, a full lymph node dissection is mandatory. If negative, it is highly unlikely that other lymph nodes in that group will harbour cancer cells, and the patient may be spared the additional morbidity of the larger operation.

Radical excision of nodes is not indicated for:

- lymphomas (Hodgkin's disease or non-Hodgkin's lymphoma) or leukaemias;
- metastatic involvement at visceral sites where there may be little or no improvement in quality of life by removal of enlarged lymph nodes.

Radiotherapy

Radiotherapy is indicated for surgically inoperable nodes and may succeed in rendering inoperable nodes operable. Postoperative radiotherapy following surgical dissection is recommended for those patients with multiple node involvement and extension of tumour beyond the capsule of the gland. Prophylactic radiotherapy to sites of potential microscopic disease is often given when treating a primary site (e.g. pelvic nodes for gynaecological malignancy or neck nodes for head and neck tumours).

Chemotherapy

Chemotherapy may be indicated for enlarged lymph nodes caused by germ cell tumour, lymphoma, metastatic breast cancer or small cell lung cancer.

PALLIATIVE SURGERY

Even when cure is no longer a realistic aim, surgery may have an important role in the palliation of local symptoms. Specific examples where surgery should be considered include:

- palliation of obstructive symptoms;
- control of haemorrhage;
- palliation of tumour fungation;
- fracture reduction and fixation.

PALLIATION OF OBSTRUCTIVE SYMPTOMS

- Palliative resection of a bowel tumour or a simple bypass procedure such as a gastrojejunostomy will avoid symptoms of intestinal obstruction.
- Laser or cryotherapy resection of an obstructing tumour mass will restore the lumen of an obstructed bronchus or oesophagus.
- Intubation of the oesophagus using a prosthesis or stent provides rapid and effective relief of dysphagia.
- Nephrostomy or passage of ureteric catheters will relieve obstructive hydronephrosis.
- Biliary stents or choledochojejunostomy will relieve obstructive jaundice caused by extrahepatic bile duct obstruction, as in carcinoma of the pancreas.

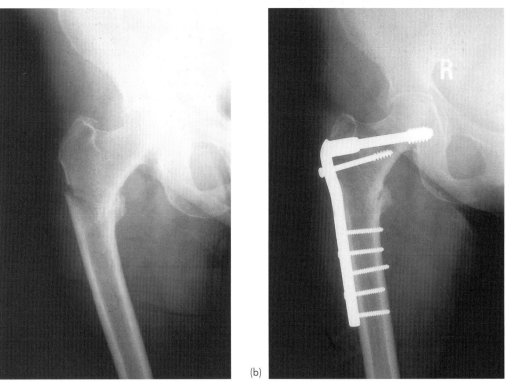

(a)

(b)

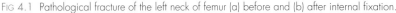

FIG 4.1 Pathological fracture of the left neck of femur (a) before and (b) after internal fixation.

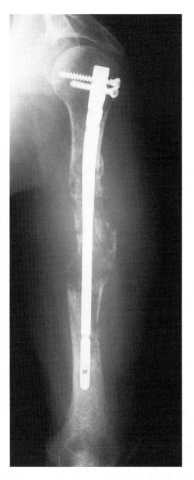

FIG 4.2 This woman had internal fixation for a pathological fracture of the mid-shaft of the humerus. This was not followed by radiotherapy. She has now developed significant bone lysis compromising the mechanical integrity of the bone.

- Gastroenterostomy will relieve gastric outflow obstruction.
- Rectal stents for rectal obstruction.
- Ventriculoperitoneal shunting of hydrocephalus may result in dramatic improvement of headache and neurological deficits even though the underlying tumour may be incurable.

CONTROL OF HAEMORRHAGE

- Diathermy at bronchoscopy or cystoscopy will control haemoptysis or haematuria.
- Bleeding tumours in the oesophagus, stomach or in the large bowel may be controlled using diathermy or laser coagulation at endoscopy.

PALLIATION OF TUMOUR FUNGATION

Local resection, even if not complete, may be of value for a locally advanced tumour mass that is necrotic and breaking down. Toilet mastectomy for a progressive breast cancer is perhaps the most common example of this.

FRACTURE REDUCTION AND FIXATION

Pathological fracture of a weight-bearing bone is best dealt with by internal fixation, as shown in Fig. 4.1, followed by postoperative radiotherapy. Radiotherapy consolidates the surgical fixation, maximizing the probability of its security in the longer term (Fig. 4.2). In certain circumstances, prophylactic fixation may also be indicated; specific indications for this include diffuse lytic bone disease in a weight-bearing area and destruction of more than 50 per cent of the cortex by a lytic deposit.

5 PRINCIPLES OF RADIOTHERAPY

Radiotherapy is the use of ionizing radiation to treat disease. Ionizing radiation may be delivered by X-ray beams, beams of ionizing particles (e.g. electrons) or by beta or gamma irradiation produced in the decay of radioactive isotopes.

TYPES OF RADIOTHERAPY

External beam radiotherapy

External beam radiotherapy is the most common form of treatment in clinical use. A range of X-ray beams is available, varying according to their energy.

SUPERFICIAL VOLTAGE

These X-ray beams are of 50–150 kV energy and are, as their name implies, suitable for the treatment of superficial lesions in the skin; their useful treatment energy penetrates no more than 1 cm beneath the surface.

ORTHOVOLTAGE MACHINES

These produce X-rays of 200–300 kV energy and penetrate to a depth of approximately 3 cm. These are therefore useful for treating structures such as ribs, scapula or sacrum but are not sufficiently powerful to reach deeper internal organs.

MEGAVOLTAGE MACHINES

These are either linear accelerators producing high energy X-ray beams of 4–20 MV or cobalt machines containing a source of cobalt-60 in their head,

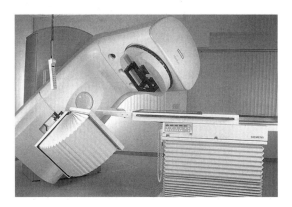

FIG 5.1 A modern linear accelerator.

which decays spontaneously to nickel-60 releasing gamma rays of 1.2 MV and 1.3 MV.

Linear accelerators form the mainstay of modern clinical radiotherapy and are gradually superseding older cobalt machines as they come to the end of their working life. A modern linear accelerator is shown in Fig. 5.1.

Electron beams are also produced by linear accelerators and have the advantage that as a particulate radiation beam they have a defined range in tissue with a sharp cut-off at the point where they deliver their energy. This is of value where a tumour is superficial and particularly when it is overlying a radiosensitive structure such as the spinal cord.

Brachytherapy

This is the use of radioactive sources placed either on or within a site involved with tumour. The great advantage of this form of treatment is the rapid fall off in dose at only a short distance from the source (obeying the inverse square law). Three types of brachytherapy are in common use:

- mould treatment – this uses sources placed directly over a superficial tumour of the skin fixed in a plastic mounting (the mould);
- intracavitary treatment – involves the placing of radioactive sources within a body cavity; intrauterine tubes and vaginal sources in the treatment of gynaecological tumours are a common application of this technique;
- interstitial treatment – involves the direct placing of radioactive needles or wire in the area of interest. This technique is used for cancer of the tongue, floor of mouth or breast.

The first isotope to be employed was radium. This is no longer used because it constitutes a major radiation hazard having a long half-life (1620 years) and decaying to a radioactive gas (radon). It was superseded initially by cobalt sources and currently by caesium and iridium as the principal isotopes used for brachytherapy.

LIVE SOURCE IMPLANTS

Direct handling of live sources is most commonly used now when iodine or palladium seeds are used for prostate implants or iridium wire hairpins are inserted directly into the tumour area, typically the tongue or floor of mouth. While the radiation from iodine-125 is short range and poses no major radiation hazards, that from iridium is more penetrating and its use has the major disadvantage of exposure of staff and others within the hospital to radiation from the time of insertion to the time of removal, which may be several days. This means that careful monitoring is required and that there are limits to the time that individuals can spend caring for the patient. It also means that friends and family are not permitted to be with the patient.

MANUAL AFTERLOADING

In this, inactive source carriers are used initially to enable accurate siting of the treatment, and so that the patient can be moved within the hospital from theatre or the X-ray department without radioactive sources in place. The active isotope is introduced manually once the patient has returned to their protected room and their postoperative recovery is complete.

REMOTE AFTERLOADING

Following placement of the source carriers, the radiation sources are introduced by remote control

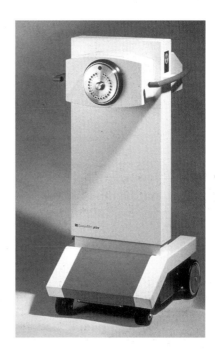

Fig 5.2 A modern brachytherapy afterloading machine which uses a small iridium source located in the head of the machine, which will pass out by remote control through the series of channels seen to deliver radiation into applicators within a tumour area connected to these outlets (courtesy of Varian).

via pneumatic pipes or a cable connected to the source carriers within the patient. This system minimizes exposure to staff and in practice means that only the patient is exposed to radiation. It is also possible to interrupt the treatment so that the patient can receive attention without further exposing hospital personnel and with no time limits on their stay. A modern afterloading machine is shown in Fig. 5.2.

All such treatments require the patient to be isolated in a protected room with thickened or shielded walls, floors and ceilings. Treatments may last from 3 to 4 minutes for a high-dose rate gynaecology treatment to several days for a radical low-dose rate interstitial treatment.

Internal isotope treatment

Internal isotope treatment involves the administration of a radioactive isotope systemically; these are then concentrated within the body at certain sites. Specific examples of this form of treatment are the use of radioiodine (^{131}I) for thyroid cancer and also neuroblastoma when conjugated in meta-iodobenzyl guanidine (mIBG), phosphorus (^{32}P) for polycythaemia rubra vera and strontium (^{89}Sr) for bone metastases.

OTHER FORMS OF RADIATION

There has been interest in forms of radiation other than X-rays or gamma rays for therapeutic use. These are either radiation which causes greater biological damage along each path track it traverses – high linear energy transfer (LET) radiation – or beams that have a highly focused deposition of radiation (Bragg peak).

NEUTRONS

Neutrons have been evaluated extensively in a number of centres across Europe and the USA. Their advantages are that they have less dependence on oxygen for cell killing and cause more direct damage to the cellular DNA. While there is little doubt that they are more effective at achieving cell kill, they are not selective for cancer cells and their use has been accompanied by unacceptably high levels of normal tissue damage and severe late side-effects.

PROTONS

Protons are available in a few high-energy cyclotron units around the world. Their advantage is the production of a highly localized, high-energy peak in their beam which, by manipulation of the beam energy and the use of absorbing materials, can be focused to a defined position in a patient. Biologically they are similar in action to X-rays. They have been used particularly for tumours in inaccessible sites such as the back of the eye and pituitary and are also under evaluation in the treatment of prostate cancer. Their limitation is the technology required to produce a beam for routine medical use.

BIOLOGICAL ACTIONS OF IONIZING RADIATION

Ionizing radiation causes damage to cellular DNA both directly and indirectly through toxic free-radicals produced from the interaction of radiation with water within the cell. This results in single- and double-strand breaks in the DNA and, unless repair occurs, these will accumulate, resulting in reproductive death of the cell.

Other factors which are important in the response to radiation include:

- Reoxygenation – hypoxic tissues are considered relatively radioresistant; fractionation of treatment allows reoxygenation to occur between each treatment as the tumour shrinks and blood flow improves;
- Repopulation – both tumour tissue and normal tissues continue to divide during a course of radiotherapy and there is even some evidence to suggest that repopulation may increase during this time as cells are lost; gaps of days between radiotherapy treatment should therefore be avoided wherever possible to prevent significant repopulation undoing any effects from irradiation in the previous days;
- Repair – much of the damage produced by X-rays and gamma rays is not sufficient to kill the cell immediately and if repaired the cell can retain its viability. This capacity in normal tissues is relied on to establish differential cell kill between tumour and normal cells.
- Redistribution – with redistribution within the cell cycle, radiosensitivity varies as cells progress through the cell cycle, being maximum during the periods of active DNA synthesis in G2 and early M phases and least during late G1 and S.

There is a spectrum of radiosensitivity for both tumour and normal cell types. Few, if any, tumours are truly radioresistant, although some may require a larger dose of radiation to achieve the same effect as others. There is also a wide spectrum of sensitivity in normal tissues. Particular care is required with certain normal tissues when delivering irradiation:

- central nervous system (CNS) tissue has a relatively low threshold for damage and has little or no capacity for repair; radiation damage to the CNS is therefore often irreversible and can result in catastrophic morbidity if, for example, necrosis of the spinal cord or brainstem results;
- the small bowel is also relatively sensitive and doses well below those required to sterilize an epithelial tumour will cause serious damage;
- the lens of the eye will develop cataract after exposure to only small doses and must therefore be carefully shielded whenever possible;
- bladder and rectum are often dose-limiting tissues when treating pelvic tumours;

■ lung damage can result, which, if it involves a large volume of lung, can cause considerable respiratory distress and even death.

The balance between causing serious normal tissue damage and curing a malignant tumour is termed the 'therapeutic ratio' and is the major limitation to the success of radiotherapy in achieving local cure of malignant tumours.

CLINICAL USE OF RADIOTHERAPY

The patient attending for radiotherapy treatment will pass through a series of steps to ensure that treatment is given as accurately and safely as possible. These include:

■ patient positioning and immobilization;
■ tumour localization;
■ treatment planning;
■ verification;
■ treatment.

Positioning of a patient is very important in order to enable an X-ray beam to reach a certain site. This is particularly the case in the head and neck region where small changes in the position of the neck or chin can greatly affect the tissues included in an X-ray beam.

In order to be able to reproduce a particular position accurately, some form of immobilization may be designed, such as a plastic head shell to hold the head in a fixed position.

Tumour localization may be achieved by simple clinical examination, as in the case of a skin tumour, plain X-rays (e.g. a bone metastasis) or computed tomography (CT) scan for tumours in the thorax, abdomen or pelvis. Alongside this it is important to identify vital structures to be avoided, such as the spinal cord or kidney. Identification of the area to be treated and structures to be avoided must be related to the direction of an X-ray beam on that site. This is usually achieved by indelible marks on the skin placed at the time of taking the localization X-ray or scan.

Treatment planning involves designing the optimal arrangement of X-ray beams in order to cover the treatment area as evenly as possible, while avoiding structures around it. At its simplest level, this may be a single direct X-ray beam on a skin tumour;

for internal tumours a more complex arrangement of two, three or four X-ray beams approaching from different directions may be required. Treatment plans of multiple beams are drawn up using computerized data describing the characteristics of the beam and enabling rapid addition of their effects at a point.

Conformal radiotherapy using external X-ray beams seeks to shape the high-dose treatment area as closely as possible to that of the tumour volume, even where this may be a highly irregular shape, while avoiding adjacent sensitive normal structures. This requires accurate three-dimensional reconstruction of the volume to be treated and irregular beam shaping using lead blocks or more commonly a multileaf collimator shaping the beam by typically 80 or 120 interleaved projections into the beam, which can be adjusted as required.

Intensity-modulated radiotherapy (IMRT) is a further development on conformal planning by varying the dose delivered within a tumour volume so that a central high-dose area may be surrounded by a lower dose region all within the same treatment.

Stereotactic radiotherapy is a means of treating a small spherical volume to a high dose typically used for localized lesions in the brain. It can be achieved in two ways. The first uses a standard linear accelerator which, using a small focused field, builds up the high-dose volume using a series of rotating arc movements. The alternative is to use the 'Gamma-knife'. This is a machine containing multiple cobalt sources, each with its independent shield, which can be opened to focus on the treatment volume in a spherical pattern. Such machines are only available in a few specialized units.

Verification entails ensuring that the treatment plan can be translated back to the patient in the defined treatment position. This is usually done on a machine called a treatment simulator, which reproduces precisely the movements of the treatment machine but produces only a diagnostic X-ray beam so that an X-ray picture of the proposed treatment beam can be taken.

Further verification may also be performed when the actual treatment is started, particularly if complex beam shapes or lead shielding are to be employed. Megavoltage images can be taken using the linear accelerator beam. Their disadvantage is that because they interact in a different manner to low-energy X-rays, there is no differential absorption between bone and soft tissue resulting in poor anatomical definition.

Treatment only proceeds once it is certain that the defined area to be treated can be encompassed using the planned X-ray beams. During treatment the patient will be continually monitored by the radiographers and seen regularly by the medical staff. Specific additional measurements of radiation exposure may be taken using dosimeters placed on vital areas such as the eyes or testes and further verification X-rays may be taken during the course of treatment.

Treatment duration

There is considerable variation in the dose and duration of radiotherapy treatment given to patients, which can appear confusing. Neither the total number of treatments nor the total dose given are necessarily a guide to the biological dose of radiation delivered. There are three components to biological radiation dose:

- total dose;
- number of treatments (fractions) that dose is given in;
- overall time of treatment.

The following general principles can be applied:

- the same total dose given in a short time or fewer fractions has greater effect than the same dose given over a longer time in many fractions;
- fraction size is an important determinant of normal tissue damage – small fractions minimize normal tissue effects (however, it follows from the previous point that, if used, small fractions demand a longer course of treatment with a higher total dose to have the same effect);
- overall treatment time is important in achieving tumour control – delays and interruptions in a course of treatment should be avoided, as should overall treatment times of greater than 6–7 weeks.

The unit of radiation dose used is the Gray (Gy) which is a measure of absorbed energy (1 Gy = 1 J/kg). This has replaced the rad but the conversion is simple: 1 Gy = 100 rads. In some centres, in order to keep the actual numbers the same, doses are described in centigray since 1 cGy = 1 rad.

Precise radiation schedules vary from centre to centre and between individual clinicians, however, some generalizations can be made. A fundamental difference lies between palliative and radical doses.

RADICAL TREATMENTS

These require high doses of radiation to eliminate the tumour but are divided into smaller fractions to minimize side-effects and remain within the tolerance of normal tissues. Examples of radical schedules include: 60–65 Gy in 30–32 fractions in 6–6.5 weeks; 55 Gy in 20 fractions in 4 weeks and 50 Gy in 15 fractions in 3 weeks.

PALLIATIVE TREATMENTS

These require short schedules with few acute side-effects. The ideal palliative treatment is a single dose; many centres use this routinely, while others treat over 1–2 weeks. Examples include: 8–10 Gy in a single dose; 20 Gy in five daily fractions over 1 week and 30 Gy in 10 daily fractions over 2 weeks.

SIDE-EFFECTS OF RADIOTHERAPY

The toxicity of radiotherapy is divided into two distinct groups: the early effects, which occur during treatment, and the late effects, which appear months or years following treatment.

Early effects

These develop during treatment usually in the second to third week of a course of radical irradiation. They may be divided as follows.

- *Non-specific effects* Many patients feel tired and lack energy during treatment. There may be many factors in addition to radiation exposure to account for this, including depression, anxiety, travelling daily to treatment and concomitant medication.
- *Specific local effects related to the area being treated* It is important to note that areas outside the irradiation field do not exhibit acute toxicity: examples are shown in Table 5.1, together with suggested treatment. As a general principle, these are all self-limiting effects that resolve spontaneously after treatment, their pathogenesis being related to temporary loss of cell division at an epithelial surface.

Late effects

These are potentially the most serious effects of treatment since, unlike the acute effects, they are not self-limiting and indeed tend to be progressive and irreversible. They arise because of the loss of stem cell recovery potential and progressive damage to

TABLE 5.1 Acute effects after radical radiotherapy

Site	Effect	Treatment
Skin	Erythema leading, if severe, to desquamation	Minimal; avoid irritants, trauma Aqueous or weak hydrocortisone cream
Bowel	Diarrhoea/colic	Low residue diet Codeine or loperamide
Bladder	Frequency/dysuria	Exclude infection
Scalp	Hair loss	Order wig in advance. Will regrow after palliative but not radical doses
Mouth/pharynx	Mucositis	Avoid irritants and alcohol. Treat candidiasis. Topical chlorhexidine or benzydamine

TABLE 5.2 Late effects after radical radiotherapy

Site	Effect	Treatment
Skin	Fibrosis, telangiectasia Rarely necrosis	Usually none
Bowel	Stricture, perforation Bleeding fistulae	If severe resection of affected segment
Bladder	Fibrosis causing frequency Haematuria, fistulae	If severe surgical resection
CNS	Myelitis causing paraplegia Cerebral necrosis	None
Lung	Fibrosis	None

small blood vessels resulting in their occlusion (endarteritis obliterans).

Fortunately, in practice they are rare but any radical treatment dose will carry a risk of late damage becoming apparent in the months and years ahead. They are not usually seen before 6 months after treatment but there is an ongoing risk which is never entirely lost. Examples of late effects are given in Table 5.2.

Finally, the risk of inducing second malignancy should be considered. In practice, this is exceedingly rare and invariably outweighed by risk from the established malignancy for which radiation is given. A clear pattern is recognized with leukaemia or lymphoma seen in the first few years after exposure, reaching a peak incidence around 3 years and not seen after 10 years. In contrast, solid tumours have an increasing risk with time; they are rarely seen before 10 years and may occur 30 years or more after exposure.

The greatest risk may be associated with low-dose exposure and there are many examples after treatment of benign disease such as tinea capitis, goitre and ankylosing spondylitis. After therapeutic radiation the risk is small but there is some evidence that this may be increased in patients that receive combined modality treatment with the addition of chemotherapy. This has recently become apparent in long-term survivors of lymphoma treatments in whom the risk after 20 years of a second tumour is around 15 per cent.

RADIATION PROTECTION

Indiscriminate use of radiation is dangerous. There are strict regulations surrounding its use for medical purposes to ensure that exposure to staff, visitors and patients is kept to an absolute minimum. This is achieved by physical separation and protection from the sources of radiation and subsequent monitoring of exposure in those at particular risk.

Separation and protection

Radiotherapy machines are localized in one area or even in a separate hospital. Their design incorporates shielding of scattered radiation to produce a defined beam, the penetration and qualities of which are carefully measured and maintained. They are housed within a room designed to contain the radiation, using lead barriers within the walls for low-energy beams and thick high-density concrete walls for high-energy beams.

Similarly, radioisotopes are stored under carefully controlled conditions in a radiation safe and administered to the patient in a designated area, again designed to contain any radiation exposure. Patients having implants or high levels of radio-iodine will be isolated in single rooms, which have additional shielding to prevent radiation reaching other areas of the ward, and staff are given strict time limits to be spent with the patient. Visitors are usually not permitted while there are high levels of radioactivity present.

Radiation monitoring

All staff involved in the direct care of patients receiving radiation treatment will be designated as workers that require regular monitoring for radiation exposure. The mainstay of monitoring is the film badge worn by these staff, which, when processed, will detect those that may have been inadvertently exposed to radiation. There are clearly defined exposure limits for adults within which all personnel must remain. All departments must have local rules regarding the handling and use of radiation sources and staff must be fully acquainted with these.

It is important to keep the dangers of radiation as used under controlled medical conditions in context, while not relaxing the rules governing its use. There is no evidence that hospital workers are at greater risk than the general population from malignant disease. The entire population is exposed to levels of background radiation and many other common daily activities carry a greater risk than low-level exposure. For example, it has been estimated that all of the following activities carry a one in a million risk of death:

- driving for 65 miles;
- flying in civil aircraft for 400 miles;
- smoking less than one cigarette;
- drinking half a bottle of wine.

6 PRINCIPLES OF SYSTEMIC TREATMENT

Cancer chemotherapy is the treatment of malignant disease with drugs rather than radiation or surgical removal. The drugs used are often highly toxic since they are rarely, if ever, selective for cancer cells and are therefore best given within an oncology unit by those experienced in their use.

Systemic therapy may be used alone, but is more often used in combination with surgery or radiotherapy as an adjuvant to locoregional treatment to enhance local control and attack potential sites of metastases.

CHEMOTHERAPY AGENTS

Cancer chemotherapy agents act upon cell division, interfering with normal cell replication. They can be broadly classified into five main groups:

- antimetabolites;
- alkylating agents;
- intercalating agents and topoisomerase inhibitors;
- spindle poisons;
- other agents.

ANTIMETABOLITES

These function at the level of DNA synthesis, interfering with the incorporation of nucleic acid bases (cytosine, thymine, adenine and guanine). Two types of drug are currently available.

One type of drug is based on chemical modification of a nucleic acid so that the drug rather than the true nucleic acid is incorporated into the DNA, thereby preventing accurate replication of the complementary base sequence, for example, 5-fluorouracil (5-FU) and its new prodrug capecitabine, gemcitabine, cytosine arabinoside and fludarabine. These drugs may also have additional modes of inhibiting DNA synthesis for example the inhibition of thymidine synthetase by 5-FU and of ribonucleotide reductase by gemcitabine.

The other type of drug inhibits reduction of folic acid (essential for the transfer of methyl groups in DNA synthesis) from its inactive dihydrofolate form to the active tetrahydrofolate (e.g. methotrexate).

ALKYLATING AGENTS

These directly interfere with the DNA double strand of base pairs by chemically reacting with the structure, forming methyl cross-bridges. These then prevent the two DNA strands coming apart in mitosis to form daughter DNA fragments and division therefore fails. Drugs in this group include cyclophosphamide, chlorambucil, melphalan and the nitrosoureas BCNU and CCNU.

INTERCALATING AGENTS

These act in a similar way to the alkylating agents but rather than directly forming cross-strands in the DNA molecule they bind between the base pair molecules, i.e. binding adenine to thymine and cytosine to guanine, again preventing the DNA double strand from dividing in order to replicate and thereby stopping cell division. Platinum compounds (cisplatin, oxaliplatin and carboplatin) act by binding specifically to guanosine, forming DNA adducts that crosslink either within one DNA strand or across strands. Other compounds active through DNA intercalation are the anthra-cycline group of drugs (Adriamycin, epirubicin and idarubicin).

Topoisomerases are enzymes that control the tertiary coiling of DNA molecules. Two main classes are recognized; topoisomerase I and II. The podophyllotoxins etoposide (VP-16) and teniposide (VM-26) are topoisomerase II inhibitors, as are the newer camptothecin group of drugs including topotecan and irinotecan.

SPINDLE POISONS

These act by preventing spindle formation, which is essential in the sorting and moving of chromosomes following replication at the end of mitosis. The drugs in this group are the vinca alkaloids: vincristine, vinblastine and vindesine. Microtubule formation is also affected by podophyllin, and the taxane group of drugs (paclitaxel and docetaxel), which are cytotoxic through promoting the polymerization of tubulin, which is the building block of the microtubule, resulting in abnormal spindle formation and thereby cell death.

OTHER AGENTS

Other drugs which are active but whose precise mode of action is unknown include mitomycin C and bleomycin.

Because of their mode of action, certain drugs require cells to be in specific phases of the cell cycle to have any effect. For example, those acting on synthesis of DNA will only act on cells actively synthesizing at the time they are exposed to the drug. Cytotoxic drugs are therefore further classified into:

- phase-specific drugs, which act only in a specific phase of the cell cycle (e.g. antimetabolites during S phase and vinca alkaloids in M phase);
- cycle-specific drugs, which require that cells are only dividing and passing through the cell cycle rather than being in the resting G_0 phase – these include the alkylating agents.

EFFICACY AND TOXICITY OF CHEMOTHERAPY

Although in principle all cycling cells should be sensitive to drugs acting upon their replication, in practice chemotherapy for most cancers is only modestly effective. This is due to a variety of reasons related to drug delivery to the cell and activation or deactivation within the target cells. Precise indications for the use of chemotherapy are detailed in the following chapters but, in general, the common malignant diseases can be broadly classified into three groups: those extremely sensitive to chemotherapy where this is the treatment of choice; those with modest sensitivity where chemotherapy may play a part in their management but usually in combination with other treatment as an adjuvant or for recurrent disease; and finally those where chemotherapy is rarely of value. Examples of the classification are given in Table 6.1.

TABLE 6.1 Classification of common malignant diseases according to their sensitivity to chemotherapy

Group 1: Highly sensitive	Group 2: Modest sensitivity	Group 3: Low sensitivity
Leukaemias	Breast	Prostate
Lymphomas	Colorectal	Kidney
Germ cell tumours	Bladder	Primary brain tumour
Small cell lung cancer	Ovary	Adult sarcomas
Myeloma	Cervix	Endometrium
Neuroblastoma		
Wilms' tumour		
Embryonal rhabdomyosarcoma		

Response and survival

In describing the efficacy of chemotherapeutic agents there are clearly defined response criteria as follows.

■ Complete response (CR) – complete resolution of all clinically detectable disease for a period of at least 1 month.
■ Partial response (PR) – a reduction in tumour dimensions of at least 50 per cent maintained for at least 1 month (the dimension usually referred to is the maximum diameter of a tumour mass).

TABLE 6.2 Scales for performance status

Score	Status
Karnofsky	
100	Normal; no complaints; no evidence of disease
90	Able to carry on normal activities; minor signs or symptoms
80	Normal activity with effort, some signs or symptoms of disease
70	Cares for self; unable to carry on normal activity or do active work
60	Requires occasional assistance but able to care for most needs
50	Requires considerable assistance and frequent medical care
40	Disabled; requires special care and assistance
30	Severely disabled; hospitalization indicated although death not imminent
20	Very sick; hospitalization necessary; active supportive treatment necessary
10	Moribund; fatal processes progressing rapidly
0	Dead
World Health Organization (WHO)	
0	All normal activity without restriction
1	Restricted in physically strenuous activity but ambulatory and able to do light work
2	Ambulatory and capable of all self care but unable to carry out any work. Up and about >50% of waking hours
3	Capable of only limited self care, confined to bed or chair more than 50% of waking hours
4	Completely disabled. Cannot carry on any self care. Totally confined to bed or chair

■ Stable disease (SD) – no change or a response that is less than a partial response or progression less than a 25 per cent increase in measurable disease during the period of observation.
■ Progressive disease (PD) – an increase in measurable disease of at least 25 per cent during the period of observation, or the development of any new lesions.

It is important to interpret with care any response data derived from clinical trials. Unless an agent or drug combination achieves a complete response in a significant proportion of patients it is unlikely to have any impact on overall survival when used to treat that disease in the general population. Partial responses may be of value in delaying progression of a disease but since they represent only a very small decrement in total cancer cell burden, significant effects on overall survival are unlikely.

With this in mind, performance status and quality of life measures are becoming an increasingly important measure of the efficacy of cancer treatment. Numerous scales of performance status have been devised, the most widespread of which is perhaps the Karnofsky scale shown in Table 6.2. Quality of life measures are more complex and usually involve some form of structured questionnaire into the patient's activities and interests.

CLINICAL USE OF CHEMOTHERAPY

Cytotoxic drugs may be given as single agents but are more usually given in combination with other cytotoxic drugs. The major limitation in using these agents lies in their toxicity to normal tissues. Because they are all non-specific in their action, both malignant and normal cells are damaged when exposed to a cytotoxic drug. When used within their defined dose limits the normal cells will recover and it is the need for this 'window' of normal cell recovery that results in the typical intermittent scheduling of these agents, most being given at 3- to 4-weekly intervals.

Common limiting toxicities are bone marrow suppression, bowel toxicity, and renal and neurological damage. Agents for which these are major limiting factors are shown in Table 6.3.

Combination chemotherapy

For many conditions combinations of drugs are used. Effectiveness results from a balance of adding together modestly active agents to give greater overall activity and spreading different toxicities. Combinations are also designed to incorporate drugs from different classes, thereby attacking cells with both phase- and cycle-specific agents with the intent

TABLE 6.3 Major toxicities for chemotherapeutic agents

Tissue affected	Toxic agents
Bone marrow[1]	All drugs, in particular Vinblastine Etoposide Carboplatin Cyclophosphamide Melphalan Ifosfamide Paclitaxel
Bowel	Melphalan Cisplatin 5-Fluorouracil (5-FU) Irinotecan Methotrexate
Renal	Methotrexate Cisplatin Ifosfamide
Neurological	Cisplatin Vincristine Ifosfamide Paclitaxel
Cardiac	Adriamycin 5-FU
Bladder	Cyclophosphamide

[1] In practice, bone marrow toxicity is becoming less important as a limiting toxicity as techniques for bone marrow support, such as autologous marrow or peripheral stem cell transplantation, become available.

of targeting as many cells in the population as possible. An example of spreading limiting toxicities is shown in Table 6.4 with CHOP used for non-Hodgkin's lymphoma.

Combination therapy may also involve the use of a non-chemotherapy agent with a cytotoxic drug to enhance its activity. The most common example of this in clinical use is the addition of folinic acid to 5-FU, which approximately doubles its response rates in the treatment of colorectal cancer. This works because folinic acid administered increases intracellular concentrations of folate, which is an essential cofactor in the incorporation of 5-FU into RNA and also its action in inhibiting thymidylate synthetase, an important enzyme in DNA synthesis.

RESISTANCE

Resistance to chemotherapy drugs can be an intrinsic property of a malignant cell but can also be acquired after exposure to individual drugs. Mechanisms of resistance include:

- altered biochemical pathways to avoid specific pathway blocks (e.g. modified folate use to avoid dihydrofolate reductase block with methotrexate);
- altered cell transport mechanisms to prevent drug concentration in cancer cell by either reduced uptake or enhanced efflux;
- altered drug metabolism increasing clearance or reducing drug activation; and
- impaired mechanisms of apoptosis (programmed cell death).

It is often found that resistance to a number of drugs develops together, a phenomenon called multi-drug resistance (MDR). This is thought to result from

TABLE 6.4 Drugs in CHOP

Drug	Action	Main toxicity
Cyclophosphamide	Alkylating agent	Bone marrow Bladder
Adriamycin	Intercalating	Bone marrow Cardiac
Vincristine	Spindle poison	Neurological (peripheral neuropathy)
Prednisolone	Unknown	Fluid retention and weight gain Gastric irritation Hyperglycaemia

common molecular mechanisms related to specific DNA sequences. Identification of one particular genetic change in drug resistance has led to isolation of the *MDR1* gene and the protein for which it codes a transmembrane glycoprotein important in cell transport. As mechanisms of resistance are elucidated, strategies to overcome them are emerging. For example, transmembrane transport can be modified by drugs such as verapamil and cyclosporin inhibiting the efflux of drugs away from the cell.

ADMINISTRATION

Chemotherapy should only be administered in specialized units with the experience and support to do so safely. Most of the agents used can be harmful if there is continuous contact with the skin and even more so if accidentally ingested through contamination of hands and work surfaces. Agents should therefore be prepared by a specialized chemotherapy pharmacist under strictly controlled conditions and gloves should be worn by the clinical staff when administering the drugs.

Prior to administration all patients should have a full blood count measured. As a general rule, chemotherapy should only be given if the following parameters are met:

- haemoglobin >10 g/dl, although this is rarely a limiting factor and it is acceptable to proceed at lower levels and transfuse if necessary;
- total white count $>3.0 \times 10^9/l$, or total neutrophil count $>1.5 \times 10^9/l$;
- platelets $>80 \times 10^9/l$.

For certain drugs renal function must also be carefully checked prior to administration. It is not usually sufficient to rely on serum urea or creatinine, and a creatinine clearance or ethylenediaminetetraacetic acid (EDTA) clearance should be performed. This applies in particular to the following:

- cisplatin;
- methotrexate (particularly at high doses);
- ifosfamide;
- carboplatin.

Because of the close relation between serum levels and creatinine clearance, the dose of carboplatin is usually defined by a formula (the Calvert formula) which relates the predicted area under the serum concentration vs. time curve (AUC) to the clearance. This enables the drug to be given relatively safely even where renal function is impaired, with a predictable AUC after administration.

Chemotherapy drugs may be given orally, by intravenous or intramuscular bolus injection or by intravenous infusion. Examples of these are shown in Table 6.5. Many chemotherapy drugs are severe irritants when injected outside a vein and extreme care must be taken during intravenous injections. These should be performed ideally by experienced staff working in a dedicated chemotherapy administration unit. Large visible veins should be chosen as far as possible and it is safest to administer the drugs into a running intravenous drip.

Where venous access is difficult, for schedules requiring lengthy infusions or when continuous infusion pumps are to be used and in procedures likely to require the administration of many intravenous drugs and transfusions, such as bone marrow

TABLE 6.5 Routes of administration[1]

Oral	Intravenous injection	Infusion	Intrathecal
Chlorambucil	Cyclophosphamide	Cisplatin	Methotrexate
Busulphan	Methotrexate	Carboplatin	Cytosine arabinoside
Melphalan (ld)	5-Fluorouracil	Mitozantrone	
Procarbazine	Adriamycin	Ifosfamide	
Etoposide	Vincristine	Methotrexate (hd)	
Capecitebine	Vinblastine	Melphalan (hd)	
Temozolamide	Vinorelbine	Paclitaxel	
		Oocetaxel	
		Gemcitabine	
		Oxaliplatin	
		5-Fluorouracil	

[1]ld, low dose; hd, high dose.

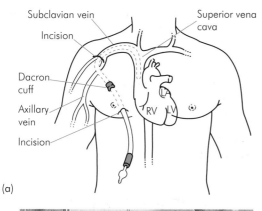

(a)

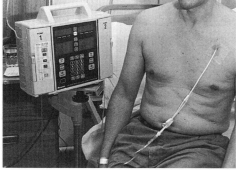

(b)

FIG 6.1 Central Hickman line shown (a) diagrammatically and (b) *in situ* in a patient. LA, left auricle; LV, left ventricle; RV, right ventricle.

transplantation or high-dose chemotherapy, an indwelling central venous catheter has many advantages. A common type is the Hickman catheter as shown in Fig. 6.1. These can be inserted under radiological control with local anaesthetic and remain *in situ* for many months. Regular flushing with heparinized saline at least weekly is required and some also recommend continuous low-dose warfarin 1 mg daily while the line remains to prevent thrombotic complications. An alternative type of central line, which may be less robust but is simpler to insert, is a line such as a PICC line which enters through the antecubital vein and is then directed through the brachial and subclavian veins into the vena cava; an example is shown in Fig. 6.2. In addition to subclavian vein thrombosis, the other major complication from central lines in chemotherapy patients is that of infection, and infected lines or subcutaneous tracts require immediate removal of the catheter together with high-dose antibiotic cover.

If extravasation of chemotherapy does occur then there should be clear guidelines for its management.

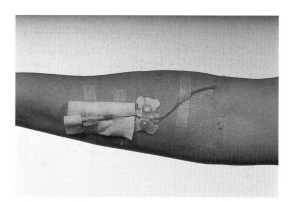

FIG 6.2 A PICC line *in situ* entering an antecubital vein.

The following principles apply:

- the chemotherapy injection or infusion must be stopped immediately;
- the cannula is left *in situ*, residual drug is aspirated and the area flushed with saline;
- ice packs may be applied and some recommend administration of local steroids or hyaluronidase.

In severe cases, with irritant drugs such as Adriamycin or epirubicin, there may be extensive soft tissue damage, as shown in Fig. 6.3, particularly if the problem is not identified immediately and action taken. Liaison with a plastic surgery unit for such eventualities is of great value. Occasionally, damage may be such as to require surgical repair.

Avoiding side-effects

As a general rule side-effects are best anticipated and prevented. Chemotherapy agents vary in their emetic potential but all may cause nausea and some severe vomiting. Antiemetics should therefore be considered for all but the most gentle of agents. A three-stage antiemetic policy will work for most patients.

Emetic potential of common chemotherapy agents

Chlorambucil and vincristine/vinblastine, used as single agents, rarely cause significant nausea and either antiemetics are not required or simple oral agents are sufficient. Other drugs or combinations fall into the groups shown in Table 6.6.

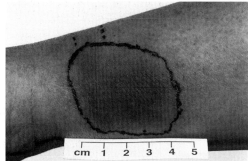

(a)

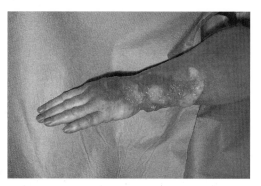

(b)

FIG 6.3 Erythema following minor extravasation of epirubicin (a) and more severe soft tissue damage following extravasation of chemotherapy given intravenously into the back of the hand (b).

The use of antiemetic drugs varies considerably among different units. A simple antiemetic protocol is given below.

- Low emetogenic schedule: metoclopramide 10 mg or prochlorperazine 25 mg rectally with chemotherapy.
- Moderately emetogenic schedule: dexamethasone 8 mg and metoclopramide 10 mg intravenously with chemotherapy followed by dexamethasone 2 mg t.d.s. orally for 2–3 days with metoclopramide 10 mg t.d.s. orally.
- Highly emetogenic schedule: dexamethasone 8 mg and ondansetron 8 mg intravenously with chemotherapy followed by dexamethasone 4 mg b.d. and ondansetron 8 mg b.d. daily for 2 days by mouth.

Anticipatory nausea and vomiting may be a particular problem for some patients when they experience symptoms with any visit to the hospital without exposure to the drugs. Lorazepam may be helpful in these instances. It is also often easier for inpatients to receive chemotherapy in the evening

TABLE 6.6 Classification of chemotherapy drugs according to their potential to provoke emesis

Low	Moderate	High
5-Fluorouracil	Cyclophosphamide	Cisplatin
Bleomycin	Methotrexate	Carboplatin
Gemcitabine	Adriamycin	Ifosfamide
Vincristine	Mitozantrone	Mustine
Vinblastine	Etoposide	Dacarbazine
Vinorelbine	Paclitaxel	

when they may have added sedation and sleep through the administration.

Other side-effects must also be anticipated and steps taken to prevent them. For example:

- diarrhoea (e.g. cisplatin, 5-FU or irinotecan) – prescribe codeine phosphate;
- mucositis (e.g. 5-FU, methotrexate) – use regular chlorhexidine and benzydamine mouthwashes;
- alopecia (e.g. Adriamycin) – use of scalp cooling and provision of wig.

Scheduling

Chemotherapy schedules vary from simple single oral drugs to complex multiple drug regimes. The design of drug schedules is based on a consideration of the effects on both normal tissues and the tumour cells.

Normal tissues are inevitably damaged by chemotherapy agents. Particularly sensitive are the dividing cells of the bone marrow and mucosal epithelial cells lining the oropharynx, gut and bladder. The general principle of scheduling chemotherapy is that each successive course should only be given when damage from the previous drug exposure has been repaired. Fortunately, both bone marrow and epithelial lining cells have a large capacity for tolerating and recovering from damage to them and usually do so within 2–3 weeks. On this basis, most chemotherapy is given at 3- to 4-weekly intervals.

Damage to tumour cells may depend on both the absolute levels of drug which can be achieved within them and the duration of exposure. In order to achieve the maximum levels possible a fine line may be drawn between serious side effects and maximizing tumour cell kill. In some circumstances where there is evidence that very high doses of drugs not normally tolerated will achieve more (e.g. acute leukaemia), then bone marrow may be removed prior to chemotherapy and stored to be used as an autograft once high-dose therapy has been given. However, these are, at present, exceptional procedures.

In order to achieve maximum levels for a suitable duration a knowledge of the pharmacokinetics of the drug is important. Drugs with short half-lives may have a greater effect when given by infusion or in divided doses (e.g. 5-FU); there also is increasing interest in the use of 5-FU as a continuous infusion over many weeks.

The design of chemotherapy drug schedules is often a combination of elegant hypothesis, serendipity and pragmatism. However, when assessing the results of chemotherapy trials and translating them into general oncological practice, careful attention to the drug dosing and scheduling is important. There is some evidence that patients who fail to receive full doses of drugs at the designated minimum intervals have a reduced benefit from the treatment and this is a strong argument for chemotherapy being managed only in experienced units familiar with the complications and tolerance for each schedule.

HORMONE THERAPY

A small number of tumours are influenced by therapeutic changes in their hormone environment. In practice, hormone therapy is of value for breast and prostatic cancer and, to a lesser extent, endometrial cancer. Occasional responses with other tumour types have been reported, particularly to the drug tamoxifen, but their basis remains uncertain. The response of breast cancer is based primarily upon the influence of oestrogen, and that of prostate cancer upon the influence of androgens.

Breast cancer

Oestrogen exerts its effect by binding to a receptor within the cell nucleus called the 'oestrogen receptor'. This process is thought to be fundamental to the way in which oestrogen can influence the development of breast cancer. Drugs which alter the balance of activity at the oestrogen receptor are therefore often of value in the treatment of breast cancer. Such drugs may act directly by binding to the receptor, thereby blocking its activity, as typified by tamoxifen, or indirectly on the production and peripheral activation of oestriol and oestrone

to oestradiol by inhibiting the enzyme aromatase. Commonly used drugs now include anastrozole and letrozole, which have largely replaced older drugs of this group such as aminoglutethimide and 4-hydroxyandrostenedione, because they have a more favourable side-effect profile.

The presence of oestrogen receptors in an individual tumour is important in predicting the likelihood of response to hormonal treatments such as tamoxifen; on first exposure to tamoxifen (or any other hormone treatment) around 50 per cent of patients with breast cancer will respond but this figure reflects a response rate of up to 80 per cent when oestrogen receptors are positive compared with around 10 per cent where they are negative. Oestrogen receptors can be demonstrated histologically on sections of a breast cancer using immunohistochemistry.

The observation that some patients will respond who have no demonstrable receptors is puzzling; one explanation may be that the receptors in these cancer cells have a slightly different structure not detected by the routine methods of assay.

Characteristically, hormone responses have a finite duration and it would seem that all breast cancers eventually become resistant to the first hormone treatment to which they are exposed. This may, however, be followed by second, third and even fourth responses to further hormone manipulations. The basis for resistance is often thought to be changes in the characteristics of the oestrogen receptor, varying from complete loss of receptor to alterations in its binding sites or in its transcriptional properties within the nucleus. In other cases, access to the receptor may be denied because of alterations of transport mechanisms and metabolism within the cell. Exposure to an alternative hormone therapy may, in many cases, achieve a second response, seen in 45 per cent of patients responding initially to tamoxifen. It is notable that around 20 per cent of patients failing to respond to tamoxifen will respond to a second exposure to an alternative endocrine therapy.

Progestogens may also be effective in breast cancer. The basis for this is less clear than that for drugs acting upon the oestrogen system. Drugs such as megestrol and medroxyprogesterone do indirectly affect activity at the oestrogen receptor causing downregulation (i.e. making them less sensitive to stimulation by oestrogen) but, in addition, specific progestogen receptors have been identified in breast cancers and found to correlate with response to treatment.

An overview of hormone therapy in breast cancer is given in Table 6.7.

TABLE 6.7 Hormone therapy in breast cancer

Drug	Mode of action	Other actions and common side-effects
Tamoxifen Toremifene	Anti-oestrogen	Oestrogen agonist in bone, uterus and on lipid metabolism Flushes, nausea, weight gain, vaginal discharge or bleeding
Aminoglutethimide	Aromatase inhibitor	Inhibits other adrenal enzymes causing 'medical adrenalectomy' Skin rashes, nausea, malaise, fatigue, liver dysfunction
Formestane	Aromatase inhibitor	Irritation around injection sites – requires intramuscular administration
Exemestane	Aromatase inhibitor	Oral administration, fewer side-effects than aminoglutethimide
Anastrozole	Aromatase inhibitor	Skin rashes and flushing, nausea, hair thinning, diarrhoea, drowsiness
Lentrozole	Aromatase inhibitor	Hot flushes, nausea, gastrointestinal upset, rash, headache, muscle pains
Medroxyprogesterone Megestrol	Progestogen	Nausea, weight gain, depression, fluid retention
Durabolin	Androgen	Virilization, increased libido, requires intramuscular injection

Prostate cancer

The basis of hormone therapy in prostate cancer is the dependence on androgen for its growth. The drugs used to treat prostate cancer therefore are anti-androgens working either directly by antagonism at the androgen receptor or indirectly on the hypothalamic–pituitary axis regulation of androgen release. Similar effects are also achieved by surgical orchidectomy removing the main site of androgen production. The possibilities for androgen blockade are shown in Fig. 6.4. The relative clinical merits of the available anti-androgen therapies are shown in Table 10.2 (see Chapter 10).

None of the individual anti-androgen treatments offer complete blockade of both testicular and adrenal androgens. This may be achieved by combining a centrally acting gonadotrophin-releasing hormone agonist/antagonist (e.g. goserelin) with a peripherally acting drug (e.g. cyproterone or bicalutamide) and is known as 'total androgen blockade'. There is, however, no evidence that this is much more effective than single-drug therapy.

An important distinction between the hormone response of prostate cancer and that of breast cancer is seen on relapse to first-line anti-androgen therapy; second responses with prostate cancer are seen only occasionally.

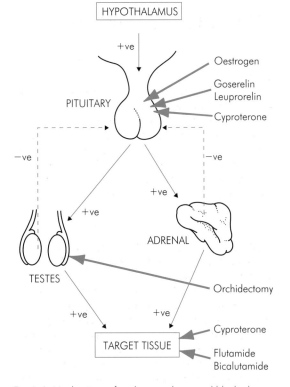

FIG 6.4 Mechanisms of androgen release and blockade.

Endometrial cancer

Endometrial cancer is recognized as a tumour which is stimulated by high levels of circulating oestrogen. Both oestrogen and progesterone receptors can be demonstrated in cells of endometrial cancer and treatment with progestogens or gonadotrophin-releasing hormone agonists/antagonists can be effective in metastatic disease. Response is predicted by the presence of oestrogen or progestogen receptors, with around 65 per cent of patients with positive receptors responding to treatment. A reduction in oestrogen receptor concentration has been demonstrated after progestogen treatment, suggesting that the efficacy of hormone treatment in endometrial cancer reflects inhibition of oestrogenic stimulus at the tumour cell in a way analogous to that seen in breast cancer.

BIOLOGICAL THERAPY

A number of the chemicals produced by the body in response to injury or infection have been explored as potential new treatments to eradicate cancer cells. Unfortunately, only limited success has so far been achieved. Invariably, such preparations are immunogenic and are therefore associated with side-effects such as malaise and low-grade fever. These are often debilitating but major toxicities are rare with commercially available compounds. In clinical practice only two agents, α-interferon and interleukin 2 appear to have any significant tumour responses.

α-Interferon

This is the treatment of choice in the rare haematological malignancy hairy cell leukaemia (Chapter 17) and has an increasing role in the management of chronic granulocytic leukaemia (Chapter 17). It may also be of value as maintenance therapy in multiple myeloma once patients have reached plateau phase (Chapter 17). Other potential roles in renal cancer and melanoma remain under investigation. In each of these instances interferon is believed to function by enhancing the natural defences available within the body, facilitating removal of malignant cells.

α-Interferon is given by subcutaneous injection three times per week. In doses above 3 MU, side-effects of fever and malaise can be dose-limiting. Treatment in the haematological malignancies mentioned may be continuous for many months or even years.

Interleukin 2

This has been extensively investigated, particularly in the management of advanced melanoma, renal cell carcinoma and colorectal cancer. Its activity against these tumours is enhanced by administering it with lymphokine-activated killer (LAK) T-cells, but even so only modest response rates of 20–30 per cent are seen, and usually only in those patients with very limited disease. No convincing evidence for the usefulness of interleukin 2 in terms of improved survival or quality of life has yet emerged and its use remains confined to strict protocols evaluating its possible role. It may be most promising in combination with interferon and chemotherapy, as used in some schedules under investigation for renal cell cancer.

Administration is similar to that for interferon with regular subcutaneous injections being required.

Monoclonal antibody treatments

Monoclonal antibodies (MABs) are the equivalent of the magic bullet, their principle being to carry a toxic agent to a cell defined by specific surface antigens against which the targeting antibody is raised. In recent years this approach has resulted in new clinical agents becoming available in particular rituximab against the CD20 antigen on B cell lymphomas and Herceptin against the HER2 antibody on breast cancer cells. Rituximab has been shown to improve results of standard combination chemotherapy when given as part of a combined schedule in high-grade diffuse B cell lymphomas. Herceptin is now a valuable additional treatment option for patients with metastatic breast cancer which is Her-2 positive; this can be demonstrated immunohistochemically and the extent of staining can be graded to predict the likelihood of response, as shown in Fig. 6.5.

Clinical trials are underway to define the precise role of these new agents in the management of these diseases; they will probably be incorporated into existing chemotherapy regimes both in the adjuvant setting and in primary treatment. Experimental work in colorectal cancer and prostate cancer is also underway.

GROWTH FACTORS

One of the major dose-limiting toxicities encountered in the use of chemotherapy is that of bone

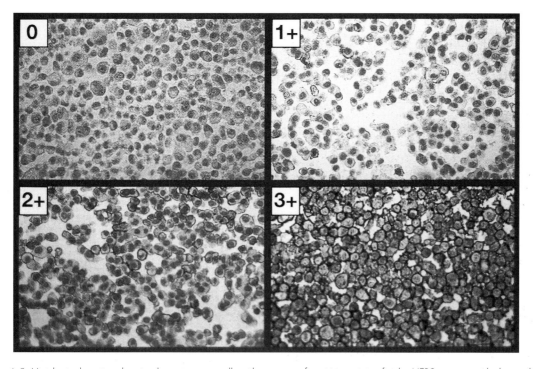

FIG 6.5 Histological section showing breast cancer cells with a range of positive staining for the HER2 receptor, which may be seen, predicting varying degrees of response to the monoclonal antibody Herceptin.

marrow toxicity. In recent years the availability of colony-stimulating factors (CSF), in particular granulocyte colony-stimulating factor (G-CSF) and granulocyte/macrophage colony-stimulating factor (GM-CSF), has enabled chemotherapy dose to be intensified within the limits of tolerance of bone marrow. These are analogues of naturally occurring growth factors, given by subcutaneous injection following exposure to chemotherapy, which stimulate the granulocyte production lines in the bone marrow, reducing the period of neutropenia after intensive chemotherapy. The factors currently available have no significant effect upon platelet and red cell lines. Their use has also facilitated the process of peripheral blood progenitor cell (PBPC) harvesting, thereby simplifying the use of ultra high-dose chemotherapy, which is being increasingly applied to the treatment of solid as well as haemopoietic tumours.

EXPERIMENTAL CHEMOTHERAPY

The chemotherapy drugs and combination regimes which are widely used in routine oncological practice today have arisen out of carefully designed and regulated drug development programmes. From discovery of a promising new drug in the laboratory, a lengthy and expensive period of evaluation starting with animal pharmacology and toxicology studies and ending in successful drug marketing has to be embarked on. The clinical studies within which new drugs may be given are outlined below and discussed in greater detail in Chapter 3.

- Phase 1 studies – these are studies in which the new agent is first tried in patients. Such agents are offered only to patients for whom there is no other recognized effective treatment and that may wish to try other drugs in the slim hope of benefit. In phase 1 studies, activity against the tumour is not an end-point but these studies are designed to assess the maximum tolerated doses and define the toxicity profile in humans.
- Phase 2 studies – these are the earliest studies in which anti-tumour activity is sought, giving the drug in doses and schedules defined from the phase 1 studies to patients that have failed previous conventional therapy or for whom there may be no effective recognized treatment.
- Phase 3 studies – having established activity in phase 2, the new agent is compared with the

standard best treatment (or, if there is none, with placebo) in a large prospective randomized trial. Large numbers of patients are entered into such trials in order to achieve statistically robust results and most of these studies are therefore multi-centre studies.

Only following satisfactory passage through the above steps is a drug incorporated in the routine treatment of cancer; this may be many years after the first identification of the compound and will be followed by further evaluation of the drug to establish its full potential and application in adjuvant and primary treatment and its role in palliation both alone and in combination. Its toxicity in wider use must also be continuously monitored and notified (postmarketing surveillance).

Current areas of research in drug development alongside the more conventional classes of chemotherapy drugs include:

- matrix metalloproteinase inhibitors designed to block the actions of this important enzyme, which facilitates cancer cell entry into tissues;
- vascular targeting agents exploiting the different characteristics of tumour vasculature from normal blood vessels to selectively damage tumour blood supply;
- anti-angiogenic agents inhibiting the development of tumour vasculature;
- bioreductive agents selectively metabolized in areas of hypoxia which are characteristic of a growing tumour;
- drugs targeted against specific receptors involved in cellular growth control, for example the epithelial growth factor receptor (EGFR).

LUNG CANCER

Epidemiology

There are 190 000 new cases of lung cancer and 180 000 deaths in the European Union per annum. It is the major cause of cancer mortality in Europe, with a peak incidence of 60–70 years. It is three times more common in men, in whom it is the most common cancer. The mortality is declining in men, but increasing in women owing to changes in smoking habits in recent decades.

Aetiology

The majority of cases of lung cancer can be attributed to exposure of the bronchial epithelium to inhaled carcinogens. There is a strong causal relationship between smoking and lung cancer, with 90 per cent of cases attributable to the use of tobacco. The bronchial tree and alveoli are directly exposed to the inhaled smoke and it is the hydrocarbon carcinogens, such as benzpyrene, liberated by the combustion of tar that are responsible rather than nicotine. These lead to metaplasia of the bronchial epithelium from a columnar pattern to a squamous one, eventually leading to dysplasia and carcinoma. The risk of developing lung cancer is related to the duration and intensity of smoking, increasing with the rise in number of cigarettes or weight of tobacco smoked per day, increasing tar content, shorter cigarette stubs and use of non-filter brands. The tumours tend to be found adjacent to the larger airways of the lung comprising mainly squamous cell carcinoma and small cell lung cancer. Evidence suggests that passive smoking leads to an increased risk if a partner smokes 20 cigarettes per day or more. The lung cancer risk declines towards that of non-smokers after 10–20 years of abstinence although there is a persistent risk in those who have smoked more than 20 per day. It is important to elicit a history of occupational asbestos exposure in patients with lung cancer as they may be eligible for industrial injuries compensation. The carcinogenic potential of asbestos is synergistic with that of tobacco smoking and of the many types of asbestos the blue variant is the most powerful carcinogen. Asbestos-induced cancers are more common in the lower lobes, usually squamous carcinomas, and may be multicentric. During the nineteenth century, cobalt miners in Eastern Europe were noted to have a very high mortality from lung cancer because of high levels of radon gas released from the granite-bearing rocks by the radioactive decay of naturally occurring uranium, which in turn led to exposure of the bronchial tree to high doses of radiation and eventual malignant transformation. There is evidence that the level of radon in dwellings may account for a small proportion of deaths from lung cancer each year, and an increased incidence of lung cancer has also been noted in patients that have had previous spinal irradiation for ankylosing spondylitis. Nickel, arsenic and chromates have all been implicated as causes of lung cancer. Tuberculous scars, subpleural blebs/bullae or the site of a previous pulmonary embolus may occasionally account for peripheral carcinomas, particularly adenocarcinoma. Cytogenetic studies have shown loss of a tumour suppressor gene on part of the short arm of chromosome 3 in some cases of small-cell lung cancer.

Pathology

Macroscopically, lung cancers arise within the bronchial epithelium and therefore usually have an endobronchial component. They may be multifocal and may arise anywhere in the bronchial tree, although squamous- and small-cell carcinomas often arise centrally in the larger airways while adenocarcinomas usually arise peripherally, particularly at the apices. Central necrosis leads to cavitation in the larger tumours. Microscopically, lung cancers may be divided into two groups:

- small cell carcinoma (SCLC) (25 per cent);
- non-small cell lung cancer (NSCLC) – squamous cell carcinoma (50 per cent), adenocarcinoma (15 per cent) and large cell anaplastic carcinoma (10 per cent).

Squamous cell carcinoma may be preceded by the stepwise progression from squamous metaplasia to dysplasia followed by carcinoma *in situ* and frankly invasive cancer. The tumour cells have the morphology of squamous epithelial cells, stain for keratin and intercellular bridges are visible under the electron microscope (these features being more evident in well-differentiated tumours).

Small cell carcinoma arises from the Kulchitsky cells of the basal layer of the bronchial epithelium and is characterized histologically by small, uniform cells containing neurosecretory granules and staining for neurone-specific enolase (NSE), reflecting their origin from cells derived from the neural crest of the fetus. The ectopic production of peptides and hormones will be reflected in their immunocytochemical staining. There are several subtypes, the best known of which is the oat cell carcinoma, which is composed of sheets of fusiform cells.

Adenocarcinoma cells stain for mucin, reflecting their glandular origin, and may be arranged in an acinar pattern. Large cell anaplastic carcinoma is poorly differentiated and cannot be recognized under the light microscope as belonging to any of the other subgroups. Clear cell and giant cell tumours are included in this group.

Natural history

The pattern of growth of a lung cancer is related to the histological subtype. The anaplastic carcinomas are the most rapid-growing, while adenocarcinomas grow slowly and may be seen to have been present over several years prior to diagnosis. Small cell carcinoma has a propensity to early and widespread metastatic dissemination, with 80–90 per cent having spread beyond the thorax by the time of diagnosis.

Lung cancer spreads circumferentially and longitudinally along the bronchus of origin, eventually leading to bronchial occlusion, which causes lobar or segmental pulmonary collapse owing to resorption of air distal to the tumour. Stasis of pulmonary secretions in turn leads to secondary infection manifesting as pneumonia and occasionally lung abscess and empyema. Proximally, the tumour may extend to the carina and trachea, while distally it may reach the visceral pleura from where it may invade the chest wall, interlobar fissures or pleural space, resulting in a blood-stained exudative pleural effusion. A pneumothorax may result from a tumour which breaches the visceral pleura and allows a direct connection between the pleural space and the bronchial tree (i.e. a bronchopleural fistula). Mediastinal structures such as the oesophagus, pericardium, heart and great vessels and occasionally the vertebral bodies and diaphragm may be invaded. The tumour frequently involves the regional lymphatics, spreading to ipsilateral peribronchial and hilar nodes, followed by subcarinal, contralateral hilar, paratracheal and supraclavicular nodes. Lung cancer has a propensity to disseminate widely via the bloodstream and virtually any site may be involved. There is an unusual and unexplained involvement of the adrenal glands in a high proportion of cases. Other common sites include the liver, skeleton, brain (especially SCLC), skin and contralateral lung, when a solitary lesion may be difficult to distinguish from a synchronous second primary lung cancer (Fig. 7.1).

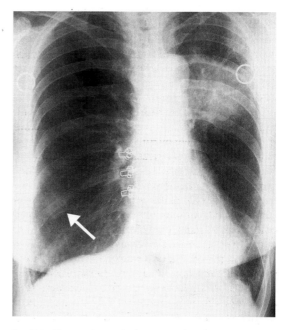

FIG 7.1 Chest radiograph demonstrating a large carcinoma arising in the left upper lobe. There is a smaller mass in the right lower lobe (arrowed) which could represent a second primary lung cancer or a metastasis.

Symptoms

A small proportion of patients will present with no symptoms, having been diagnosed on a chest X-ray either as part of a routine screen or as part of the investigation of another disease. Most, however, present due to intrathoracic symptoms:

- cough;
- haemoptysis;
- dyspnoea;
- chest pain;
- recurrent chest infections.

Cough is caused by bronchial irritation by the tumour and is often unproductive unless associated with secondary infection. Broncho-alveolar tumours (see Rare tumours, p. 64) characteristically result in the expectoration of large quantities of mucoid sputum. The cough will have a 'bovine' character if there is also a vocal cord palsy.

Haemoptysis varies in severity from slight streaking of the sputum with blood to frank haemorrhage where there is a large intrabronchial component to the tumour with mucosal ulceration. Massive intrapulmonary haemorrhage may occasionally lead to the death of the patient.

Dyspnoea reflects a deficiency in pulmonary ventilation caused by a restrictive defect (e.g. pleural effusion, diffuse parenchymal infiltration), obstructive defect (e.g. bronchial obstruction by tumour or secondary infection) or a combination of the two. It will first be noted on mild exertion, progressing to dyspnoea at rest.

Chest pain may be pleuritic or aching in nature and localized to the involved hemithorax, reflecting pleural involvement by tumour, secondary infection of the pleura or direct invasion of the chest wall.

Recurrent chest infections are a common presenting feature and carcinoma of the lung should be considered in anyone of the appropriate age who has had recurrent chest infections for no apparent cause or an infection that has failed to resolve following one or more courses of the appropriate antibiotic.

Dysphagia may result from extrinsic compression from the primary tumour, particularly if the tumour is arising from the left main bronchus as the oesophagus is a close anatomical relation posteriorly. A large mass of involved lymph nodes (usually subcarinal) should also be considered as a cause. A hoarse voice suggests invasion of the recurrent laryngeal nerve, giving rise to a vocal cord paralysis which in turn results in a hoarse voice and 'bovine'

cough due to failure to adduct the vocal cords. Indirect laryngoscopy in the clinic or visualization of the cords at bronchoscopy will be diagnostic. Tumours arising at the lung apex may cause nerve root pain as they lead to direct invasion of the T1 nerve root leading to pain radiating down the ipsilateral arm to the medial aspect of the forearm, and may lead to infiltration of the spinal cord itself. Non-specific extrathoracic symptoms include anorexia, weight loss, malaise and lethargy.

Signs

No physical signs at all may be elicited, particularly in those presenting without symptoms after a routine chest X-ray. Pulmonary collapse and/or consolidation is the most frequent finding. Examination of the hands frequently reveals clubbing, characterized by an increase in nail convexity in the transverse and longitudinal planes, loss of the nail fold angle and sponginess of the nail bed on compression of the nail (Fig. 7.2). There may be nicotine staining of the fingers. The supraclavicular lymph nodes should be checked as these are the only palpable nodes that are in continuity with the regional lymphatics. The syndrome of superior vena cava obstruction deserves special mention (see Chapter 22). Involvement of the cervical sympathetic nerves at the level of T1 leads to Horner's syndrome (Fig. 7.3) characterized by partial ptosis, miosis (pupillary constriction), enophthalmos (indrawing of the globe of the eye relative to the orbit) and anhydrosis (loss of sweating on the ipsilateral side of the face). The ipsilateral hand may be warmer due to vasodilation, and there will be wasting of the small muscles of the hand, as these are partly innervated by the T1 nerve root (Fig. 7.4).

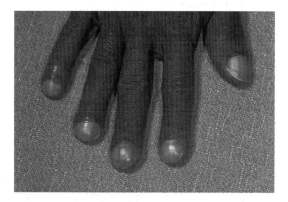

FIG 7.2 Clubbing of the fingers. This is a common non-metastatic manifestation of squamous carcinoma. There are many non-malignant causes (e.g. chronic pulmonary and cardiac disease).

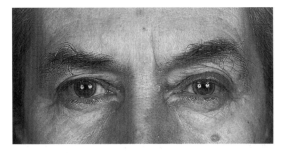

FIG 7.3 Horner's syndrome affecting the left eye. There is a partial ptosis, enophthalmos and miosis of the pupil.

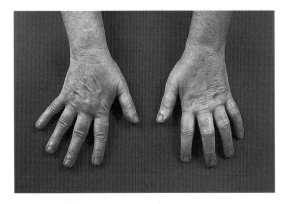

FIG 7.4 The hands of the patient in Fig. 7.3. Note the clawing of the left hand due to a T1 nerve root lesion. This has weakened the extensor muscles of the fingers leading to unopposed action of the muscles which causes finger flexion.

A small proportion will present with one or more of a variety of clinical syndromes which are unassociated with metastases. These are the so-called non-metastatic manifestations of malignancy (Table 7.1). Other signs will depend on the tumour burden and sites of spread.

Differential diagnosis

Differential diagnosis includes:

- benign tumours – papilloma, hamartoma, carcinoid, fibroma, leiomyoma;
- other malignant primary tumours – mesothelioma, bronchial gland carcinomas, soft tissue sarcomas;
- metastases;
- non-neoplastic diseases (e.g. aspergilloma, chronic lung abscess, Wegener's granulomatosis);
- radiographic artefact (e.g. nipple shadow).

TABLE 7.1 Non-metastatic manifestations of lung cancer

Cutaneous
  Dermatomyositis
  Acanthosis nigricans
  Erythema gyratum ripens
  Hypertrichosis languinosa
  Clubbing
  Hypertrophic pulmonary osteoarthropathy
  Scleroderma
  Herpes zoster
  Urticaria

Neuromuscular
  Myositis
  Proximal myopathy
  Peripheral neuropathy
  Mononeuritis multiplex
  Cortical degeneration
  Progressive multifocal leucoencephalopathy
  Transverse myelitis
  Cerebellar degeneration
  Eaton–Lambert myasthenic syndrome

Ectopic hormone production
  Hypokalaemia and water retention
    (antidiuretic hormone)
  Hyperpigmentation and hypokalaemic
    alkalosis (adrenocorticotropic hormone)
  Hypercalcaemia (parathyroid hormone)
  Carcinoid (serotonin)
  Hypoglycaemia (insulin-like peptides)
  Hyperglycaemia (glucagon, growth hormone)
  Gynaecomastia and testicular atrophy
    (gonadotrophins, β-human chorionic
    gonadotrophin)
  Hypertension (renin)

Haematological
  Anaemia (may be sideroblastic)
  Disseminated intravascular coagulation
  Eosinophilia
  Thrombocytosis
  Thrombocytopenia
  Leucocytosis/leukaemoid picture
  Red cell aplasia
  Bone marrow plasmacytosis

Miscellaneous
  Murantic endocarditis
    (may lead to systemic emboli)
  Membranous glomerulonephritis
  Hypo-uricaemia
  Hyperamylasaemia
  Migratory thrombophlebitis
    (Trousseau's syndrome)

Investigations

Chest X-ray

This has the advantage of providing a relatively rapid, non-invasive, widely available means of ascertaining the position, size and number of tumours. For optimal assessment, a postero-anterior and lateral view should always be requested. Common features of lung cancer include a discrete opacity (Fig. 7.5) which may be cavitating, hilar lymphadenopathy, pulmonary collapse, consolidation, and pleural effusion. Associated intrathoracic complications due to local invasion may be assessed, with special care being taken to look for rib erosion in peripherally placed tumours. The hemidiaphragms should be inspected, looking for excessive elevation – the right is usually slightly higher than the left because of the underlying liver. An elevated hemidiaphragm suggests palsy of the ipsilateral phrenic nerve, which in turn suggests mediastinal infiltration and therefore an inoperable tumour.

Sputum cytology

This is a rapid means of obtaining a tissue diagnosis with minimal patient inconvenience and distress; it has the advantage of being suitable for outpatients awaiting a definitive investigation such as a bronchoscopy. The sensitivity of the test increases with the number of sputum specimens collected, so at least three specimens are desirable. Samples should represent bronchial secretions rather than saliva and the best time for collection is early in the morning. Prior to collection, 5 ml of nebulized saline and physiotherapy may help a patient that has a non-productive cough. Central tumours are most likely to be detected in this way, particularly those associated with a large endobronchial component, e.g. squamous carcinoma. It should be noted that sputum containing squamous carcinoma cells could be related to an underlying primary cancer of the upper respiratory tract (e.g. larynx).

Bronchoscopy

This should be performed whenever active treatment is indicated. A fibre-optic bronchoscope is passed down the respiratory tract via the nose after topical anaesthesia, although rigid bronchoscopy under general anaesthesia is sometimes performed by the thoracic surgeon. Detailed anatomical information is gained of the precise location of the tumour within the bronchial tree, which is of value when surgery or radiotherapy is contemplated; vocal cord palsy also may be confirmed on entry into the lower respiratory tract with the scope. Once visualized, the tumour can be biopsied or if the tumour is located too peripherally for the bronchoscope to reach it, saline can be injected and aspirated and the 'washings' sent for cytology; a small brush can be used to obtain 'brushings' from the epithelial lining of the bronchi. Bronchoscopy may also allow emergency procedures to be performed, such as diathermy or laser of a bleeding tumour.

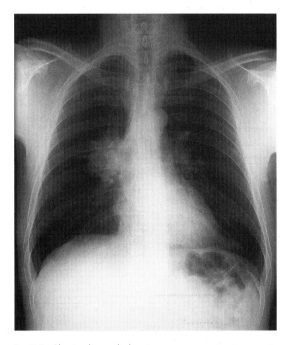

FIG 7.5 Chest radiograph showing a squamous carcinoma arising adjacent to the right hilum. In this example, there is no associated pulmonary collapse, suggesting patency of the bronchi.

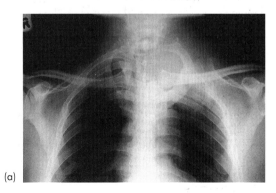

(a)

FIG 7.6a Pancoast tumour. Chest radiograph showing an apical tumour arising from the apex of the left lung. Note the soft tissue swelling in the supraclavicular fossa. There is pulmonary collapse leading to narrowing of the intercostal spaces and destruction of the underlying posterior ribs.

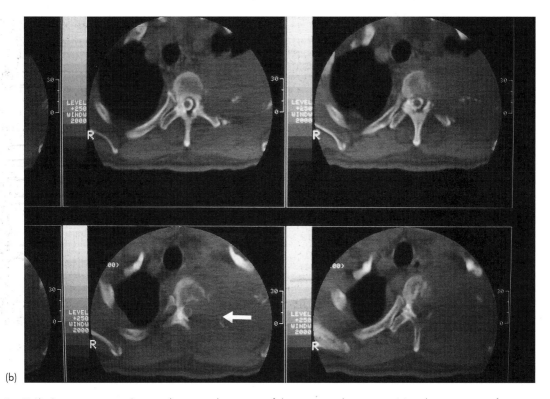

(b)

FIG 7.6b Pancoast tumour. Computed tomography images of the corresponding region. Note the enormous soft tissue mass destroying the rib and vertebral body. Such patients are at high risk of spinal cord compression (arrowed).

Computed tomography

Computed tomography (CT) is indicated whenever curative treatment is contemplated. It is the investigation of choice for detecting chest wall invasion, particularly in the case of apical tumours which may not be well visualized with plain radiographs (Fig. 7.6), and for detecting mediastinal lymphadenopathy, both of which individually are contraindications to surgical resection. The thorax is scanned to supplement the findings on plain X-rays and bronchoscopy as the superior soft tissue contrast of CT more precisely defines the local extent of the tumour and distinguishes tumour from collapsed/consolidated lung tissue (Fig. 7.7). The liver and adrenals (Fig. 7.8) are included to exclude distant metastases. A limited CT scan can also be used to facilitate percutaneous needle biopsy in those patients in whom a tissue diagnosis cannot be obtained by less invasive means.

Magnetic resonance imaging

Magnetic resonance imaging (MRI) may be used in staging, providing images that are complementary to those obtained by CT. It is of particular value in

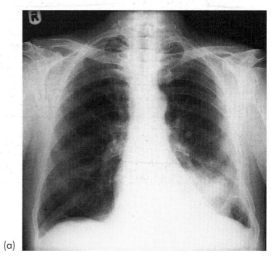

(a)

FIG 7.7a Chest radiograph in a patient with a carcinoma causing obstruction of the left lower lobe bronchus leading to collapse and consolidation distally.

providing high-resolution images of soft tissues, which may clarify the extent of local tumour invasion (e.g. when CT has suggested equivocal large blood vessel infiltration).

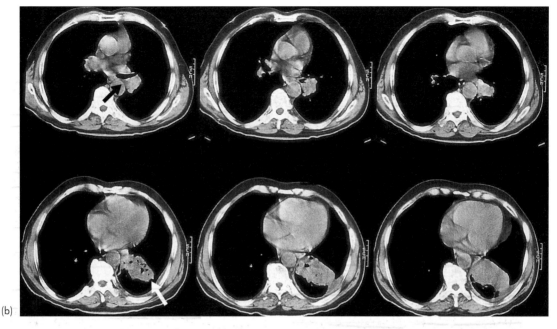

(b)

Fig 7.7b Computed tomography (CT) images of the thorax from the same patient demonstrating the primary tumour near the left hilum (top left arrow). The collapse and consolidation can be seen distal to this (bottom left arrow). There is also a left basal pleural effusion. These images demonstrate the greater detail seen with CT compared with plain radiographs.

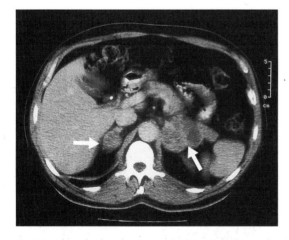

Fig 7.8 Bilateral adrenal metastases. Computed tomography image of the upper abdomen.

Isotope bone scan

This is performed to exclude bone metastases in those that are being considered for radical therapy.

Biopsy/aspiration of palpable metastases

Biopsy or fine-needle aspiration of palpable metastatic deposits such as a supraclavicular lymph node or a cutaneous nodule is a relatively atraumatic means of obtaining a tissue diagnosis.

Mediastinotomy and/or mediastinoscopy

These are invasive surgical investigations to determine whether the tumour is operable by allowing the surgeon to visualize and sample the mediastinal lymph nodes. Such procedures have been superseded by the CT scan.

Thoracotomy

This is the most invasive means of obtaining tumour tissue for histopathology, and is reserved for the very small proportion of patients that are not diagnosed after routine investigations. Unless the tumour has been shown to be inoperable during preoperative assessment, the surgeon will aim to proceed to radical resection after frozen section has been performed, particularly for non-small cell lung cancer (NSCLC).

Lung function tests

These are performed to assess the patient's ventilatory capacity with regard to the compliance of the lungs and degree of airway obstruction and are only required prior to definitive lung resection as a guide to how disabled the patient would be postoperatively. A simpler guide is the patient's exercise tolerance – inability to climb a flight of stairs without stopping would be considered a contraindication to surgery.

Indirect laryngoscopy

This is indicated if the patient has an unexplained vocal abnormality and entails visualization of the position and mobility of the two vocal cords using a laryngeal mirror in the ear, nose and throat (ENT) clinic. Partial or complete palsy suggests pressure on the recurrent laryngeal nerve.

Staging

The TNM staging (see Chapter 2) is the most frequently used and can be used as a guide to management and prognosis.

- TX – primary tumour cannot be assessed, or tumour proven by the presence of malignant cells in sputum or bronchial washings but not visualized by imaging or bronchoscopy.
- T0 – no evidence of primary tumour.
- Tis – carcinoma *in situ*.
- T1 – a tumour that is 3 cm or less in greatest dimension, surrounded by lung or visceral pleura, and without bronchoscopic evidence of invasion more proximal than the lobar bronchus (i.e., not in the main bronchus).
- T2 – a tumour with any of the following features of size or extent:
  - More than 3 cm in greatest dimension;
  - involves the main bronchus, 2 cm or more distal to the carina;
  - invades the visceral pleura;
  - associated with atelectasis or obstructive pneumonitis that extends the hilar region but does not involve the entire lung.
- T3 – a tumour of any size that directly invades any of the following: chest wall (including superior sulcus tumours), diaphragm, mediastinal pleura, parietal pericardium; or tumour in the main bronchus less than 2 cm distal to the carina but without involvement of the carina; or associated atelectasis or obstructive pneumonitis of the entire lung.
- T4 – a tumour of any size that invades any of the following: mediastinum, heart, great vessels, trachea, oesophagus, vertebral body, carina; or separate tumour nodules in the same lobe; or tumour with a malignant pleural effusion.

- NX – regional lymph nodes cannot be assessed.
- N0 – no regional lymph node metastasis.
- N1 – metastasis to ipsilateral peribronchial and/or ipsilateral hilar lymph nodes, and intrapulmonary nodes including involvement by direct extension of the primary tumour.
- N2 – metastasis to ipsilateral mediastinal and/or subcarinal lymph node(s).
- N3 – metastasis to contralateral mediastinal, contralateral hilar, ipsilateral or contralateral scalene, or supraclavicular lymph node(s).
- MX – distant metastasis cannot be assessed.
- M0 – no distant metastasis.
- M1 – distant metastasis present.

American Joint Committee on Cancer (AJCC) stage groupings, based on TNM, are frequently used in lung cancer.

- Stage 0 – Tis, N0, M0.
- Occult – TX, N0, M0.
- Stage IA – T1, N0, M0.
- Stage IB – T2, N0, M0.
- Stage IIA – T1, N1, M0.
- Stage IIB – T2, N1, M0; T3, N0, M0.
- Stage IIIA – T1, N2, M0; T2, N2, M0; T3, N1, M0; T3, N2, M0.
- Stage IIIB – any T, N3, M0, T4; any N, M0.
- Stage IV – any T; any N, M1.

With SCLC, a two-category staging system is still used which correlates well with prognosis and serves as a guide to determining the most appropriate therapy in clinical trials.

- Limited (30 per cent) – extent of tumour as defined by physical examination and radiological investigations is confined to the ipsilateral hemithorax and ipsilateral supraclavicular nodes; most 2-year survivors will be in this group.
- Extensive (70 per cent) – defined as disease other than limited stage.

Management

RADICAL TREATMENT OF NSCLC
Surgery

Complete surgical excision is desirable and offers the best chance of cure, although only about 25 per cent of patients will be suitable candidates. Surgery will involve either lobectomy or pneumonectomy,

TABLE 7.2 Contraindications to radical surgery for lung cancer

Patient parameter	Preoperative investigation
Poor lung function	Routine lung function testing
Phrenic nerve palsy	Diaphragmatic screening
Recurrent laryngeal nerve palsy	Indirect laryngoscopy
Invasion of trachea, aorta, heart, superior vena cava, oesophagus	Computed tomography scan of thorax
Distant metastases	Relevant imaging studies and/or biopsies

depending on the site of the tumour, its size and the patient's respiratory reserve. Both procedures have a significant mortality of approximately 5 per cent and 10 per cent, respectively. A more conservative segmental resection may be considered for those with very small tumours or limited respiratory reserve although the rate of local recurrence is higher than lobectomy, especially for larger cancers. Only 25 per cent of those selected for radical resection will be cured owing to either occult persistence of local disease or distant metastases at the time of surgery. The survival rate following surgery varies greatly from series to series but is in the region of 20–30 per cent at 5 years and reflects the selection criteria used by the surgeon to determine which patients undergo surgery and the skill of the surgeon concerned. Table 7.2 outlines the contraindications to surgery.

Radiotherapy

Comparisons of radiotherapy versus surgery have often been confounded by the majority of poor performance status patients being treated with radiotherapy. This is partly because radiotherapy has the advantage of treating tumours adjacent to or directly involving vital thoracic structures which cannot be sacrificed at operation. Five-year survivals of 10–30 per cent (or even higher for T1N0 tumours) have been achieved with radiotherapy alone. Preoperative and postoperative radiotherapy has not produced any significant prolongation of survival and is not routinely practised. Indeed, meta-analysis of the randomized trials of postoperative radiotherapy suggest a 7 per cent 2-year survival disadvantage for this approach; this should therefore be used only within the context of further clinical trials. The greatest advance in recent years has been the development of CHART (continuous, hyperfractionated, accelerated radiotherapy). This regime was developed to exploit the radiobiological advantages conferred by rapid completion of treatment and avoidance of breaks in radiotherapy at weekends. This entails treatment three times daily,

7 days a week for 2.5 weeks (54 Gy in 36 fractions). In the pivotal randomized trial of CHART which enrolled over 500 patients with NSCLC, the 2-year survival was 29 per cent for CHART versus 20 per cent for conventional (2 Gy/day) radiotherapy. The acute side-effects were similar, except for a rapid onset of severe dysphagia in the CHART group.

Chemotherapy

Cisplatin is still considered the cornerstone of chemotherapy for NSCLC. Meta-analysis indicates that cisplatin-based chemotherapy leads to small but consistent improvements in overall survival in all patient groups. In early NSCLC, chemotherapy in combination with surgery or radiotherapy yields a 13 per cent reduction in the odds of death at 2 years (4 per cent absolute survival advantage at 2 years; 2 per cent at 5 years). The optimal sequencing of modalities and schedule of drug administration remains to be determined and is under study in ongoing clinical trials. Chemotherapy is being used increasingly in a preoperative (neo-adjuvant) role to try to downstage disease to facilitate surgery or high-dose radiotherapy, again with promising results. As with other solid tumours, synchronous chemoradiotherapy (CRT) protocols are in widespread use to maximize loco-regional control and to treat occult metastatic disease at distant sites.

RADICAL TREATMENT OF SCLC
Surgery

There is no proven role for radical surgery in the treatment of SCLC.

Radiotherapy

Thoracic radiotherapy is of value as the combined modality treatment of those with limited stage disease. It has also gained wider acceptance in decreasing the risk of intrathoracic recurrence in those who have had a complete or near-complete response to induction chemotherapy.

Of those with controlled local, regional or visceral disease, 60 per cent will sustain an intracerebral relapse within 2 years. This is often the sole site of disease relapse and frequently proves to be a fatal manifestation of their disease. Prophylactic cranial irradiation (PCI) decreases the incidence of cerebral metastases by around 50 per cent. Meta-analysis data suggests a 6 per cent absolute survival advantage for PCI. There is some retrospective evidence suggesting the possibility of neuropsychiatric sequelae from PCI, but this has not been seen in prospective studies addressing this issue.

Chemotherapy

The propensity for SCLC to disseminate early and its inherent chemosensitivity means that systemic treatment with chemotherapy is the most appropriate initial management for both limited and extensive stages of disease. Median survival for untreated limited SCLC is only 14 weeks, falling to 7 weeks for extensive disease. Chemotherapy improves the median survival significantly. Combination therapy is more efficacious than single-agent chemotherapy. Objective responses in the order of 70–90 per cent have been reported for a variety of schedules, the active drugs being cisplatin/carboplatin, cyclophosphamide, ifosfamide, etoposide, vincristine and doxorubicin. Complete responses of 30–40 per cent can be expected in limited disease, and 20–30 per cent in those with extensive disease. There is no benefit in prolonging chemotherapy beyond 6 months duration. In recent years, published data has emerged suggesting a benefit for chemotherapy (e.g. etoposide and cisplatin) given concurrently with thoracic radiotherapy for limited stage disease. Chemotherapy drugs do not cross the blood–brain barrier to a substantial degree, hence the need for PCI in complete responders.

PALLIATIVE TREATMENT

The priority of treatment is to relieve symptoms for the patient's remaining lifespan with as little inconvenience and discomfort as possible. There is published evidence confirming that immediate chemotherapy confers a survival advantage for patients with metastatic disease versus best supportive care.

Radiotherapy

Radiotherapy is employed for local symptoms of both NSCLC and SCLC when chemotherapy is deemed inappropriate, and is very effective at relieving cough, chest pain and haemoptysis, with palliation lasting for much of the patient's remaining lifespan. Dyspnoea may be helped if it is caused by bronchial obstruction. Treatment may be delivered using external beam radiotherapy or high-dose rate brachytherapy using an endobronchial catheter placed adjacent to the tumour under bronchoscopic guidance. Large single doses of thoracic radiation are as effective as a more prolonged course (e.g. 10 fractions in 2 weeks) in terms of onset, quality and duration of response, at least for patients in poor general condition. Median survival in such cases is only 6 months, with a 1-year survival of 20 per cent falling to 5 per cent at 2 years. Palliative thoracic irradiation can be repeated if symptoms recur, provided that care is taken not to exceed the radiation tolerance dose of the spinal cord.

Chemotherapy

A rather pessimistic aura has pervaded the management of advanced NSCLC for too long. The emergence of new drugs and the resulting combination therapy has led to increased response rates, disease-free survival and overall survival prolongation. Cisplatin remains the standard treatment for NSCLC. In advanced NSCLC, cisplatin-based chemotherapy reduces the risk of death at 1 year by 27 per cent (10 per cent absolute survival advantage; increase in median survival of 6 weeks). Combination chemotherapy yields an approximate doubling in response rates compared with single agents, but is significantly more toxic. In recent years, a number of other agents used alone or in combination with cisplatin have demonstrated activity in NSCLC:

- vinorelbine;
- gemcitabine;
- paclitaxel/docetaxel.

Objective responses are often lower than the rate of symptom relief in lung cancer patients. Combinations are associated with higher response rates than single-agent therapy. A randomized trial comparing five cisplatin-containing regimens showed no significant difference in response, duration of response, or survival. Controversy therefore still exists over the optimum combination of these drugs.

For SCLC, the drug regimes are similar to those used for primary treatment. It is sound practice to use drug combinations with constituent drugs to which the patient has not previously been exposed.

OTHER TREATMENT MODALITIES
Endobronchial laser therapy

This is particularly useful for proximal endobronchial tumours in relieving haemoptysis by permitting direct coagulation of the bleeding tumour and in relieving bronchial obstruction by acting as a cutting diathermy. It is frequently used in patients that have already received a maximal dose of radiation to the thorax.

Vocal cord apposition

Teflon injection into the posterior two-thirds of the vocal cord leads to approximation of the vocal cords and is indicated for recurrent laryngeal nerve palsy when there is persistent aspiration of food and pharyngeal secretions into the bronchial tree, leading to recurrent chest infections or respiratory distress.

Pleuro-pericardial aspiration

Drainage of pleural and pericardial effusions will rapidly relieve dyspnoea and sometimes any associated chest pain or dry cough. Talc or bleomycin may be instilled into the pleural cavity to obliterate the pleural space (pleurodesis) and thereby prevent further fluid accumulation.

Other medical measures

Other medical measures include:

- antibiotics for chest infections;
- codeine or methadone linctus as a cough suppressant;
- analgesics for chest pain;
- treatment of biochemical abnormalities resulting from non-metastatic manifestations.

Tumour-related complications

Complications can be divided into thoracic and extrathoracic. Thoracic complications include:

- atrial fibrillation;
- broncho-oesophageal fistula;
- dysphagia;
- empyema;
- Horner's syndrome;
- lung abscess;
- massive pulmonary or pleural haemorrhage;
- pericardial effusion;
- pleural effusion;
- pneumonia;
- pneumothorax;
- spinal cord compression;
- sudden death from rupture of one of the great vessels;
- superior vena cava obstruction (Fig. 7.9).

Extrathoracic complications can be inferred from Table 7.1. Ectopic hormone production is most common with SCLC although squamous carcinomas may produce a parathyroid hormone-like peptide leading to hypercalcaemia or a syndrome of inappropriate anti-diuretic hormone secretion (SIADH).

Treatment-related complications

Radiotherapy

Radiation oesophagitis is characterized by a feeling of retrosternal discomfort on swallowing food or fluids, particularly if hot or spicy, and beginning 2 weeks after commencing radiotherapy. Symptoms are rarely severe enough to interfere significantly with the patient's nutrition and usually subside within 2 weeks of completing radiotherapy. Radiation pneumonitis has an acute phase beginning 6 weeks to 3 months after radiotherapy and is characterized by dry cough, fever, dyspnoea and chest pain. Radiologically, there is a diffuse opacification of the lung corresponding to the applied radiation fields, which is often more severe than the symptoms would suggest. Mild cases resolve spontaneously but more severe cases will require treatment with a broad-spectrum antibiotic together with prednisolone, 20–40 mg daily. Some will progress to a chronic phase characterized by increasing pulmonary fibrosis, leading to a restrictive defect and some degree of permanent respiratory compromise. The probability of pneumonitis can be minimized by using a small radiation dose per fraction and treating as small a lung volume as possible. As a consequence of the large doses per fraction used for palliative radiotherapy, some patients surviving long enough may be at risk of developing radiation myelitis.

Surgery

Potential complications of surgery include:

- empyema due to infection within the pleural space;
- decrease in respiratory reserve due to resection of lung tissue;
- persistent bronchopleural fistula;
- seeding of the tumour into the thoracotomy scar and subcutaneous tissues; and
- discomfort related to the scar, which may lead to an unremitting neuralgia.

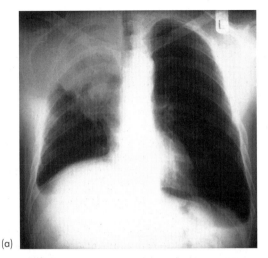

(a)

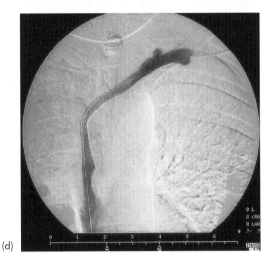

(b)

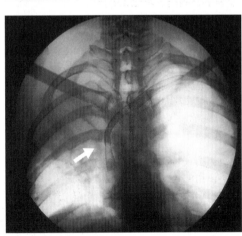

(c)

(d)

(e)

Fig 7.9 Superior vena cava (SVC) obstruction. (a) Chest radiograph showing collapse of the right upper lobe. (b) Computed tomography image of the same patient showing a soft tissue mass in the medial segment of the right upper lobe. It is impinging on the SVC. (c) SVC venogram. The left brachiocephalic vein is patent. Blood flow is obstructed at the SVC. (d) Flow in SVC restored. (e) SVC stent *in situ*.

Case history: lung cancer

A 65-year-old female smoker with no prior history of pulmonary disease presents to her general practitioner during the winter months with a chest infection manifesting as cough productive of purulent sputum and mild shortness of breath on exertion. She receives a course of amoxycillin to good effect but remains slightly short of breath which she attributes to her age. Four weeks later, the cough and sputum return. Once again she responds to a broad-spectrum antibiotic but this time the cough persists. She attributes this to her smoking. She then presents 6 weeks later with increasing cough, sputum with some blood streaking and more significant shortness of breath. Auscultation of the chest is inconclusive. In view of persistent pulmonary symptoms in a smoker, a chest X-ray is arranged and this reveals collapse and consolidation of the right middle lobe. An urgent referral is made to a chest physician. Bronchoscopy is performed and this indicates a polypoid tumour almost completely obstructing the right middle lobe bronchus with some ulceration and bleeding. Biopsies are taken and laser resection used to restore patency to the bronchus and achieve haemostasis. Histology confirms small cell carcinoma.

She is staged with a computed tomography (CT) scan of the brain, thorax and abdomen which shows bulky right hilar lymphadenopathy but no evidence of distant metastatic disease. Following the scan, she complains of headache and lethargy. Serum biochemistry profile indicates a sodium level of 118 mmol/l. Serum osmolarity is low at 230 mOsm/l (normal range 275–295 mOsm/l) and urine osmolarity inappropriately low at 300 mOsm/l (normal range 400–1000 mOsm/l). A diagnosis of inappropriate antidiuretic hormone secretion is made and she is commenced on fluid restriction and demeclocycline to good effect.

Once well, she commences systemic chemotherapy with doxorubicin, cyclophosphamide and etoposide. After three cycles, a CT scan of the thorax shows re-expansion of the right middle lobe and a dramatic reduction in the size of the hilar lymphadenopathy. After a further three cycles, there is no further measurable disease. The demeclocycline is withdrawn and the fluid restriction successfully relaxed. Her excellent response to induction chemotherapy is therefore consolidated by a course of radiotherapy to the site of the original bronchial tumour and adjacent hilum, given concurrently with a course of prophylactic cranial irradiation.

She remains well until 8 months later when she experiences further cough and dyspnoea. This is now associated with malaise and lethargy, and her performance status is rapidly deteriorating. Chest X-ray confirms recurrent bronchial obstruction and CT scan indicates liver metastases. She declines further chemotherapy. She requires two bronchoscopic laser treatments within a 2-week period. In order to reduce the need for continual bronchoscopies, she is treated with endobronchial brachytherapy as a day-case procedure. This successfully palliates the local symptoms of her disease. She is referred to the community multidisciplinary team affiliated to her local hospice and dies 6 weeks later.

Chemotherapy

Many of the drugs used for SCLC cause alopecia. Radiotherapy may increase the toxicity of drugs such as cyclophosphamide, leading to pulmonary fibrosis, and Adriamycin, leading to heart failure.

Prognosis

The prognosis from lung cancer remains poor and despite advances in surgery, radiotherapy and chemotherapy it has not changed for several decades. The three main poor prognostic factors include:

- advanced stage (e.g. large tumour size, extrathoracic disease);
- small cell histology;
- poor performance status.

Patients with disease not amenable to radical therapy have a median survival of 6 months or less. Only about 5 per cent of SCLC patients survive 5 years. The pretreatment prognostic factors which consistently predict for prolonged survival include good performance status, female gender and limited stage disease. Patients with involvement of the central nervous system or liver at the time of diagnosis have a significantly worse outcome. Median survival with current treatment of limited stage SCLC is 18–24 months, compared with 6–12 months for those with extensive disease. Approximately 10–20 per cent of patients with NSCLC survive 5 years. Stage at presentation is the most important prognostic factor in this disease.

Among surviving smokers, there is a significant risk of second primary cancers of 3–4 per cent per annum, about half of which will be second lung primary cancers.

Screening

Several large prospective screening projects have been completed which have entailed regular chest X-rays or sputum cytology. These have not shown early detection by screening to improve survival in the screened population. Lung cancer survivors may be screened to reflect their risk profile for second malignancies.

Prevention

Lung cancer is predominantly caused by smoking tobacco. Better health education, legislation to reduce cigarette advertising and punitive taxes on tobacco may decrease consumption and in turn reduce the incidence significantly. Ventilation of dwellings in regions where radon gas levels are high and avoidance of industrial carcinogens may also contribute to a reduction in lung cancer incidence. Retinoids and antioxidant compounds such as β-carotene may have a role as chemopreventative agents. There is some evidence that vitamin A may prevent second malignancies in long-term survivors.

Rare tumours

Bronchoalveolar carcinoma

This arises more often in women, with a peak incidence of 40–50 years. A higher proportion will be non-smokers compared with other lung cancer types. The cell of origin is the type 2 pneumocyte of the alveoli. It arises peripherally and the expectoration of large quantities of mucus is characteristic.

Carcinoid

Bronchial carcinoids are the most common benign tumours, arising in the major bronchi. They are more common in the right lung and usually metabolically inactive but may produce carcinoid

syndrome without liver metastases. They may occasionally be the site of ectopic adrenocorticotropic hormone (ACTH) production.

MESOTHELIOMA

Epidemiology

There are 850 new cases and approximately 600 deaths in the UK per annum from pleural tumours, almost all of which are mesotheliomas. They may arise at any age but are most common in the 50–70 year age-group. There is a male predominance (5:1), reflecting occupational exposure to asbestos (e.g. in miners, builders, naval dockyard workers). Only three-quarters of patients actually give a history of asbestos exposure. Case clustering has been described around asbestos mines (e.g. central Turkey, Cyprus and Greece) and in those that used to live near the asbestos-processing factories of East London.

Aetiology

Mesothelioma is not caused by smoking. It is now recognized that asbestos exposure is the main risk factor for both pleural and peritoneal mesothelioma. Blue asbestos (crocidolite) is more carcinogenic than white and brown types, and this is because of the size and shape of the asbestos fibres. Not only are asbestos workers at risk, but also their spouses, since the fibres are carried on clothing. There is a long latent period (often 30–40 years) between asbestos exposure and development of mesothelioma, and cancer risk is dependent on duration and intensity of fibre exposure. Most patients have no evidence of asbestosis. About half will give a history of occupational exposure to asbestos. Patients with a possible occupational history of asbestos exposure should be identified as they may be eligible for industrial injuries compensation. Such patients should have a post-mortem examination.

Pathology

Mesothelioma arises from mesothelial cells of the pleura, much less commonly the peritoneum, and very occasionally the pericardium or tunica vaginalis around the testicle. Pleural tumours are slightly more common on the right, probably owing to the greater surface area of pleura at risk. Evidence of pulmonary asbestosis is more common in those with peritoneal mesothelioma, who often have a history of heavy asbestos exposure. Macroscopically, there are multiple, small, pale tumour nodules diffusely involving visceral and parietal layers of the pleura, particularly at the cardiophrenic angle medially. These nodules coalesce to form plaques that encase the underlying lung and infiltrate into the fissures and intralobular septae. Eventually, the pleural space is obliterated. There may be an associated pleural effusion, usually rich in protein and blood stained.

Microscopically, the tumours contain varying proportions of epithelial and spindle cell elements (resembling adenocarcinoma and sarcoma, respectively). Approximately two-thirds are epithelial and one-quarter are mixed epithelial/sarcomatous. Asbestos bodies may be found in the underlying lung and asbestos fibres may be identified in the tumour by electron microscopy.

Natural history

Mesothelioma relentlessly invades adjacent thoracic structures such as the underlying lung, overlying chest wall, pericardium and contralateral hemithorax. The tumour eventually invades through the diaphragm to involve the peritoneum and abdominal viscera. It also has a propensity to invade the chest wall and skin at the site of a previous thoracocentesis due to direct implantation of tumour cells. Sarcomatous tumours have a more rapidly progressive natural history compared with epithelial types. Lymphatic spread is uncommon. Symptomatic distant metastases are also uncommon, even during the terminal phase of the disease, but are a greater problem in those with sarcomatous histology and the very few, highly selected patients treated by radical surgery.

Symptoms

Ninety per cent of patients with pleural mesothelioma present with increasing dyspnoea on exertion and/or chest discomfort on the affected side. Seventy per cent will have symptoms less than 6 months in duration at presentation. Dry cough and systemic symptoms such as anorexia, weight loss and fever may occur. In contrast to lung cancer, haemoptysis is very uncommon.

Signs

Finger clubbing and signs of chronic respiratory compromise may be seen if there has been prior asbestosis. There is usually reduced expansion, dullness to percussion and reduced breath sounds over the affected region of the chest. This can be difficult to distinguish from a pleural effusion.

Differential diagnosis

Asbestos may also cause a primary lung cancer which may present with similar symptoms and signs. Others cancers, particularly adenocarcinomas, occasionally demonstrate a pleural pattern of spread and are difficult to distinguish on pleural fluid cytology alone or on analysis of small fragments of pleura.

Investigations

Chest X-ray

This usually shows a lobulated pleural mass with loss of volume of the affected hemithorax and there may be an associated pleural effusion (Fig. 7.10). The changes are commoner in the lower zones and may be bilateral. An underlying asbestosis may be seen. The chest X-ray is best taken after drainage of an effusion, which may obscure the subtle signs of pleural thickening.

Pleural fluid cytology

This can be performed in the outpatient clinic by inserting a hypodermic needle into an intercostal

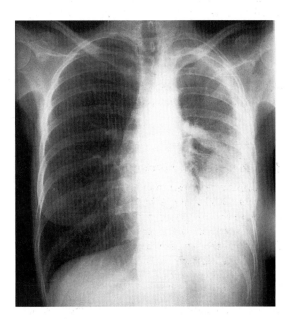

FIG 7.10 Chest radiograph showing encasement of the left lung by a mesothelioma. There is an associated pleural effusion.

space under local anaesthetic. The fluid is often heavily blood-stained and high in protein. A high (>50 ng/l) level of hyaluronic acid is common. Cytological examination may reveal malignant mesothelial cells, although the sensitivity is not high (approximately 40 per cent).

Pleural biopsy

This is more invasive than obtaining fluid for cytology. It does, however, give a more reliable tissue diagnosis. A needle technique can usually be performed under local anaesthetic. Ultrasound or CT can be used to obtain better localization of pleural plaque for sampling. In difficult cases, an open biopsy at thoracoscopy or thoracotomy is necessary. Surgical biopsy has the advantage of yielding a larger specimen for histological analysis, drainage of pleural fluid and even simultaneous talc pleurodesis.

Ultrasound of thorax

This is a useful investigation for localizing the best place to perform a percutaneous pleural biopsy or aspiration of a loculated pleural effusion.

Computed tomography scan of thorax and abdomen

This is much better than plain radiographs for demonstrating pleural plaques (Fig. 7.11) and assessing the degree of local invasion. It may be useful for localizing a suitable site for needle biopsy. It is also useful in excluding gross involvement of the peritoneum.

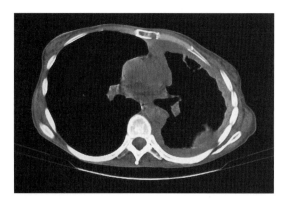

FIG 7.11 Computed tomography image of the patient in Fig. 7.10 after drainage of the pleural effusion. Note the thick layer of tumour surrounding the edge of the lung.

Staging

There is no formal staging system in widespread clinical use. The modified Butchart staging classification shown below is an example.

- Stage I – disease confined within the capsule of the parietal pleura, ipsilateral pleura, lung, pericardium, and diaphragm.
- Stage II – all of stage I with positive intrathoracic (N1 or N2) lymph nodes.
- Stage III – local extension of disease into the following: chest wall or mediastinum; heart or through the diaphragm, peritoneum; with or without extrathoracic or contralateral (N3) lymph node involvement.
- Stage IV – distant metastatic disease.

Treatment

Comparative studies show a survival advantage for active treatment versus observation only. Very few patients are suitable for radical surgical resection. Pleuropneumonectomy (excision of lung, pleura, hemidiaphragm and ipsilateral half of pericardium) followed by high-dose hemithoracic radiotherapy in selected patients has yielded promising results but is yet to be tested in a randomized trial. Mortality (20–30 per cent) and morbidity are high. The less radical procedure of pleurectomy (mortality 2 per cent) may palliate selected patients with severe, recurrent pleural effusions. Patients may derive much symptomatic relief from simple drainage of a pleural effusion.

Radiotherapy is of value in palliating chest pain. Treatment is usually given to the involved hemithorax. Two-thirds of patients will respond symptomatically, although it is difficult to demonstrate any objective tumour response to the moderate doses used.

Adriamycin is an active chemotherapy agent with an objective response rate of 15–20 per cent. Cisplatin is also active in this disease. Vinorebine has also shown promising activity either as a single agent or in combination with cisplatin.

Tumour-related complications

Many patients succumb to respiratory failure from uncontrolled local disease. Pericardial constriction may occur due to extrinsic tumour pressure and malignant pericarditis may cause atrial fibrillation. Direct invasion of the myocardium may also compromise cardiac function. Mediastinal compression may lead to dysphagia and superior vena cava obstruction. Seeding of tumour cells along the path of an intercostal needle is common and may lead to subcutaneous and skin nodules. Peritoneal involvement may lead to intestinal obstruction and ascites. Non-metastatic manifestations include hypercoagulability of the blood, autoimmune haemolytic anaemia, phlebitis, hypoglycaemia and SIADH.

Treatment-related complications

Pleuropneumonectomy has a mortality of approximately 20 per cent. Treatment of the whole hemithorax with radiotherapy may lead to oesophagitis, nausea due to irradiation of the stomach and/or liver, and pneumonitis due to the large volume of lung irradiated.

Prognosis

The disease runs a variable natural history, and therefore prognosis is unpredictable. In a retrospective series of pleural mesothelioma patients, important prognostic factors have been found to be stage, age, performance status and histology. Epithelial variants have a better prognosis than sarcomatoid ones. For patients treated with aggressive surgical approaches, factors associated with improved long-term survival include epithelial histology, negative lymph nodes, and negative surgical margins. Prognosis is usually very poor, with a mean survival of 9 months; only 30 per cent survive to 1 year, falling to <5 per cent at 2 years.

Screening/prevention

The dangers of asbestos exposure are now appreciated. Asbestos is used much more sparingly in industry. Care must still be taken when older buildings are renovated, with careful isolation of the working area and use of respirators. High-risk individuals should be offered regular chest radiographs.

8 BREAST CANCER

The breasts are hormonally responsive organs. Their only purpose is to produce milk (lactation) in women. In men, they are vestigial, serving as a remnant of the common embryological development of males and females.

Epidemiology

There are 210 000 new cases of breast cancer and 76 000 deaths recorded in the European Union per annum. It is the most common malignancy in females, the average woman having a one in 12 chance of developing the disease at some point during her lifetime. Left-sided cancers are slightly more common than right-sided ones (relative risk 1.05). The peak age incidence is 50–70 years and only 0.5–1 per cent of cases arise in men. It is a disease of the Western world, being much less prevalent in the Far East, particularly Japan. There is an increased incidence in higher socio-economic groups.

Aetiology

As many as 5 per cent of cases may result from inheritable genetic abnormalities. The relative risk (RR) of breast cancer is significantly increased when first-degree relatives have previously been affected:

- one maternal first degree relative (RR 2);
- first-degree relative diagnosed <40 years (RR 3);
- two first-degree relatives (RR 4);
- bilateral breast cancer (RR 4).

Some familial cases have been found to have a mutated gene located on chromosome 17, *BRCA1*. *BRCA1* carriers also have an increased risk of developing carcinoma of the ovary. Female and male breast cancer may also be associated with another breast cancer gene, *BRCA2*, on chromosome 13. Inheritance of either of these mutated genes confers an 80–90 per cent lifetime risk of breast cancer. Other genetic abnormalities associated with familial breast cancer include *P53* mutations in Li Fraumeni families (associated with leukaemia, gliomas, adreno-cortical carcinomas and soft tissue sarcomas) and heterozygotes for the ataxia telangiectasia gene.

Epidemiological studies implicate hormonal factors in the causation of breast cancer. Breast cancer is more common in women with an early menarche or a late menopause. An artificial menopause (surgical oophorectomy or radiation ovarian ablation) before the age of 35 years, increasing parity, young age (<30 years) at first pregnancy and breast feeding are protective.

Japanese women have a low risk of developing breast cancer. Japanese migrants to the USA eventually acquire the risk of the indigenous population, suggesting that there is an unknown environmental cofactor involved.

An increased incidence of breast cancer has been reported in atomic bomb survivors, women treated with radiotherapy for postpartum mastitis, Hodgkin's disease or ankylosing spondylitis and women that have undergone regular chest fluoroscopies to monitor the progress of iatrogenic pneumothorax as treatment for tuberculosis. The carcinogenic effect of radiation on the breast varies inversely with age at time of exposure and is dependent on radiation dose.

Bittner demonstrated that a virus transmitted via breast milk in mice led to the development of mammary tumours. A viral cause has not been demonstrated in humans with breast cancer.

Common benign lumps such as fibroadenomata do not progress to carcinoma, but atypical ductal hyperplasia confers an increased risk of breast cancer and such patients should be kept under regular surveillance.

Ductal carcinoma *in situ* (DCIS) and lobular carcinoma *in situ* (LCIS) are both precursors to invasive malignancy (see below).

Pathology

Macroscopically, most carcinomas arise in the upper outer quadrant of the breast and are usually solitary although multifocal tumours may occur in the same or opposite breast. The tumour may be well circumscribed or diffusely infiltrating. The cut surface and texture will vary depending on the tumour type. For example, a scirrhous tumour will have a gritty texture and grey/white cut surface, while a colloid carcinoma will have a more gelatinous texture. Conversely, a diffusely infiltrating lobular cancer may be invisible to the naked eye.

Microscopically, breast cancers may be classified as 'lobular' arising in the lobules at the termination of the duct system of the breast or 'ductal' which arise from the extralobular ducts themselves. *In situ* carcinoma is diagnosed when all the malignant cells are confined to the lumen of the duct or lobule and do not breach the basement membrane. This contrasts with invasive carcinoma where malignant cells breach the basement membrane. The vast majority are ductal carcinomas but there are a number of variants, including papillary, scirrhous, colloid, medullary and comedo carcinomas. Oestrogen and progesterone receptors are detectable, reaching high levels in well-differentiated tumours.

There are several variants worthy of special mention.

- *Ductal carcinoma in situ* This is more common than LCIS, with a peak incidence 5–10 years later. Seventy to eighty per cent are symptomatic with a lump palpable in 60 per cent. Ten per cent present with nipple discharge, usually blood stained. Central necrosis leads to calcium deposition and therefore 50 per cent can be detected by mammography. Two per cent of surgically staged patients will have spread to the axilla due to areas of unrecognized invasive carcinoma, and 40 per cent will progress to invasive carcinoma after biopsy alone.

- *Lobular carcinoma in situ* This may be an incidental finding in a biopsy performed for benign breast disease or associated with an invasive cancer. Seventy per cent of cases arise in premenopausal women and it is frequently bilateral. It is usually undetectable clinically and may not be seen on a mammogram owing to the lack of necrosis (and therefore calcification) in the lesion. It is a marker of a high probability of subsequent invasive cancer. About one-third will develop invasive cancer in the same or contralateral breast within 20 years of diagnosis. The rate of progression to carcinoma after biopsy alone is approximately 1 per cent per annum.

- *Inflammatory carcinoma* This comprises only 2 per cent of all cases of breast cancer. Clinically, there is ill-defined erythema, tenderness, induration and oedema (Fig. 8.1). It may be misdiagnosed as a breast abscess. Microscopically there is invasion of dermal lymphatics by tumour cells. It behaves aggressively with a high rate of local recurrence and distant metastases.

- *Paget's disease of the breast* This is a premalignant condition affecting the nipple and areola and arises in older women. Clinically, there is erythema, dryness and fissuring of the nipple, sometimes with exudation of fluid, resembling eczema (Fig. 8.2). Unlike eczema, it is very rarely bilateral, confined to the nipple/areola, less itchy and not associated with vesicle formation. It is microscopically characterized by large, pale Paget cells within the epidermis, which do not invade the dermis. All patients have an associated ductal carcinoma. Half have an associated lump, more than 90 per cent of which are invasive carcinomas. If no lump is palpable, 30 per cent will have an underlying invasive carcinoma and 70 per cent DCIS.

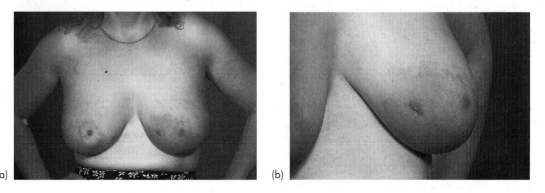

(a) (b)

FIG 8.1 (a) Inflammatory breast cancer. (b) Note the small skin biopsy scar. The tissue removed confirmed dermal lymphatic invasion by carcinoma cells.

- *Bilateral breast cancer*   This is more common in those with a strong family history of breast cancer and those diagnosed at an early age. Synchronous primaries (i.e. two tumours occurring simultaneously) are rare, occurring in less than 1 per cent of cases, while a metachronous primary (i.e. diagnosed 6 months or more after the original tumour) has an incidence of 1–2 per cent per year on follow-up. A second primary tumour is suggested by its being of a different histological type and differentiation to the original tumour with surrounding *in situ* changes.
- *Male breast cancer*   This is rare. Recent data suggests an association with *BRCA2* mutations. The tumours are morphologically the same as those seen in women. There is a high incidence of oestrogen receptor positivity and therefore hormonal therapy, analogous to that used in women, plays a useful role in management.

Natural history

The primary tumour enlarges and invades adjacent breast tissue, eventually leading to fixation to the pectoral fascia, serratus anterior muscle and ribs. The parietal pleura may be breached in neglected cases leading to transcoelomic spread within the pleural cavity. The dermal lymphatics may be invaded leading to 'peau d'orange' or satellite lesions. The dermis and epidermis may become infiltrated directly leading to nodules (Fig. 8.3), plaques, ulceration or inflammatory changes (Fig. 8.4). In neglected cases, the whole breast may be replaced by tumour, with tumour growing externally as an exophytic mass (Fig. 8.5).

The likelihood of lymph node involvement increases with increasing tumour size, decreasing tumour differentiation and lymphatic channel invasion within the primary tumour. Approximately

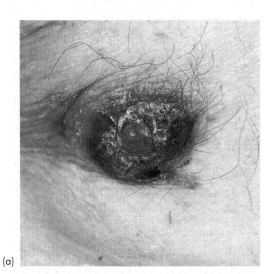

(a)

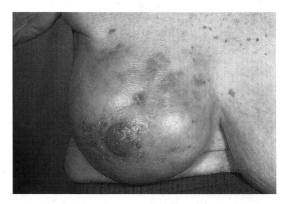

FIG 8.3 Locally advanced breast cancer. The breast is diffusely infiltrated by tumour. Multiple nodules are erupting over the surface of the breast.

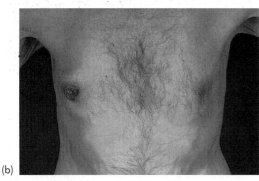

(b)

FIG 8.2 (a) Paget's disease of the nipple (male patient): note the resemblance to eczema. (b) Same patient: note the large breast mass suggestive of the underlying carcinoma.

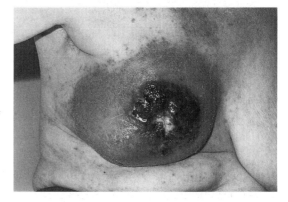

FIG 8.4 Locally advanced breast cancer. There is ulceration of the overlying skin and inflammatory changes in the surrounding skin, suggesting invasion of the dermal lymphatics.

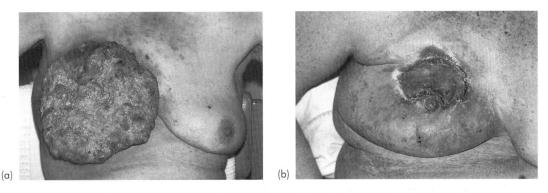

(a) (b)

FIG 8.5 (a) An enormous fungating breast cancer. This patient suffered from schizophrenia, which contributed to the late presentation. (b) Same breast after a course of radiotherapy. The odour and discharge have reduced. However, a tumour of this size is difficult to eradicate with radiotherapy alone.

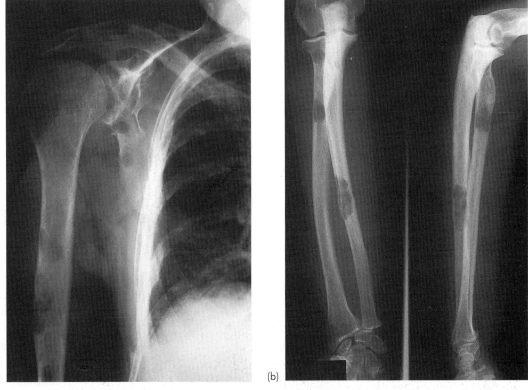

(a) (b)

FIG 8.6 Lytic bone metastases. Such lesions are at particular risk of pathological fracture. (a) Humerus, scapula and clavicle. (b) Anterior–posterior and lateral views of forearm.

one-third will have macroscopic or microscopic spread to the axillary nodes at the time of diagnosis. Involvement of the supraclavicular nodes is of particularly poor prognostic significance and is classified as a distant metastasis in the TNM staging. Medial tumours may involve the internal mammary nodes in the parasternal region, particularly if large and if the axillary lymph nodes are involved.

The most common sites for distant metastases include bone, liver, lung, brain and skin. Bone metastases may be predominantly lytic (Fig. 8.6), sclerotic (Fig. 8.7) or a mixture of the two types.

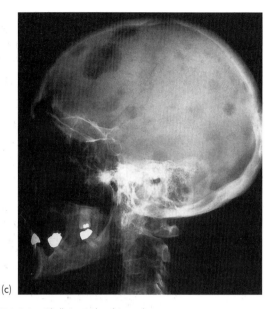

(c)

FIG 8.6c Skull. Lateral radiograph.

Breast cancer occasionally spreads to both ovaries, giving rise to 'Krukenberg tumours', a phenomenon also seen in stomach cancer. Lobular cancers have a particular propensity for gastrointestinal and genitourinary involvement.

Symptoms

The majority present with a painless breast lump or distortion of the breast which may be associated with a blood-stained nipple discharge. Patients detected by screening are likely to be asymptomatic. Less frequently the presentation is with diffuse enlargement or reddening of the breast, and occasionally lymphadenopathy or symptoms from distant metastases.

Signs

The lump is usually non-tender, well defined and most likely to be located in the upper outer quadrant, which contains the majority of the breast tissue. Breast

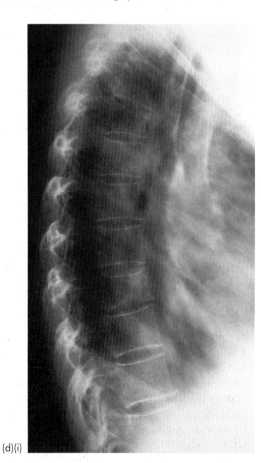

(d)(i)

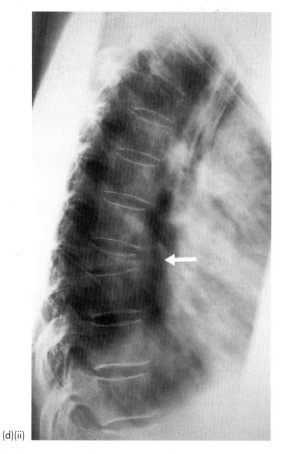

(d)(ii)

FIG 8.6d (i) and (ii) Vertebrae. Sequential lateral radiographs of the thoracic spine taken nearly two months apart showing development of a wedge collapse.

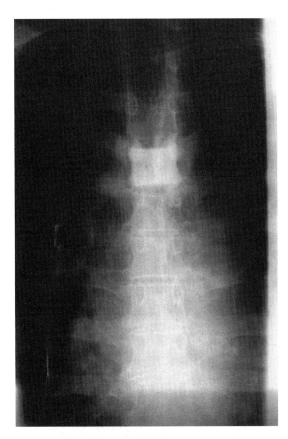

FIG 8.7 Plain radiograph of the thoracic spine showing a sclerotic metastasis from breast cancer.

discomfort is occasionally a presenting symptom. In advanced cases, the overlying skin may be dimpled or frankly invaded by tumour leading to reddening, induration and nodular irregularity. Fixation to the skin or chest wall will limit mobility of the lump, and this should be sought by the clinician during physical examination. A very large lump will lead to obvious asymmetry of the breasts. There may be enlargement of the ipsilateral axillary lymph nodes, the mobility of which should be assessed as part of the clinical staging, and less frequently enlargement of the supraclavicular lymph nodes. Hepatomegaly may suggest metastatic infiltration while intrathoracic signs of collapse, consolidation or pleural effusion may suggest pulmonary or pleural metastases. Bone metastases are most frequent in the thoracic and lumbar spine and may lead to tenderness when pressure is applied to the affected vertebrae.

Differential diagnosis

A number of benign breast lumps may be clinically indistinguishable from carcinoma, including fibroadenoma, duct papilloma, breast abscess, fat necrosis, haematoma and galactocele. Many such cases will be diagnosed as non-malignant during preoperative investigations. Rarer malignant tumours of the breast may occasionally cause confusion ('rare tumours').

Investigations

'Triple assessment' comprises physical examination, mammography and ultrasonography.

Mammography

This comprises radiographic examination of the breasts using low-energy X-rays to allow definition of the soft tissue detail and breast architecture. Two views are taken of each breast, usually in craniocaudal and oblique projections. It may substantiate the clinical diagnosis of carcinoma, detect DCIS in both the affected and contralateral breast, and localize the tumour to assist the planning of a biopsy or definitive surgical procedure. Carcinoma is suggested by an irregular mass lesion containing areas of microcalcification, sometimes with distortion of the surrounding breast architecture (Fig. 8.8).

Breast ultrasound

Breast ultrasound enables the radiologist to determine whether a lump is solid or cystic, the former being more likely to be malignant, and facilitates fine-needle aspiration (FNA) or needle biopsy of small lumps under direct vision, reducing the risk of a 'geographical miss' and thereby increasing the sensitivity of the procedure. It provides images that are complementary to those obtained by mammography.

Magnetic resonance imaging

This is reserved for the investigation of more difficult cases, for example a suspicious lump arising in a breast augmented with a tissue expander or a silicon implant where mammography can be difficult to interpret.

Fine-needle aspiration cytology

This is a rapid, safe, relatively non-traumatic procedure which can be performed at an outpatient consultation and can provide a tissue diagnosis within hours. It should be performed whenever a palpable lump or suspicious area of induration is found, and is applicable to the primary tumour, regional lymph nodes or suspicious skin lesions. Small, impalpable lesions may have to be localized using a stereotactic mammogram or ultrasound. It cannot however distinguish a focus of *in situ*

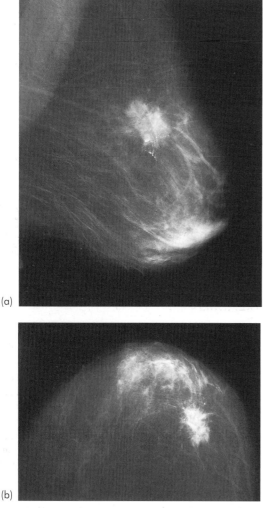

(a)

(b)

FIG 8.8 Two-view mammogram showing a spiculate density with associated microcalcification typical of carcinoma. (a) Oblique view; (b) cranio-caudal view.

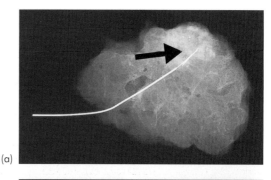

(a)

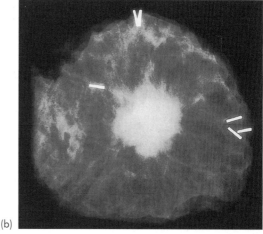

(b)

FIG 8.9 (a) Specimen radiograph of a wire localization breast biopsy. Preoperatively, the tip of the wire was placed adjacent to the impalpable, mammographic abnormality. The lesion is close to one of the resection margins. (b) Specimen radiograph showing more satisfactory margin of excision. The radio-opaque markers allow the pathologist to orientate the specimen.

carcinoma from invasive carcinoma, and does not allow accurate grading of the tumour.

Needle biopsy

This is performed under local anaesthetic and is a little more traumatic than FNA but gives a core (or cores) of tissue for histological analysis. This may allow a preoperative diagnosis of *in situ* versus invasive carcinoma, a preliminary grading and determination of hormone receptor status.

Excision biopsy

An excision biopsy is mandatory when it is not possible to obtain a tissue diagnosis by FNA or core

biopsy. The procedure is usually performed under general anaesthetic and the specimen can be sent for instant frozen section so that if a more radical operation is deemed necessary it can be performed immediately. Small, impalpable lesions are first localized with a 'guidewire' under radiological control which can be used to determine which piece of tissue should be excised (Fig. 8.9). A specimen radiograph is useful to confirm peroperatively that the area under suspicion has been fully excised.

Exclusion of metastatic disease

The results of the following investigations may influence the treatment planned, offer useful prognostic information and provide a valuable baseline assessment which may be of assistance in the future care of the patient:

- chest X-ray;
- computed tomography (CT) scan of the thorax and abdomen;
- isotope bone scan;
- serum CA 15-3 breast cancer tumour marker assay (persistently high level after surgery may suggest distant metastatic disease).

However, there is little evidence that routinely performing such screening investigations in asymptomatic patients is either clinically useful or cost effective, but they should be performed if there is any clinical suspicion of metastases at these sites and considered in high risk individuals (e.g. those with four or more axillary lymph nodes). Suspicious areas on bone scan should be assessed further by plain radiographs, particularly if in weight-bearing bones. Equivocal results may warrant further assessment using magnetic resonance imaging (MRI).

Staging

The TNM staging (see Chapter 2) is the most frequently used and can be used as a guide to management and prognosis.

- T0 – no evidence of primary tumour.
- TX – primary tumour cannot be assessed.
- Tis – carcinoma *in situ*.
- T1 – 2 cm or less in greatest dimension:
  la – 0.5 cm or less in greatest dimension;
  lb – >0.5 cm but not >1 cm in greatest dimension;
  1c – >1 cm but not >2 cm in greatest dimension.
- T2 – >2 cm but not >5 cm in greatest dimension.
- T3 – >5 cm in greatest dimension.
- T4 – tumour of any size with extension to chest wall and/or skin:
  4a – invasion of chest wall (ribs, serratus anterior, intercostal muscles);
  4b – oedema/peau d'orange, ulceration, satellite nodules confined to same breast;
  4c – both 4a and 4b;
  4d – inflammatory carcinoma.
- N0 – no lymphadenopathy.
- N1 – ipsilateral mobile axillary nodes.
- N2 – ipsilateral axillary nodes fixed to one another or to adjacent structures.
- N3 – ipsilateral internal mammary node metastases.
- M1 – involvement of supraclavicular nodes or distant metastases.

Treatment

The aims of treatment are:

- loco-regional control with optimal cosmesis;
- reduction of risk of developing distant metastatic disease;
- minimization of short- and long-term treatment-related morbidity

The treatment of breast cancer for an individual depends on the clinical stage of the disease, menopausal state and performance status of the patient. Ideally, the patient should be assessed in a multidisciplinary breast clinic by both the surgeon and the oncologist prior to any definitive treatment, so that the optimum treatment can be instituted at the outset.

TREATMENT OF LOCAL DISEASE

Ductal carcinoma *in situ* (DCIS)

Ductal carcinoma *in situ* is curable in the vast majority of patients. However, local treatment must ensure that it is eradicated as there is a high risk of local recurrence, which may be invasive in potential. Traditionally, simple mastectomy was the treatment of choice, and this is still the case for multifocal disease or when clear surgical margins cannot be attained. However, in recent years, the experience of breast conservation for invasive cancers has been extrapolated to DCIS. While small foci of low/intermediate grade DCIS can be treated with excision alone if adequate margins of clearance are attained, local excision and adjuvant radiotherapy to the breast alone is now standard treatment in many centres for unifocal DCIS that has been completely excised. Tamoxifen reduces the risk of local recurrence within the breast after breast-conserving treatment. Pure DCIS should not spread to regional lymph nodes and therefore no axillary surgery is necessary. Similarly, DCIS has no potential for systemic spread and therefore there is no role for chemotherapy in its management.

Invasive cancer

Surgery

Surgery facilitates total clearance of the primary tumour and pathological examination of the primary tumour and regional lymph nodes. The operation used will depend on the size of the lump, its location within the breast, the size of the breast, the presence of multifocal disease or extensive carcinoma *in situ* in the surrounding breast tissue, and the surgeon's own practice and prejudices. Options for treating the primary tumour include:

- wide local excision; /lumpectomy
- simple mastectomy;
- modified radical mastectomy;
- radical mastectomy.

With lumpectomy/wide local excision, the tumour is excised with a small (approximately 1 cm) margin of apparently uninvolved surrounding breast tissue. This gives an excellent cosmetic result as it preserves the breast bulk and nipple/areola complex, even in women with small breasts. It is unsuitable for very large tumours (>5 cm in maximum dimension), particularly if located centrally, or diffusely infiltrating carcinomas, particularly inflammatory carcinomas. Surrounding *in situ* disease will be left behind. Even if the excision margins are clear after microscopic examination of the specimen, there is a risk of local recurrence in the order of 30 per cent without further local treatment.

Simple mastectomy involves complete removal of the involved breast. The pectoral muscles are preserved. Although a prosthesis will be required, the physical appearance of the chest wall will be far superior to that after a more radical mastectomy.

Modified radical (Patey) mastectomy comprises a simple mastectomy and axillary lymph node dissection. Radical (Halstead) mastectomy involves *en bloc* removal of the breast, pectoralis major and minor muscles, and the axillary contents. The cosmetic result is poor but the local control rate is as high as conservative surgery and post-operative radiotherapy.

In recent decades, there has been an increasing trend towards a philosophy of breast conservation, which has been attributable to an improvement in the techniques of postoperative radiotherapy and an appreciation of its complementary role in the management of breast cancer. For a tumour 4 cm or less in maximum dimension, there is strong evidence that complete excision by lumpectomy combined with postoperative radiotherapy is as effective in obtaining local control as mastectomy alone, with 5-year disease-free survival rates of about 80 per cent. For tumours greater than 4 cm in maximum dimension, lumpectomy may still be performed and followed by radiotherapy. Because of the uncertainty and the poorer cosmetic result when a large tumour is treated conservatively, many surgeons will perform mastectomy for these larger tumours. Mastectomy is still the treatment of choice in certain situations:

- when the patient wishes to have the breast removed;
- extensive ductal carcinoma *in situ*;
- Paget's disease of the nipple, with an occult primary;
- multifocal primaries;
- inflammatory carcinoma;
- treatment of malignant phyllodes tumour or sarcoma;
- a very large tumour in a small breast, particularly if centrally located;
- salvage treatment after failure of conservative therapy;
- as a toilet procedure for a fungating tumour.

The psychosexual trauma and disturbance of body image that breast surgery can inflict should be considered. Patients for whom a mastectomy is planned should have the opportunity to see a trained breast-care nurse counsellor prior to their surgery so that the implications of the operation can be sympathetically and skilfully discussed. Patients may wish to be fitted with a prosthesis to maintain their chest contour or undergo immediate/subsequent surgical reconstruction of the breast using either a tissue expander or autologous muscle flap transposition (Fig. 8.10). Patients undergoing conservative treatment should also be offered counselling, as studies suggest that these patients experience psychological trauma similar to that of mastectomy patients.

The axilla is frequently a site for lymph node metastases, which in many cases cannot be detected clinically. The risk increases with increasing tumour size and grade, and the presence of lymphovascular invasion. The presence of lymph node metastases is a valuable prognostic factor, and correlates with the risk of the patient subsequently developing distant metastases. A surgical procedure to obtain lymph nodes for pathological analysis is therefore important in determining the need for adjuvant systemic therapy. An axillary procedure should be performed in all breast cancer cases as the results will help determine the optimal adjuvant therapy strategy. There are three possible procedures:

- sentinel lymph node mapping;
- axillary sampling;
- axillary dissection.

Sentinel lymph node mapping is increasingly being used in breast cancer patients. This entails

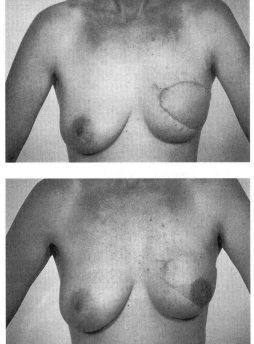

(a)

(b)

FIG 8.10 Reconstruction of the left breast using a latissimus dorsi flap. (a) The breast mound after flap reconstruction; (b) after nipple reconstruction.

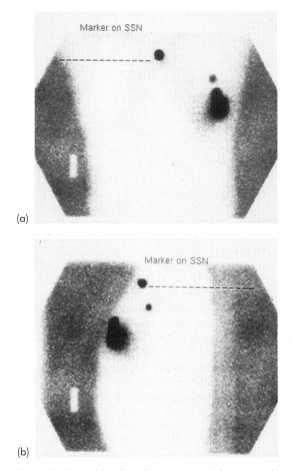

(a)

(b)

FIG 8.11 Sentinel lymph node scintigram. Radioactive technetium has been infiltrated around the breast cancer. The sentinel lymph node is shown (the midline spot is a sternal notch reference marker). (a) Front view; (b) lateral view.

preoperative injection of a vital dye and/or radio-labelled technetium colloid around the tumour. These markers are then taken up by the regional lymphatic vessels and concentrated initially within the sentinel lymph node(s) (Fig. 8.11). The rationale is that if this node (or nodes) is removed alone and found histologically not to contain malignant cells, it is highly (>90 per cent) likely that no other regional lymph nodes are involved and therefore no further surgery is necessary. This procedure has the advantage of being a far less traumatic form of lymph node surgery which should be associated with a faster recovery and less compromise of the shoulder, arm and hand. Conversely, involvement of the sentinel lymph node(s) suggests that full axillary dissection is necessary.

Axillary sampling entails removal of the lower lymph node group up to the level of the lower border of the pectoralis minor muscle. At least four nodes should be obtained for histological examination. If these nodes are clear of cancer, it is likely that nodes higher in the axilla will also be clear. Conversely, if a node is positive, a full axillary lymph node dissection will be necessary.

Axillary dissection is a more extensive surgical procedure comprising removal of the axillary contents at least up to the level of the upper border of the pectoralis minor muscle (level 2) or even axillary vein (level 3). Twenty to 30 nodes may be retrieved for the pathologist, giving more detailed prognostic information. It also has the advantage of being a one-stop therapeutic manoeuvre in its own right, lessening the risk of axillary recurrence. It has the disadvantage of increasing the surgical morbidity, resulting in local sensory loss, stiffness of the shoulder and a risk of lymphoedema of the ipsilateral arm.

Radiotherapy

Radiotherapy is indicated in all patients treated by breast-conserving surgery. Such an approach produces long-term survival equivalent to that of

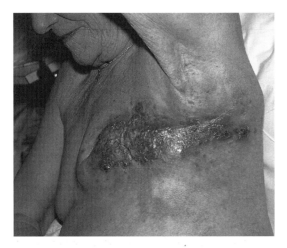

FIG 8.12 Chest wall recurrence after mastectomy.

mastectomy. External beam radiotherapy to the breast alone typically comprises a 5-week course of treatment to the whole breast to reflect the increased risk of recurrence at the site of the original primary but also the possibility of recurrence elsewhere within the breast owing to occult foci of DCIS and LCIS. An extra 'boost' may be delivered specifically to the tumour bed when the margins of excision are narrow or focally involved. Despite data from studies initiated prior to 1975 indicating an excess risk of cardiovascular death for women treated with radiotherapy, this has not been shown to be the case for more recent studies, presumably reflecting more careful planning to exclude the myocardium and a lower dose per fraction. Simple mastectomy alone is associated with a local recurrence rate of 5–10 per cent. Radiotherapy reduces the risk of chest wall recurrence (Fig. 8.12) but is used more selectively for those at particularly high risk of chest wall relapse. The following are recognized risk factors for local recurrence after mastectomy:

- incomplete microscopic excision, usually at the deep margin;
- T3 and T4 tumours;
- poorly differentiated tumours;
- lymphovascular invasion;
- involved axillary lymph nodes.

The axilla should not be routinely irradiated after axillary dissection irrespective of node status as there will be a considerable risk of lymphoedema of the arm and stiffness of the shoulder, which in some cases will be incapacitating. External beam radiotherapy may be given to the axilla in those patients who have not undergone axillary surgery and in whom the risk of lymph node involvement is significant:

- any poorly differentiated tumour;
- primary tumour of 20 mm or more;
- evidence of lymphovascular permeation.

The supraclavicular fossa may be irradiated after a significantly positive (four or more involved nodes) axillary node dissection or if the apical node is involved.

Chemotherapy/hormone manipulation as initial (neo-adjuvant) treatment for locally advanced disease

Inoperable tumours are initially treated with systemic therapy. Chemotherapy is the treatment of choice for most women with hormone therapy in addition for those shown to have hormonally sensitive tumours on biopsy. Those unfit or unsuitable for chemotherapy will be considered for hormone therapy alone. Once maximal response to systemic therapy has been attained, if there is no evidence of metastatic disease, the breast may be treated by appropriate surgery followed by radiotherapy. Neo-adjuvant chemotherapy has been established as a means of decreasing the mastectomy rate, although it has no significant survival advantage over postoperative chemotherapy.

ADJUVANT SYSTEMIC THERAPY

Adjuvant systemic therapy complements the role of radiotherapy or surgery to the breast. The former acts upon cancer cells which have already metastasized outside the breast and its regional lymphatics, while the latter reduces the local relapse rate. It is now widely accepted that adjuvant systemic therapy is of proven benefit in reducing the risk of distant relapse due to metastatic spread, and that this translates into a significant benefit in disease-free and overall survival. Breast cancer is statistically an important cancer accounting for much morbidity and mortality among women, and so only a small increase in these parameters will be worthwhile. There are two main types of adjuvant systemic therapy:

- tamoxifen/ovarian ablation
- chemotherapy.

Tamoxifen/ovarian ablation

Tamoxifen is an anti-oestrogen which acts by blocking the action of oestradiol on its receptors within the cytoplasm and nucleus of the tumour cells. The dose is 20 mg once daily. There is no evidence that a higher dose is any more effective. It has been proven to be an effective adjuvant agent in women with cancers that are oestrogen receptor positive. It may also confer benefit to those women with progesterone receptor positive cancers, and should not be used in women whose cancers have been shown to be hormone receptor negative. In oestrogen receptor positive cases, 5 years of tamoxifen reduces:

- the odds of recurrence by approximately 40 per cent, an absolute reduction of approximately 13 per cent by 15 years of follow up;
- the odds of dying from breast cancer by approximately 30 per cent, an absolute reduction of approximately 9 per cent by 15 years of follow up.

In the same group of patients, the addition of chemotherapy to tamoxifen produces a further benefit in terms of recurrences and deaths from breast cancer versus tamoxifen alone. These benefits are also independent of age and nodal status. Tamoxifen also halves the risk of developing a contralateral primary breast cancer over the 5 years it is taken and for up to 5 years afterwards. All patients should be prescribed tamoxifen for 5 years. Randomized trials are in progress to determine whether prolonging tamoxifen beyond 5 years confers any advantage. Other trials are in progress to determine whether aromatase inhibitors have a role in the adjuvant setting.

Women <50 years of age benefit from ovarian ablation. Surgical oophorectomy produces castrate levels of oestrogen permanently and instantaneously. It is particularly useful for those women who are *BRCA* gene carriers who may be at high risk of developing ovarian cancer. As an alternative, gonadotrophin-releasing hormone analogues act by downregulation of the hypothalamo–pituitary axis, resulting in a complete cessation of ovarian oestrogen production. Either goserelin or leuprorelin is suitable. They are given once monthly as a subcutaneous injection and their effect is reversible. In the absence of chemotherapy, ovarian ablation reduces:

- the odds of recurrence by approximately 30 per cent, an absolute reduction of approximately 13 per cent by 15 years of follow up;
- the odds of dying from breast cancer by approximately 30 per cent, an absolute reduction of approximately 10 per cent by 15 years of follow up.

A premenopausal woman with a node positive, oestrogen receptor positive tumour should be offered ovarian ablation if their adjuvant chemotherapy does not lead to permanent amenorrhoea.

Chemotherapy

The criteria used to determine whether a patient should receive adjuvant chemotherapy vary from centre to centre and should be considered flexible rather than rigid. The Nottingham prognostic index is the only validated, objective way of combining the important prognostic variables of tumour size, grade and nodal status. However, it has not found widespread favour in Europe and the USA. A typical set of criteria are presented, any one of which would be sufficient to recommend chemotherapy as standard treatment.

Premenopausal woman:

- age <35 years;
- moderately differentiated (grade 2) tumour 20 mm or greater in maximum microscopic diameter;
- poorly differentiated (grade 3) tumour of any size;
- axillary lymph node involvement.
- oestrogen receptor negativity

Postmenopausal women 50–69 years:

- oestrogen receptor negativity;
- axillary lymph node involvement;
- poorly differentiated tumours >20 mm.

For women ≤50 years of age, adjuvant chemotherapy has been proven to reduce:

- the odds of recurrence by approximately 35–40 per cent, an absolute reduction of approximately 11 per cent by 15 years of follow up;
- the odds of dying (breast cancer and other causes) by approximately 25–30 per cent, an absolute reduction of approximately 5 per cent for node negative cases and 11 per cent for node positive cases by 15 years of follow up.

For women 50–69 years of age, adjuvant chemotherapy has been proven to reduce:

- the odds of recurrence by approximately 20 per cent, an absolute reduction of approximately 5 per cent by 15 years of follow up;
- the odds of dying from breast cancer by approximately 10 per cent, an absolute reduction of approximately 2–4 per cent by 15 years of follow up.

Adjuvant chemotherapy therefore confers greater benefit to younger patients. Its effect is independent of hormone receptor status. There is comparatively little data available for the use of adjuvant chemotherapy in the >70 year age group. Women of this age group should only be offered chemotherapy if their cancer is hormonally insensitive and very adverse risk factors are present (e.g. four or more involved axillary lymph nodes).

There is still no consensus as to what should be considered as the optimum chemotherapy regime. There is evidence that 6 months of chemotherapy using a combination of at least two drugs is to be preferred. The most tried and tested regime is 'classical' CMF comprising:

- cyclophosphamide 100 mg/m^2 p.o. day 1 to day 14;
- methotrexate 40 mg/m^2 i.v. day 1 and day 8;
- 5-fluorouracil 600 mg/m^2 i.v. day 1 and day 8;
- repeat cycle 4-weekly for 6 cycles.

The pooled results from randomized trials suggests that an anthracycline (doxorubicin or epirubicin) containing regime may yield an extra 4–5 per cent absolute survival advantage after 10 years of follow up compared with CMF. AC is an example of an anthracycline regime:

- adriamycin (doxorubicin) 60 mg/m^2 i.v. day 1;
- cyclophosphamide 600 mg/m^2 i.v. day 1;
- repeat cycle 3-weekly for 4–6 cycles.

There is increasing interest in using a taxane (paclitaxel or docetaxel) in the adjuvant setting because of encouraging results from preliminary studies suggesting superiority to a standard anthracycline regime alone, particularly for oestrogen receptor negative women. This approach is currently being tested in a number of randomized

clinical trials. It should therefore still be considered experimental.

TREATMENT OF METASTATIC DISEASE

The disease is incurable at this stage, and treatment is aimed to palliate symptoms and keep the patient as active as possible with minimal side effects and the least inconvenience. As for other solid tumours, active treatment will have a superior outcome to best supportive care.

Surgery

There is no role for breast surgery in the patient with metastatic disease provided that a tissue diagnosis has already been obtained and satisfactory local control of the breast tumour can be achieved by other treatment modalities. Toilet mastectomy is occasionally performed for symptomatic locally uncontrollable disease. Thoracoscopic talc pleurodesis is sometimes of value in the treatment of recurrent malignant pleural effusions, and internal fixation is indicated if fracture of a weight-bearing bone has occurred or is imminent. In highly selected patients that are fit, with a long disease interval and a solitary cerebral metastasis as sole site of disease, craniotomy, excision and postoperative radiotherapy should be considered.

Radiotherapy

The natural history of breast cancer dictates that most patients with metastatic breast cancer will have symptomatic bone metastases leading up to the terminal phase of the disease, although some will also be troubled by brain, cutaneous or choroidal metastases. Radiotherapy is the treatment of choice for metastases causing local symptoms.

Hormone therapy

Tamoxifen is the agent of first choice in women who are not taking it as adjuvant therapy. The response rate is greatest in those with high levels of oestrogen receptor, usually those with well-differentiated tumours and the elderly, with an objective response in 40 per cent of oestrogen receptor positive tumours and 10 per cent of oestrogen negative ones. Median duration of response is 10 months. Unless already performed as adjuvant therapy, premenopausal women with metastatic disease should undergo some form of artificial menopause (surgical oophorectomy or regular treatment with a gonadotrophin releasing hormone analogue).

Case history: breast cancer

A 43-year-old premenopausal woman presents with a 6 cm diameter lump arising within a small breast with no axillary lymph node enlargement. Mammography and ultrasound are suspicious for carcinoma. Fine-needle aspiration confirms malignant cells and a core biopsy indicates a grade 3 invasive ductal carcinoma, which is hormone receptor negative. Staging investigations indicate no evidence of metastatic disease. The tumour is therefore staged as T3N0M0. The only surgical option is mastectomy. The patient will require chemotherapy after mastectomy so opts to receive it as neo-adjuvant (i.e. preoperative) treatment. A radio-opaque marker is inserted under ultrasound guidance to mark the site of the tumour radiologically. After three cycles of chemotherapy using doxorubicin and cyclophosphamide (60 mg/m^2 and 600 mg/m^2 repeated every 21 days), the lump clinically measures 2 cm in diameter. By six cycles, it is almost impalpable clinically but still visible on mammography. A breast-conserving operation is now feasible and she undergoes a wire localized excision of the residual disease and axillary lymph node dissection. Histopathological examination confirms a 1 cm diameter area of residual grade 2 ductal carcinoma and ductal carcinoma *in situ* (DCIS), representing tumour that has been downgraded by chemotherapy. Two of 12 axillary lymph nodes sampled are involved. The tumour is confirmed as negative for oestrogen receptors, progesterone receptors and *HER2*. Postoperative radiotherapy is delivered to the breast alone. No further adjuvant therapy is given as hormone manipulation will confer no advantage. The woman remains well for 9 months after completing her treatment but then presents with a persistent aching pain in the right upper quadrant of the abdomen. Examination reveals tenderness and fullness in the right subcostal region. Liver function tests indicate a gamma-glutamyltransferase (GGT) of 470 U/l (normal <42 U/l) and alkaline phosphatase (ALP) of 350 U/l (normal range 38–126 U/l). The CA15-3 breast cancer marker is also elevated at 400 U/ml (normal range <50 U/ml). Preliminary liver ultrasound confirms multiple hypo-echoic lesions suggestive of metastases. Computed tomography (CT) scan of the thorax/abdomen and isotope bone scan are undertaken as staging investigations. These confirm multiple metastases throughout both lobes of the liver but no disease elsewhere. In view of a relapse occurring in less than 1 year after treatment with an anthracycline, chemotherapy is recommended using a taxane (Docetaxel 75–100 mg/m^2 every 21 days). Three cycles are given with resolution of the woman's presenting symptoms. Repeat examination is normal and CT of the liver shows a partial response. The CA15-3 is 75 U/ml and there has been a greater than 50 per cent decrease in GGT and ALP. A further three cycles of Docetaxel are given with further clinical, biochemical and radiological response. CA15-3 falls to 40 U/ml by the end of chemotherapy and a baseline scan 6 weeks after the last cycle shows a further response compared with the previous one. Six months later, she presents with increasing dyspnoea on exertion. Clinically, there are no signs of note. Chest X-ray shows bilateral perihilar opacification suggestive of lymphangitis. A CT scan confirms military-type metastases throughout both lung fields and a further increase in the number and size of liver metastases. Further chemotherapy is delivered using vinorelbine 25 mg/m^2 on days 1 and 8 of a 21-day cycle. Granulocyte colony-stimulating factor (G-CSF) growth factor support is necessary due to significant myelotoxicity. An interval scan after three cycles shows no response. There is no further response to treatment. It is decided that further active oncological treatment is inappropriate and that symptom control should be the priority. The woman dies approximately 2 years after presentation.

Other options include:

- an aromatase inhibitor such anastrozole, letrozole or exemestane (these are only suitable for postmenopausal women; preliminary data from a large trial comparing tamoxifen with anastrozole have shown anastrozole to be at least as effective as tamoxifen as first-line treatment of metastatic disease but with a lower incidence of side-effects);

- a progestogen such as megestrol acetate 80 mg BD or medroxyprogesterone acetate 400 mg BD.

There is good evidence that for postmenopausal women, aromatase inhibitors are superior to progestogens with respect to duration of response and survival. There is emerging evidence of an advantage in their use as first-line agents in the treatment of metastatic disease. Responses to second-line hormone therapy are more likely in those who have responded convincingly to first-line hormone therapy.

Chemotherapy

Chemotherapy is effective against soft tissue metastases but is less effective than radiotherapy for palliating bone metastases. The choice of first-line metastatic regime will depend on that used for adjuvant therapy (if any). At least six cycles are administered unless chemoresistance is demonstrated by progression during treatment. After six cycles, the treatment may be continued for as long as some objective response is obtained unless toxicity is so severe as to compromise the patient's quality of life and warrant termination of treatment.

Those patients failing CMF can be treated with an anthracycline regime: doxorubicin 75 mg/m^2 repeated every 21 days; epirubicin 90 mg/m^2 repeated every 21 days. For anthracycline refractory patients, a taxane should be considered: paclitaxel 175 mg/m^2 repeated every 21 days; docetaxel 100 mg/m^2 repeated every 21 days.

Other options include:

- vinorelbine 25 mg/m^2 days 1 & 8 of a 21-day cycle;
- capecitabine 2500 mg/m^2 divided into two oral doses per day for days 1–14 of a 21-day cycle.

Immunotherapy

The development of the monoclonal antibody Trastuzumab (Herceptin) represents a triumph of drug development and is one of the most exciting advances in oncology within the last decade. It is known that 25–30 per cent of breast cancers have overamplification of the *HER2* oncogene in the nucleus or overexpression of its protein product on the cell surface. Trastuzumab is a humanized murine antibody that specifically targets the *HER2*-positive cells, leading to cell-mediated cytotoxicity. Initial trials in patients with metastatic disease have shown single-agent response rates of approximately 30 per cent. In combination with certain cytotoxic agents such as paclitaxel, carboplatin and doxorubicin/cyclophosphamide, Trastuzumab increases overall response rates and leads to a significant improvement in median survival. It has the distinct advantage of being relatively non-toxic.

Some patients experience fever and chills after the first infusion, and cardiotoxicity is recognized, particularly in combination with doxorubicin.

Other drugs

Bisphosphonates such as disodium pamidronate, sodium clodronate and the newer more potent agent zoledronate have a role in those with skeletal metastatic disease. There is evidence from double-blind, placebo-controlled randomized trials that regular administration of bisphosphonates may reduce:

- risk of bone pain;
- risk of hypercalcaemia;
- risk of pathological fracture;
- need for palliative radiotherapy.

Tumour-related complications

Fungating tumours may become infected, causing an offensive discharge or lead to chronic blood loss. Uncontrolled disease in the axilla may lead to brachial plexopathy and/or lymphoedema of the arm. Hypercalcaemia, spinal cord compression and pathological fracture are seen in patients with widespread skeletal metastases (see Chapter 22). Pulmonary spread may lead to nodules, pleural effusion and lymphangitis (Fig. 8.13). Occasionally, pericardial invasion will lead to a pericardial effusion, which may in turn lead to cardiac tamponade (Fig. 8.14). Disseminated intravascular coagulation is a rare complication of advanced disease when the tumour burden is high and usually heralds the terminal phase of the disease. Mucin production by the tumour may activate the clotting cascade

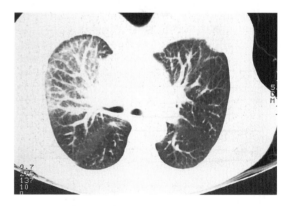

Fig 8.13 Pulmonary lymphangitis. Computed tomography image of the thorax. Note the widened lymphatic channels emanating from the hila bilaterally.

causing uncontrolled coagulation, coupled with a physiological thrombolysis leading to occlusion of both small and large blood vessels. Consumption of clotting factors deranges thrombin time and activated partial thromboplastin time resulting in a bleeding tendency, while platelet consumption leads to thrombocytopenia manifested as epistaxis, petechiae and bruising. Fibrin degradation products are elevated.

Treatment-related complications

Radiotherapy

Breast radiotherapy leads to breast erythema, swelling, skin irritation and tenderness which settle within 4–8 weeks of completing treatment. The skin may temporarily break down in areas subject to friction such as the inframammary fold. Late complications of radiotherapy are uncommon and include chronic breast/chest wall discomfort, breast shrinkage, breast swelling, breast firmness,

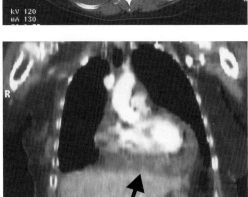

(a)

(b)

FIG 8.14 Computed tomography images of the thorax showing a large pericardial effusion in a patient with known pleural metastases. The patient presented acutely with cardiovascular collapse secondary to cardiac tamponade. (a) Transverse view; (b) coronal reconstruction.

telangiectasia of the skin, rib fractures, radiation costo-chondritis and pulmonary fibrosis. Data from randomized trials initiated prior to 1975 have suggested an increased risk of death from cardiovascular disease, confined to those women with left-sided breast cancers. Axillary irradiation (and surgery) is associated with late morbidity such as lymphoedema of the arm (Fig. 8.15), stiffness of the shoulder, radiation injury to the brachial plexus and radionecrosis of the proximal humerus, although with current techniques the incidence is very low.

Chemotherapy

Infertility, as signalled by amenorrhoea, is a frequent complication of chemotherapy. This will be permanent and associated with menopausal symptoms in many. The age at receiving chemotherapy is the most important factor for predicting the chance of spontaneous recovery of the menstrual cycle. Many studies with long-term follow up have suggested an increased risk of leukaemia and myelodysplasia in long-term survivors who have received chemotherapy. Anthracyclines such as epirubicin and doxorubicin may cause a reduction in left-ventricular function. This is more likely to manifest in those with severe hypertension or coexisting cardiac conditions, and may lead to congestive cardiac failure.

Hormone therapy

Menopausal symptoms, particularly vasomotor symptoms such as hot flushes, are the main problems with tamoxifen or ovarian ablation. Vasomotor symptoms are particularly difficult to treat. Many oncologists remain reluctant to prescribe hormone replacement therapy although there is no direct evidence of it being detrimental. Megestrol acetate, 20 mg BD, is a useful treatment. Some SSRI anti-depressants also have activity. Acupuncture is also worthwhile for some patients. Adjuvant tamoxifen is associated with a three- to four-fold increase in the risk of thrombo-embolic phenomena (deep-vein thrombosis, pulmonary embolism) and endometrial cancer in postmenopausal women.

Prognosis

The prognosis has improved significantly in recent years. Approximately one-third to half of an unselected population of women with breast cancer treated by surgery alone will die from their disease. The addition of radiotherapy and systemic therapies

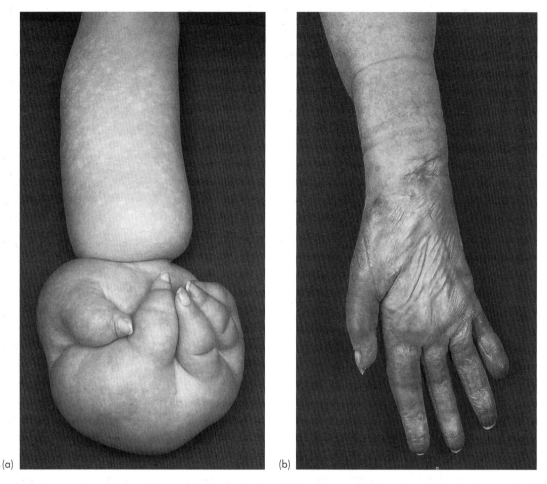

(a)   (b)

FIG 8.15 *Massive lymphoedema of the arm. This woman had a full axillary dissection followed by radiotherapy to the axilla 20 years earlier. The brachial plexus was damaged so there is no motor function in the arm or hand. (a) Before treatment. (b) After an intensive course of compression bandaging and manual lymphatic drainage. The arm is still non-functional but lighter to carry and less disfiguring.*

will lead to a significant improvement in survival by independently contributing additional odds reductions in recurrence and in turn mortality. The following should be considered as adverse prognostic factors:

- increasing TNM stage;
- poorly differentiated tumours;
- lymphatic vessel and/or vascular channel invasion;
- oestrogen and progesterone receptor negativity;
- positivity for the oncogene *HER2*;
- young age (<35 years) at diagnosis.

Screening

Screening should permit the diagnosis of a higher proportion of early stages of the disease. Since early stage at diagnosis is an important favourable prognostic factor, this should translate into a reduction in mortality from breast cancer. About 20 per cent of screen-detected cancers will be *in situ*, a further 20 per cent will be invasive cancers less than 1 cm in diameter and a similar percentage will be 1–2 cm.

Breast self-examination (BSE) should be routinely practised by women at the same time each month to take account of the variation in breast size and consistency with the menstrual cycle. However, to date, BSE has not been shown to have decreased breast cancer mortality and there has been concern as to the stress of such a practice. 'Breast awareness' has been proposed, whereby a woman has an appreciation of her breasts and reports any untoward findings to her doctor for immediate assessment.

Mammography is a sensitive means of detecting carcinomas, often before the lump is palpable by the patient or clinician, thereby facilitating the detection of early breast cancers with a particularly good prognosis. In the UK there is currently a National Breast Screening Programme in operation, with all women aged 50–64 years being offered 3-yearly mammograms. Women aged 65 years or more will be screened on request. Such a programme should result in a mortality reduction of 20–30 per cent. There is at present no consensus as to whether premenopausal women should be included in such a screening programme, as they tend to have dense breasts which may obscure the radiological signs of early breast cancers and studies to date have indicated a much smaller impact on survival than in the over-50 age-group. However, young women with a family history of breast cancer should be offered regular clinical assessments and mammographic screening. Ultrasonography is a poor substitute for mammography.

Prevention

Patients with a strong family history of breast cancer should be referred to a specialist genetics clinic for risk assessment, counselling and identification of other susceptible family members. Those shown (by gene testing or by statistical modelling) to be *BRCA* gene carriers are at sufficient lifetime risk of developing breast cancer to be considered for bilateral mastectomy, which very substantially reduces the risk but does not eliminate it completely.

Breast cancer is sufficiently common to make prevention a worthwhile exercise. Any method of prevention must be easy to comply with, free of short- and long-term adverse effects and be cost effective. The difference in dietary fat intake between the Western world and Africa and Asia contributes to the geographical variation in incidence. A reduction in the proportion of daily calories obtained from dietary fat may make a significant impact on the incidence of breast cancer. It has been estimated that a decrease in dietary fat from the average of 40 per cent to 20 per cent would decrease the incidence of breast cancer several-fold. Dietary manipulation has the advantage of being inherently cost effective, and may reduce morbidity and mortality from cardiovascular and cerebrovascular disease and colorectal cancer. Uncertainty exists as to when such a dietary adjustment should be instituted and for how long, although its other advantages make it desirable to make it a lifelong commitment.

Breast cancer is one of the few malignant diseases for which a large randomized trial has shown that chemoprevention is not only feasible but also effective. Tamoxifen, 20 mg daily, as adjuvant therapy has been conclusively shown to decrease the risk of contralateral breast cancer. This observation has been extrapolated to the prevention setting where a large (15 000 women) placebo-controlled, double-blind, randomized trial has been shown to significantly reduce the risk of developing DCIS and invasive breast cancer. There is an increased risk of thrombo-embolic disease and endometrial cancer in women receiving tamoxifen. Tamoxifen also reduces cholesterol levels and helps maintain bone mineral density in postmenopausal women, and may therefore have additional health benefits. The osteoporosis-prevention drug raloxifene has also been shown to reduce substantially the risk of developing breast cancer, and has the advantage of not causing hyperstimulation of the endometrium. The aromatase inhibitor anastrozole also reduces the risk of contralateral breast cancer in women receiving the drug as adjuvant therapy or as treatment for metastatic breast cancer. Anastrozole may therefore be a promising prevention strategy for postmenopausal women.

9 GASTROINTESTINAL CANCER

CARCINOMA OF THE OESOPHAGUS

Epidemiology

There are 25 000 new cases of oesophageal cancer and 23 000 deaths recorded in the European Union per annum. Overall, there is a male-to-female ratio of 3:1, although tumours of the upper third are much more common in females. The peak incidence is 60–70 years. The highest incidence is found in Russia, Turkey, China, Iran and Southern Africa.

Aetiology

Tobacco smoking is a strong risk factor for oesophageal cancer. The regular consumption of alcoholic spirits predisposes to cancer due to chronic irritation of the mucosa. Carcinogenic contaminants of alcoholic drinks have also been implicated in some cases (e.g. the home-made beer consumed by the Xhosa people in Transkei). Barrett's oesophagus is characterized by glandular metaplasia of the squamous epithelium of the lower third of the oesophagus, usually in response to chronic gastro-oesophageal reflux from a hiatus hernia. Patients are at risk of developing an adenocarcinoma of the oesophagus. In achalasia there is chronic stasis and pooling of food and secretions in a dilated oesophagus owing to a loss of oesophageal motility. The increased risk of cancer is due to prolonged contact of the mucosa with carcinogens within the food or produced from food by the action of bacteria. Patterson–Brown–Kelly syndrome (Plummer–Vinson syndrome) is characterized by koilionychia, iron-deficiency anaemia, the presence of an 'oesophageal web' in the upper third of the oesophagus on barium swallow, and is usually seen in women. It leads to a carcinoma of the upper third of the oesophagus typically in the post-cricoid region. Tylosis is a very rare, dominantly inherited condition characterized by palmar and plantar hyperkeratosis and a strong predisposition to oesophageal carcinoma.

Pathology

Approximately 40–50 per cent of carcinomas arise in the middle third of the oesophagus, 40–50 per cent in the lower third and less than 10 per cent in the upper third, the tumour appearing nodular, ulcerating or diffusely infiltrative. If there is oesophageal obstruction, the proximal oesophagus is frequently dilated and contains food debris. A fistula may exist between the oesophagus and trachea or bronchial tree, and there may be evidence of an aspiration pneumonia particularly in the lower lobes of the lungs. Cancers of the upper two-thirds of the oesophagus are invariably squamous cell carcinomas. Those in the lower third are most commonly squamous but one-third are adenocarcinomas, which may have arisen in an area of metaplasia such as Barrett's oesophagus. These must be distinguished from adenocarcinoma of the proximal stomach which has infiltrated the oesophagus. The histological spectrum of oesophageal cancer is changing with an increasing proportion being classified as adenocarcinomas.

Natural history

The tumour will spread within the oesophagus both longitudinally and circumferentially, eventually resulting in complete oesophageal obstruction.

Invasion through the deeper layers of the oesophageal wall will result in spread to the surrounding mediastinal structures, such as the trachea, main bronchi (especially left), pleura, lung, vertebrae and great vessels. Insidious spread along the submucosa is common and may lead to skip lesions some distance from the main tumour. The pattern of lymphatic involvement reflects the complex blood supply to the oesophagus. Tumours of the upper third will spread to the deep cervical and supraclavicular nodes, those of the middle third to the mediastinal, paratracheal and subcarinal nodes, and those of the lower third to the nodes of the coeliac axis below the diaphragm. The venous drainage of parts of the oesophagus is into the portal circulation and so the liver is the most common site of distant metastases, although the lungs and skeleton may also be involved.

Symptoms

Dysphagia is the most common presenting symptom. A middle-aged or elderly patient complaining of this symptom should be considered to have oesophageal cancer until proven otherwise and referral to a gastroenterologist is mandatory. The symptom begins insidiously as a sensation of food sticking, usually when solids such as meat have been eaten, progresses so that there is difficulty with softer foods/liquids and may be associated with retrosternal discomfort caused by stretching of the oesophagus and increased peristalsis. Regurgitation usually accompanies severe dysphagia. Retrosternal discomfort is followed by effortless regurgitation of the oesophageal contents. These do not taste sour as they have not entered the stomach. This contrasts with gastro-oesophageal reflux where there will be a strong taste of acid. Weight loss is caused by both reduced caloric intake due to dysphagia and/or regurgitation, and the non-specific effects of malignancy. Recurrent aspiration is a problem in patients with proximal tumours leading to overflow into the upper respiratory tract or with a fistula connecting the oesophagus to the lower respiratory tract. The patient experiences a severe bout of coughing within a short time of swallowing, and may expectorate solid material from the food bolus. Both predispose to recurrent chest infections, which may be fatal.

Signs

There is often evidence of malnutrition, the degree of which is dependent on the duration and severity of dysphagia and whether there has been a history of alcoholism. In cases of oesophageal obstruction the patient may even be dehydrated owing to poor fluid intake. Women with Plummer–Vinson syndrome may appear anaemic and have koilionychia, while alcoholics may have stigmata of chronic liver disease. There is usually no palpable evidence of disease, although an epigastric mass may be palpable in tumours of the lower third of the oesophagus and if there are large intra-abdominal lymph nodes. The cervical and supraclavicular lymph nodes should be palpated carefully. Hepatomegaly suggests metastatic disease but may indicate fatty infiltration or cirrhosis in heavy drinkers.

Differential diagnosis

Care has to be taken not to confuse a tumour arising from the oesophageal mucosa with a tumour arising from an adjacent structure and invading into the oesophagus, e.g. carcinoma of the left main bronchus (most often squamous or small cell carcinoma), carcinoma of the fundus of the stomach or gastro-oesophageal junction (adenocarcinoma). Other differential diagnoses include a benign oesophageal stricture due to chronic gastro-oesophageal reflux, achalasia and hysteria, although this is only a diagnosis made after excluding all other possible causes.

Investigations

Serum alkaline phosphatase, gammaglutamyl transferase and a liver ultrasound should be performed in all cases to screen for liver metastases and a chest X-ray is performed to exclude lung metastases and mediastinal lymphadenopathy.

Barium swallow and meal

A barium swallow will outline the whole oesophageal lumen, a carcinoma appearing as a stricture, filling defect or abnormal flow of barium (Fig. 9.1). It may also suggest the presence of a fistula connecting the oesophagus to the bronchial tree, although the radiologist should be warned if this is thought to be likely at the time of requesting the examination. This investigation will not give a tissue diagnosis and all patients should proceed to endoscopy.

Endoscopy

This is the investigation of choice. The oesophagus starts at the lower border of the cricoid cartilage at the level of the 6th cervical vertebra, approximately 15 cm from the incisor teeth. It is 25 cm long, entering

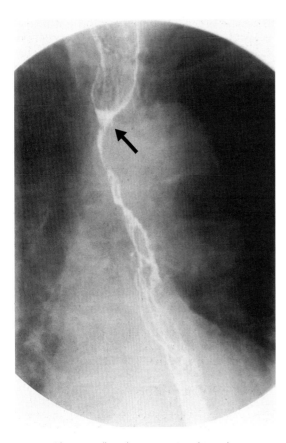

FIG 9.1 Barium swallow showing an irregular, malignant stricture of the middle third of the oesophagus. Note the small pool of barium at the top of the stricture (arrowed).

the stomach at the level of the 10th thoracic vertebra (i.e. approximately 40 cm from the incisors). Endoscopy allows a thorough assessment of the whole oesophagus. The tumour can be visualized directly, a biopsy taken for histology and brushings for cytology. It also allows a thorough evaluation of the stomach, which is particularly important in tumours of the lower third of the oesophagus, and is the most sensitive means of detecting small primary tumours and skip lesions. Endoscopic ultrasound is also a useful tool, permitting direct imaging of the tumour. It is particularly sensitive for determining the depth of invasion and involvement of immediate lymph node groups.

Computed tomography of the thorax and upper abdomen

Computed tomography (CT) provides information on the local extent of the disease with respect to invasion beyond the oesophagus and is of value in

planning radiotherapy or surgery because it will also allow an assessment of the regional lymph nodes, liver, lungs and adrenals.

Magnetic resonance imaging of the thorax and upper abdomen

Magnetic resonance imaging (MRI) will be useful in the preoperative assessment of borderline cases (e.g. when CT has indicated equivocal involvement of local structures or liver lesions of uncertain significance).

Bronchoscopy

This may be necessary to exclude direct invasion of the posterior tracheal wall and left main bronchus when considering the operability of a tumour of the upper or middle third.

Staging

The TNM staging system (see Chapter 2) is most frequently used.

- Tis – carcinoma *in situ*.
- T0 – no evidence of primary.
- TX – primary cannot be assessed.
- T1 – involving lamina propria/submucosa.
- T2 – involving muscularis propria.
- T3 – involving adventitia.
- T4 – involving adjacent structures.
- N0 – no regional lymphadenopathy.
- N1 – regional lymph node involvement.
- M0 – no distant metastases.
- M1 – distant metastases.

Treatment

Many patients will be poorly nourished, which lessens their tolerance of radical treatment and therefore referral to a dietician is advisable in all cases. A liquidizer may help the patient to continue eating food prepared at home. It may be necessary for the patient to be given liquid dietary supplements to maintain calorie intake, and enteral feeding via a nasogastric tube or via a percutaneous gastrostomy catheter may be the only means of maintaining nutrition.

RADICAL TREATMENT

Surgery

Surgery is a potentially curative treatment modality and is the treatment of choice for localized lower third tumours as this is the most surgically accessible part of the oesophagus.

Contraindications to surgery include:

- poor performance status;
- severe malnutrition;
- vocal cord palsy, which indicates infiltration/pressure on the recurrent laryngeal nerve, suggesting spread beyond the oesophagus;
- broncho-oesophageal fistula;
- invasion of great vessels (aorta, superior vena cava), pericardium;
- cervical/coeliac node involvement clinically or radiologically;
- distant metastases.

Tumours of the middle third can be treated by an Ivor Lewis two-stage oesophagectomy. The stomach is mobilized via upper abdominal incision, the oesophagus approached via the right 5th intercostal space, the tumour is resected allowing a 5 cm margin of macroscopically normal oesophagus, and the oesophagus is then reanastomosed. The operative mortality is high depending on patient selection and the surgeon's skill. For tumours of the lower third, a left thoraco-abdominal incision is made, the tumour mobilized via a trans-hiatal approach and resected with reanastomosis of the transected oesophagus. In experienced hands, and with appropriate patient selection, the operative mortality will be less than 5%.

Radiotherapy

Radiotherapy is the treatment of choice for tumours of the upper third, where surgery would be difficult, but can also be used for tumours elsewhere that are not amenable to surgery. The treatment-related mortality is much lower than radical surgery. Although distant metastases are a contraindication to radical radiotherapy, extra-oesophageal invasion may still be encompassed within the high-dose radiation zone. Treatment is given daily over 5–6 weeks.

Neo-adjuvant chemotherapy is increasingly used and is the subject of ongoing clinical trials. This typically involves the use of 5-fluorouracil (5-FU) and either cisplatin or mitomycin C, yielding objective response rates of 30–60 per cent. As with other tumour sites, most published experience has been with its use in squamous carcinomas. While there appears to be a prolongation of disease-free survival, no benefit in overall survival has been established.

In recent years, there has also been increasing interest in synchronous chemoradiotherapy (CRT),

particularly for squamous carcinomas and inoperable tumours. The advantage of combined chemotherapy and radiotherapy is that there may be synergy between the two treatments, leading to the max-imum probability of preoperative downstaging. This may in turn facilitate curative surgery for some individuals or maximize non-surgical treatment for those that remain inoperable. To date, the few randomized trials of CRT versus radiotherapy alone have shown a promising improvement in median and overall survivals for the CRT group, with 3-year survivals of 20–30 per cent. Similar trials of preoperative CRT and surgery versus surgery alone have shown pathological complete response rates of 20–30 per cent and 3-year survival rates similar in magnitude. This is a promising approach which deserves further study.

Chemotherapy

Except for synchronous CRT (see above), there is no defined role for chemotherapy in the curative treatment of oesophageal cancer. Adjuvant chemotherapy is less established as a valid approach compared with other forms of cancer.

PALLIATIVE TREATMENT

Dysphagia and regurgitation are the symptoms most often requiring treatment. Both are extremely distressing and can erode the quality of life significantly.

Radiotherapy

A short course of radiotherapy will relieve dysphagia in most patients with acceptable short-term morbidity and can usually be repeated if necessary. This may be given as a course of external beam irradiation or intraluminal brachytherapy whereby a high-activity radiation source is inserted directly into the oesophagus via a nasogastric tube.

Chemotherapy

Combinations of 5-FU and cisplatin have a role in the palliative treatment of oesophageal cancer. One such regime, which is of particular value, particularly in adenocarcinomas, is ECF:

- epirubicin 60 mg/m^2 i.v. day 1;
- cisplatin 60 mg/m^2 i.v. day 1, with full pre- and post-hydration;
- 5-FU 200 mg/m^2 i.v. daily by continuous i.v. infusion;
- repeat bolus chemotherapy 3-weekly for six cycles.

Other treatments

Fibreoptic endoscopy permits a number of procedures to be performed under direct vision. Dilatation using metal bougies allows a stricture to be stretched and relieves dysphagia to some degree in the majority, although the procedure may need to be repeated a number of times during the patient's remaining lifetime. Alternatively, an endoprosthesis such as an Atkinson tube may be inserted to maintain oesophageal patency and is particularly useful in relieving recurrent aspiration caused by a fistula. Laser therapy may be given to coagulate a bleeding tumour or to unblock an obstructed oesophagus. Administration of laser light-sensitizing agents can be used as part of a course of 'photodynamic therapy' to kill tumour cells more selectively.

Tumour-related complications

Malnutrition may be caused by chronic dysphagia. Invasion of tumour into the adjacent main bronchi may lead to a broncho-oesophageal fistula (Fig. 9.2). Aspiration of food into the respiratory

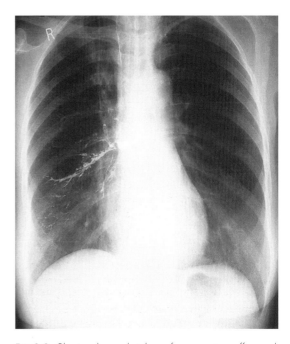

FIG 9.2 Chest radiograph taken after a gastrograffin swallow. Contrast has leaked into the right side of the bronchial tree. This is diagnostic of a broncho-oesophageal fistula.

Case history: oesophageal cancer

A 60-year-old man with a history of chronic bronchitis develops dysphagia. He experiences retrosternal discomfort when he swallows solid foodstuffs (e.g. meat, bread). He has a long history of gastro-oesophageal reflux and had a barium swallow some years earlier, which confirmed a hiatus hernia. He initially self-medicates himself with a proton pump inhibitor in addition to a mucosal surface protectant. His discomfort temporarily improves but then worsens and is accompanied by regurgitation of food.

He is referred to a gastroenterologist. Endoscopy reveals a polypoid tumour at 32–36 cm obstructing the lumen of the oesophagus, with no extension into the stomach. Biopsy confirms a poorly differentiated adenocarcinoma with some evidence of an underlying Barrett's oesophagus and chronic oesophagitis. Computed tomography (CT) scan shows no evidence of mediastinal or abdominal lymphadenopathy and no evidence of liver metastases.

He is initially treated with chemoradiation over a 5-week period, during which time his symptoms improve significantly. Repeat endoscopy 6 weeks later reveals no obvious mucosal abnormality and random biopsies show chronic inflammatory cells alone. At this time, his shortness of breath is worse than usual and he has a dry cough. Chest X-ray confirms opacification corresponding to the radiation fields, suggesting a degree of radiation pneumonitis.

In view of an apparent pathological complete response, and his respiratory compromise, he is not deemed a suitable candidate for major surgery.

Eighteen months later, he presents with recurrent dysphagia. He is referred to a dietician for dietary advice. Endoscopy confirms a recurrence at the same level as previously, which is dilated. Adenocarcinoma is confirmed histologically. Six weeks later, his symptoms have recurred. An oesophageal stent is inserted which provides good symptom control for 3 months. He then develops right upper quadrant pain and anorexia. Liver ultrasound confirms hepatic metastases. He declines further chemotherapy. There is a symptomatic improvement with dexamethasone but he dies of his disease 4 weeks later.

tract will lead to pneumonia which may be further complicated by lung abscess and empyema. Haemorrhage is a rare but potentially fatal local tumour complication.

Treatment-related complications

Surgery

Loss of oesophageal integrity after surgical resection may lead to a fistula or mediastinitis, which may be fatal, while pneumothorax, pulmonary collapse and pneumonia may complicate a thoracotomy.

Radiotherapy

During treatment, it is inevitable that the patient will experience some worsening of dysphagia owing to a radiation oesophagitis. This can be minimized by avoidance of very hot or cold food/fluids, and relieved by a mucosal protectant sipped slowly. Anorexia and nausea/vomiting are likely if stomach and/or liver is included in the radiation fields and will be helped by a regular antiemetic. Radiation pneumonitis is uncommon and usually subclinical, although it may cause a dry cough, fever and dyspnoea. Oesophageal stricture may occur from 6 months after radiotherapy, giving rise to dysphagia, and needs to be distinguished from recurrent tumour, preferably by endoscopy so that a dilatation can be performed simultaneously.

Chemotherapy

Apart from drug-specific toxicity, combined modality treatment with chemotherapy and radiotherapy leads to a severe acute oesophageal reaction which may compromise nutrition and require supportive therapy.

Prognosis

Overall 5-year survival is only 5–10 per cent and is usually a result of many cases having occult lymph node or distant metastases at presentation. For the subgroup undergoing potentially curative surgery, the 5-year survival is 20 per cent or more depending on selection criteria.

Screening/prevention

Informing the public of the risks of tobacco and alcohol could reduce the incidence of oesophageal cancer. In areas of very high prevalence, screening is a beneficial and cost-effective exercise. In the UK, patients with a Barrett's oesophagus and achalasia should be offered annual endoscopic examination because of their high risk of developing carcinoma.

Rare tumours

Adenoid cystic carcinoma

This is a tumour arising from the mucous glands of the mucosa and is of the same type as those arising in the parotid salivary gland and elsewhere.

Small cell carcinoma

Although infiltration from an underlying lung primary should be considered, a primary tumour of this type has been described.

Melanoma

This is a rare site for mucosal melanoma. Prognosis will be very poor because of advanced stage at presentation.

Carcinoid

This is an uncommon site for this rare tumour. It should be treated, as elsewhere, by surgical resection.

Leiomyosarcoma

This tumour arises from the smooth muscle fibres of the oesophageal wall. It is best treated by radical surgery combined with radiotherapy.

CARCINOMA OF THE STOMACH

Epidemiology

There are 75 000 new cases and 60 000 deaths recorded in the European Union per annum, with a peak incidence of 50–70 years and a male-to-female ratio of 1.5:1. Blood group O confers some protection against developing stomach cancer while blood group A is associated with a higher incidence of the diffuse form of stomach cancer. The incidence is very high in Japan and Chile, and increased in lower socio-economic groups.

Aetiology

The stomach is exposed to a variety of carcinogens both ingested and produced from the action of bacteria within the stomach. Nitrosamines have been implicated in stomach cancer, as has a diet rich in smoked foodstuffs. Atrophic gastritis and achlorhydria both increase the risk of developing stomach cancer, in the case of pernicious anaemia by five-fold. This may be related to bacterial overgrowth and increased production of endogenous carcinogens. A partial gastrectomy or gastroenterostomy is also associated with an increased cancer risk, probably owing a chronic reflux of bile salts into the stomach. An adenoma–carcinoma sequence is recognized but is much rarer than in the large bowel.

Pathology

Stomach cancers usually form discrete ulcerating lesions, but may be nodular or polypoid. They are occasionally diffusely infiltrating leading to obliteration of the stomach lumen. Fifty per cent arise in the pyloric region while of those arising in the body, most are found along the lesser curvature. Ninety-five per cent are adenocarcinomas, and 5 per cent are squamous carcinoma or adenoacanthoma (adenocarcinoma with areas of squamous metaplasia). There may be evidence of prior intestinal metaplasia and carcinoma *in situ* in the surrounding mucosa.

Natural history

Cancers spread longitudinally and circumferentially within the stomach, and as with carcinoma of the oesophagus insidious submucosal spread is frequent. Occasionally, this leads to diffuse infiltration of the whole stomach with luminal narrowing and rigidity of the stomach wall, and a picture known as linitis plastica. Progressive invasion into the muscle layer of the stomach wall eventually leads to invasion of the serosa and in turn invasion of adjacent viscera such as the omentum, pancreas, spleen, left kidney and adrenal. Invasion superiorly by a tumour of the fundus may result in occlusion of the lower third of the oesophagus leading to dysphagia and regurgitation. There is a propensity for transcoelomic spread with diffuse peritoneal seeding leading to ascites (Fig. 9.3) and ovarian deposits (Krukenberg tumours), particularly with the signet ring variant. Spread to the regional lymph nodes (gastric, gastroduodenal, splenic and coeliac groups) occurs early in the natural history, and Virchow's node in the left supraclavicular fossa may be involved (Troisier's sign). Distant spread occurs to the liver via the portal venous circulation, lung, bone, brain and skin.

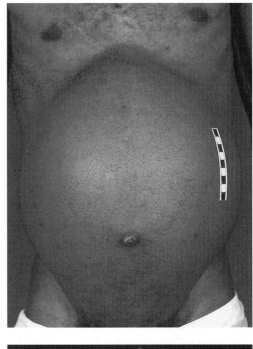

(a)

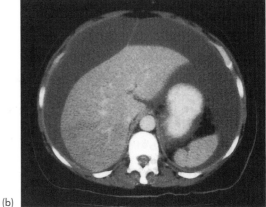

(b)

FIG 9.3 Massive ascites. (a) Frontal view of abdomen. (b) Transverse computed tomography image of abdomen.

Symptoms

The patient frequently presents with non-specific gastrointestinal symptoms such as epigastric discomfort, anorexia, nausea, vomiting and weight loss, which are frequently confused with a benign condition such as peptic ulceration or gastritis, and may even be relieved by the antacids, H_2 antagonists or proton pump inhibitors prescribed for these conditions; others present with the symptoms of an iron-deficiency anaemia. Stomach cancer should always be considered in the assessment of such patients. A more acute presentation may occur with stomach perforation, haematemesis and/or melaena.

Signs

At presentation, many will have been losing weight, and cachexia is a frequent finding. An epigastric mass may be palpable and there may be palpable lymph nodes in the left supraclavicular fossa. The liver may be enlarged, tender and knobbly, suggesting metastatic infiltration, and there may be ascites. Non-metastatic manifestations such as dermatomyositis and acanthosis nigricans may also be seen.

Differential diagnosis

This includes:

- inflammatory conditions (e.g. peptic ulcer);
- other malignant gastric tumours (e.g. lymphoma, leiomyosarcoma);
- benign gastric tumours (e.g. leiomyoma, carcinoid).

Investigations

Barium meal

Double-contrast barium meal will outline the gastric mucosa and is a sensitive investigation for detecting mucosal abnormalities. Although carcinomas often have a characteristic appearance, there may be confusion with benign peptic ulcers and therefore further investigation to obtain a tissue diagnosis is mandatory.

Fibreoptic endoscopy

This permits direct visualization of the gastric mucosa, allowing a more accurate assessment of the macroscopic appearances of an abnormality. It also permits biopsy and brushings for cytology to give a tissue diagnosis.

Computed tomography scan of the abdomen

This will provide the surgeon with information regarding invasion beyond the stomach and whether the regional lymph nodes are enlarged, and thereby help to determine whether the tumour is operable (also see below).

Tests to exclude metastatic disease

These tests include:

- baseline liver function tests;
- a CT scan of the thorax and abdomen to exclude hepatic and/or pulmonary metastases;
- serum assay of carcinoembryonic antigen, which may be elevated reflecting tumour burden; it may permit early diagnosis of distant and/or local relapse after curative treatment.

Staging

The TNM system (see Chapter 2) is widely used.

- Tis – carcinoma *in situ*.
- T0 – no evidence of primary.
- TX – primary cannot be assessed.
- T1 – involving lamina propria/submucosa.
- T2 – involving muscularis propria/subserosa.
- T3 – penetrates serosa.
- T4 – involving adjacent structures.
- N0 – no regional lymphadenopathy.
- N1 – 1–6 regional lymph nodes involved.
- N2 – 7–15 regional lymph nodes involved.
- N3 – >15 regional lymph nodes involved.
- M0 – no distant metastases.
- M1 – distant metastases.

Treatment

RADICAL TREATMENT

Surgery

This is the only potentially curative treatment but only two-thirds of patients are deemed operable after full staging investigations and a further two-thirds of these will be found to be inoperable, meaning that overall only one in five patients stand any chance of being cured. The extent of surgical resection remains an area of controversy. A partial or total gastrectomy is performed in operable cases, depending on the size and site of the tumour. Total gastrectomy in smaller tumours will have the advantage of surgically clearing occult mucosal spread and synchronous second primary cancers. A D1 resection involves removal of the first echelon perigastric lymph nodes, while a D2 resection will remove the second echelon nodes and invariably is a more substantial surgical procedure, requiring greater expertise and a higher operative mortality. Despite this, evidence is emerging particularly from Japan of the superiority of a D2 lymphadenectomy particularly for larger, more deeply penetrating tumours. There is no evidence to support routine removal of the spleen.

Radiotherapy

Radiotherapy has no curative role in treatment because of the dose-limiting toxicity induced in the stomach and adjacent structures such as the small bowel and transverse colon when a high dose of radiation is administered. Adjuvant postoperative radiotherapy does not significantly improve survival but does reduce the risk of local recurrence approximately threefold. A recent, large, randomized trial indicated that postoperative CRT substantially improved overall survival in high-risk completely resected locally advanced adenocarcinoma of the stomach and gastro-oesophageal (GE) junction. In the USA, this CRT regime is becoming the standard of care.

Chemotherapy

The role of chemotherapy in this context is not established. A meta-analysis published almost a decade ago showed no survival advantage for postoperative chemotherapy. A more recent one indicated a 17 per cent reduction in the odds of dying from gastric cancer after a curative resection.

PALLIATIVE TREATMENT

Surgery

Intestinal bypass surgery (e.g. gastrojejunostomy) is effective in relieving gastric outflow obstruction while gastrectomy may be justified in the presence of metastatic disease when massive bleeding cannot be controlled by less invasive methods.

Radiotherapy

Radiotherapy is valuable in relieving the local symptoms of inoperable disease such as dysphagia, haemorrhage or pain due to retroperitoneal infiltration.

Chemotherapy

As with other solid tumours, there is some evidence suggesting that immediate chemotherapy confers a survival advantage compared with best supportive care. This may be of value in relieving symptoms from metastatic disease, particularly for lung and liver metastases. The most active single agent is 5-FU, which may be used in combination with other drugs such as Adriamycin and mitomycin C (FAM)/ methotrexate (FAMtx) or epirubicin and cisplatin (ECF). Response rates of 30–40 per cent have been

reported with median survivals in the region of 6–12 months. As gastric cancer has some analogies with colorectal cancer with respect to 5-FU being the agent with the best track record, it is not surprising that drugs such as irinotecan are also being tested. Building on their success at other sites, the taxanes are also the subject of further study in this disease.

Endoscopic procedures

Laser therapy is particularly useful for the photocoagulation of a persistently bleeding tumour or debulking of a large tumour that is narrowing the oesophageal lumen. An oesophageal endoprosthesis is occasionally of benefit for a tumour of the upper stomach which is occluding the oesophagus from below.

Tumour-related complications

Haemorrhage may be life threatening if a major gastric vessel is eroded, while chronic blood loss will lead to an iron-deficiency anaemia with a reduced serum ferritin. Invasion through the stomach wall into the peritoneal cavity may lead to leakage of gastric contents and an acute peritonitis. Pyloric stenosis may lead to gastric outflow obstruction, eventually leading to episodes of projectile vomiting, visible peristalsis, a 'succussion splash' and obstruction. Mucin secretion by the tumour may rarely result in activation of the plasmin/plasminogen cascade, leading to a disseminated intravascular coagulation manifested by abnormal clotting, thrombocytopenia and raised fibrin degradation products (FDPs; see Chapter 8).

Treatment-related complications

Surgery

Loss of stomach volume will lead to a feeling of fullness after small portions of food, while loss of gastric acidity may predispose to iron deficiency. Impaired intrinsic factor production will lead to vitamin B_{12} deficiency secondary to impaired absorption at the terminal ileum, resulting in a macrocytic anaemia, while impaired digestion may result in malabsorption and a 'dumping syndrome' due to hypoglycaemia. Stomal ulceration and ultimately a second malignancy may occur.

Radiotherapy

During treatment, the patient will experience some degree of anorexia, nausea and vomiting. High doses of radiation to the stomach may result in a chronic gastritis. The left kidney may receive a dose sufficient to impair its function permanently, which will be relevant if the right kidney function is subnormal. Radiation enteritis is also a recognized complication.

Prognosis

The median survival for patients with unresectable disease is about 4 months and the 5-year survival is less than 10 per cent overall, rising to 15–20 per cent in those undergoing successful surgical resection. Early gastric cancer has a good 5-year survival of 70 per cent or more. In stage TisN0M0 disease confined to the mucosa, results from radical surgery are excellent with 5-year survivals of 90 per cent or more. Adverse prognostic factors include increasing tumour stage at presentation, unresectable disease, diffuse morphology and poor tumour differentiation.

Screening/prevention

A screening programme of double-contrast barium examination of the stomach and gastroscopy has been successfully implemented in Japan. This has led to a greater proportion of early cancers being detected, resulting in a decline in mortality.

Rare tumours

Gastrointestinal stromal tumour

Gastrointestinal stromal tumours (GISTs) are mesenchymal neoplasms occurring in later life. Seventy per cent arise in the stomach and 25 per cent in the small intestine. They express a growth factor receptor with tyrosine kinase activity (*c-kit*) which can be detected with CD117 immunohistochemistry. Their uncontrolled cell proliferation makes them highly malignant tumours that are relatively resistant to conventional treatments and invariably fatal. However, encouraging responses have been seen with the antibody imatinib (Glivec) which targets *c-kit*.

Leiomyoma

This is a benign tumour arising from smooth muscle of the stomach wall, often found incidentally during investigation of the upper gastrointestinal tract but it may ulcerate leading to haematemesis.

Carcinoid

The stomach is a very uncommon site for carcinoid tumours, which are best treated surgically (see Chapter 14).

Lymphoma

The stomach is a common site for extranodal lymphoma which is usually a low-grade tumour of mucosa-associated lymphoid tissue (MALToma).

CARCINOMA OF THE PANCREAS

Epidemiology

There are 38 000 new cases and almost as many deaths recorded in the European Union per annum. Most patients are aged over 50 years at diagnosis and the peak incidence is at 60–80 years; there is an equal sex distribution. It is a disease of industrialized countries.

Aetiology

Pancreatic cancer has been associated with:

- smoking tobacco;
- high dietary fat and meat consumption;
- high coffee and/or alcohol consumption;
- diabetes mellitus;
- chronic pancreatitis;
- previous surgery for peptic ulcer disease;
- industrial exposure to the insecticide DDT;
- familial cancer syndromes (e.g. multiple endocrine adenomatosis type 1, von Hippel–Lindau syndrome, ataxia telangiectasia.

Pathology

The tumour may be well circumscribed or diffusely infiltrating the pancreas. Thirty per cent arise in the head of the pancreas and are often associated with a dilated common bile duct, and 20 per cent arise in the body or tail; the remainder are more diffuse in origin. Carcinoma arises from the ducts (90 per cent) and glandular elements (10 per cent) rather than the hormone-producing cells and is invariably a mucin-producing adenocarcinoma. There may be evidence of a chronic pancreatitis distal to any blocked pancreatic ducts and the majority stain for carcinoembryonic antigen (CEA).

Natural history

The tumour infiltrates diffusely through the gland, or may grow along the pancreatic duct system, eventually reaching the common bile duct and ampulla of Vater. The capsule may be breached, leading to invasion of the stomach, duodenum, spleen, aorta and retroperitoneal tissues, and transcoelomic spread may occur with diffuse peritoneal involvement and ascites.

Regional lymph nodes are frequently involved and include the pancreaticoduodenal, gastroduodenal, hepatic, superior mesenteric and coeliac groups. The majority have distant metastases by the time of diagnosis at sites including the liver, lung, skin and brain.

Symptoms

Pancreatic cancer is notorious for presenting late in the natural history of the disease, reflecting the deep-seated anatomical position of the pancreas and high prevalence of non-specific upper gastrointestinal symptoms in the population. Tumours of the head of the pancreas most frequently present with obstructive jaundice (progressive jaundice, dark urine, pale stools, itching) due to occlusion of the common bile duct. Tumours of the body and tail of the pancreas are more likely to present with pain, usually epigastric with radiation to the back. Extensive pancreatic infiltration or blockage of the major ducts will lead to malabsorption owing to exocrine dysfunction, which will result in pale, fatty, offensive stools (steatorrhoea) which float on water and are difficult to flush down the lavatory pan. Pancreatic endocrine dysfunction will lead to impaired glucose tolerance or diabetes mellitus in 20 per cent, causing thirst, polyuria, nocturia and weight loss.

Signs

The patient often has jaundice and the gallbladder may be palpable in the right upper quadrant of the abdomen, suggesting extrahepatic biliary obstruction that is not caused by chronic gallstone disease (positive Courvoisier's sign). There will be pale stools on rectal examination and dark urine. Scratch marks on the trunk are a sign of pruritus due to bile salt retention. A mass may be palpable in the epigastrium, fixed due to its retroperitoneal location. Weight loss is common and may lead to profound cachexia. The liver may be enlarged and knobbly, consistent with metastatic infiltration. There may be petechiae, purpura and bruising in advanced disease due to disseminated intravascular coagulation (DIC).

Differential diagnosis

Gallstones are a common cause of obstructive jaundice and abdominal pain, although they are not commonly associated with systemic symptoms and are not a cause of glucose intolerance. Benign tumours such as a glucagonoma, gastrinoma or VIPoma should also be considered.

Investigations

Liver function tests

These will demonstrate the degree of obstructive jaundice, characterized by raised total serum bilirubin, elevated alkaline phosphatase and gammaglutamyltransferase.

Clotting profile

There will be derangement of vitamin K-dependent clotting factors. This will be reflected in a prolongation of the international normalized ratio (INR), and will show clinically as bruising and a tendency to prolonged bleeding. A full blood count and clotting profile should always be performed prior to invasive investigations such as an endoscopic retrograde cholepancreaticogram (ERCP) or CT-guided biopsy, and serum collected for grouping so that fresh frozen plasma or blood can be given at short notice should there be a haemorrhage after biopsy. Patients suspected of having DIC should have blood sent to measure FDPs.

CA 19-9 tumour marker assay

This is worth measuring as a baseline. It is a potentially useful marker of disease activity and response to treatment.

Chest X-ray

A chest X-ray is indicated to exclude pulmonary metastases.

Computed tomography of the abdomen

This characteristically shows dilatation of the common bile duct associated with a mass lesion in the head of the pancreas, a discrete mass in the body or tail of the pancreas, or diffuse enlargement of the pancreas. All patients considered suitable for radical surgery should undergo this investigation as it is the best way of defining the extent of local invasion, presence of enlarged regional lymph nodes and liver metastases. It also facilitates a fine-needle biopsy when a definitive diagnosis cannot be made by less invasive procedures.

Magnetic resonance imaging

The superior soft tissue resolution of MRI is best exploited when curative surgery is contemplated. It is useful for clarifying the local extent of tumour infiltration with regard to adjacent anatomical structures that cannot be sacrificed and may be of use in surgical planning.

Endoscopic retrograde cholepancreaticogram (ERCP)

A side-viewing endoscope is passed into the duodenum allowing cannulation of the ampullary duct under direct vision. Using an image intensifier, a cannula is advanced into the main pancreatic duct and contrast material injected to opacify the pancreatic duct system and extrahepatic biliary tree. Gallstones will appear as filling defects in the ducts while pancreatic carcinoma will lead to distortion and obstruction of the pancreatic ducts and extrinsic compression of the common bile duct. Duodenal and pancreatic aspirates collected through the endoscope may be sent for cytology.

Percutaneous transhepatic cholangiography (PTC)

A needle is passed through the skin into a dilated extrahepatic bile duct under ultrasound control and a cholangiogram obtained by injecting contrast material into the biliary tree. It will visualize any gallstones in the biliary tree, and in the case of carcinoma confirm blockage of the common bile duct by extrinsic compression at the level of the pancreas.

Laparotomy

Occasionally, it is not possible to make a diagnosis from less invasive investigations. If there are no metastases detected during staging and the tumour is otherwise operable, laparotomy is justified with a view to radical surgery if frozen section is positive for malignancy.

Staging

The TNM system (see Chapter 2) is widely used.

- Tis – carcinoma *in situ*.
- T0 – no evidence of primary.
- TX – primary cannot be assessed.
- T1 – limited to pancreas, 2 cms or less in greatest dimension.
- T2 – limited to pancreas, >2 cm in greatest dimension.
- T3 – direct invasion involving any of: duodenum, bile duct or peripancreatic tissues.
- T4 – direct invasion involving any of; stomach, spleen, colon, adjacent large vessels.
- N0 – no regional lymphadenopathy.
- N1 – regional lymph nodes involved.
- M0 – no distant metastases.
- M1 – distant metastases.

Treatment

RADICAL TREATMENT

Pancreatic cancer is a condition where more effective management strategies are required. Very few advances have been made over the last decade and the prognosis remains poor. Such patients should therefore be recruited to clinical trial protocols whenever possible.

Surgery

This is the only potentially curative option. Patients must be carefully selected for radical surgery as only 10–20 per cent will be suitable candidates. Improvements in imaging technology, including spiral CT, MRI, positron emission tomography (PET), endoscopic ultrasound examination and laparoscopic staging can aid in the diagnosis and the identification of patients with disease that is not amenable to resection. The operation of choice was originally described by Whipple and comprises a pancreaticoduodenectomy, although this is associated with significant operative morbidity and mortality, even in the hands of surgeons regularly performing the operation.

Radiotherapy

Carcinoma of the pancreas is incurable using current radiotherapy techniques and doses because of the high incidence of metastases at diagnosis, and the proximity of radiation dose-limiting normal tissues such as the spinal cord, small bowel and kidneys. Some of these problems can be overcome by delivering radiotherapy intraoperatively but even this has not made a significant impact on curability and survival. Newer radiotherapy techniques such as intensity-modulated radiotherapy (IMRT) may allow a higher dose delivery in the future. For the present, local recurrence remains a major problem with recurrence rates varying between 50 per cent and 80 per cent. The only treatment that has been shown to reduce this is postoperative CRT using 5-FU, which is more effective than radiotherapy alone and confers a modest survival advantage, but the problem of liver metastases is not adequately addressed with this approach and the start of treatment is invariably delayed by the recovery period after surgery. Preoperative CRT has the advantage of starting immediately following diagnosis and allowing greater selection for surgery pending the results of restaging of the local disease and liver after CRT.

PALLIATIVE TREATMENT

Surgery

Many patients are found at laparotomy to be inoperable. Rather than going on to perform an operation that will not prolong the patient's life, if the patient has obstructive jaundice or is at risk of developing it in the near future, a bypass procedure (choledochojejunostomy) to allow free drainage of bile is justified. Gastroenterostomy will relieve duodenal obstruction by a large periampullary carcinoma.

Radiotherapy

This is of value in relieving pain caused by retroperitoneal tumour extension, but is not a satisfactory treatment for the relief of obstructive jaundice.

Chemotherapy

It may not be justified to treat patients with pancreatic carcinoma with chemotherapy as most patients will already have systemic symptoms, an impaired performance status and short life expectancy. 5-Fluorouracil is the most active drug, with objective response rates of about 20 per cent. The FAM (5-FU, Adriamycin and mitomycin C) combination has been widely used. Gemcitabine has also shown activity in this disease, with disease stabilization in 40% but a low objective response rate. It may be a more useful agent in combination with other cytotoxic drugs or as part of a CRT protocol. Some of the newer agents being tested in colorectal adenocarcinoma (e.g. oxaliplatin, irinotecan, capecitabine, paclitaxel and docetaxel) may find a role in the treatment of this disease.

Hormone therapy

Initial *in vitro* experiments suggested the possible utility of hormone therapies. This stimulated clinical trials of tamoxifen. No significant advantage was proven with this approach.

Medical treatment

Endoscopic placement of a bile duct stent is of value in relieving obstructive jaundice. Cholestyramine may relieve the pruritus of intractable obstructive jaundice, while pancreatic enzyme supplements will relieve the steatorrhoea associated with the malabsorption of fats. Vitamin K administered intravenously may be indicated if there is a symptomatic coagulopathy related to a deficiency of the vitamin K-dependent clotting factors.

Tumour-related complications

There are a number of recognized vascular complications:

- renal vein thrombosis;
- portal vein thrombosis;
- splenic vein thrombosis;
- thrombophlebitis migrans;
- Disseminated intravascular coagulation (DIC).

Renal vein thrombosis results in renal congestion and a nephrotic syndrome. Portal vein thrombosis leads to a Budd–Chiari syndrome, characterized by the rapid accumulation of ascites and hepatic congestion, while splenic vein thrombosis leads to portal hypertension and oesophageal varices. Thrombophlebitis migrans is characterized by intermittent bouts of tenderness, erythema and induration of superficial veins. Disseminated intravascular coagulation is caused by mucin production by the tumour, which leads to an inappropriate activation of the clotting cascade (see Chapter 8).

Non-metastatic manifestations include:

- profound depression;
- migratory thrombophlebitis;
- hypercalcaemia (production of parathyroid hormone-like peptides);
- Cushing's syndrome (adrenocorticotropic hormone production);
- carcinoid syndrome (5-hydroxytryptamine production);
- murantic endocarditis;
- syndrome of metastatic fat necrosis.

Treatment-related complications

Surgery

Radical pancreaticoduodenectomy has an extremely high operative morbidity and mortality. The loss of exocrine and endocrine pancreatic secretions will lead to permanent diabetes mellitus requiring insulin and malabsorption of fat requiring enzyme supplements with each meal.

Radiotherapy

Radiotherapy to the pancreatic bed will result in temporary anorexia, nausea, vomiting, gastritis, colic and diarrhoea. Late complications are infrequently encountered because of the extremely poor prognosis of the disease.

Prognosis

The outlook is extremely poor, with a 5-year survival of less than 5 per cent. Of those undergoing radical surgery, there is a 5-year survival of about 10–20 per cent.

Rare tumours

Gastroenteropancreatic (GEP) neuroendocrine tumours comprise:

- carcinoid;
- gastrinoma;
- insulinoma;
- glucagonoma;
- VIPoma.

The pancreas is a rare site for carcinoid (see Chapter 14). Partial pancreatectomy will be curative unless there has been metastasis to the liver.

Gastrinoma is a gastrin-secreting tumour which leads to the Zollinger–Ellison syndrome, characterized by hypersecretion of acid in the stomach leading to intractable peptic ulceration. An elevated serum gastrin level is diagnostic and about two-thirds are malignant. It may be associated with adenomata of the pituitary and parathyroid as part of multiple endocrine neoplasia type 1 (MEN 1). After detailed staging with a CT scan and selective venous angiography, the treatment of choice is a partial pancreatectomy.

Insulinoma arises from the β-cells of the islets and secretes insulin, leading to fasting hypoglycaemia. There is an association with MEN 1. Ninety per cent are benign and 10 per cent multiple. Treatment is surgical, as for gastrinoma. Historically, diazoxide (a β-cell toxin) has been used to relieve the unremitting hypoglycaemia of advanced disease.

Glucagonoma arises from the α-cells of the pancreas and secretes glucagon, leading to a syndrome of diabetes mellitus, a migratory necrolytic erythema of the skin and stomatitis. Approximately half are malignant, with metastases in the liver. Surgery is the treatment of choice.

VIPoma leads to Werner–Morrison syndrome characterized by severe watery diarrhoea and hypokalaemia. The majority are benign.

The somatostatin analogue octreotide has shown considerable activity in GEP tumours and therefore has an important role in symptom relief and disease stabilization and has superseded streptozotocin as the systemic treatment of choice for inoperable and/or metastatic disease.

HEPATOCELLULAR CANCER

This is synonymous with hepatoma.

Epidemiology

This is one of the most common tumours worldwide, but is comparatively rare in the European Union, with 28 000 new cases and about the same number of deaths recorded per annum. The peak incidence in the developed countries is 40–60 years compared with 20–40 years in endemic areas. There is a male-to-female predominance of 2:1 in Europe and a very high incidence in areas where hepatitis B is endemic such as Africa and the Far East.

Aetiology

The hepatitis B virus is implicated, an observation supported by the geographical variation of hepatoma matching that of areas where hepatitis B is endemic in the population. Hepatoma often arises in a cirrhotic liver although the aetiological agent (e.g. alcohol, iron in haemochromatosis, autoantibodies in chronic active hepatitis) responsible for the cirrhosis is unimportant. Macronodular cirrhosis is a greater risk factor than micronodular cirrhosis, and males greatly outnumber females with this complication. Aflatoxin is a mycotoxin produced by the fungus *Aspergillus flavus*, which is found in stored cereals and is a hepatic carcinogen when ingested. Thorotrast was used as a radiographic contrast agent and contains a high level of the radioactive isotope thorium, which emits α-particles, leading to intense irradiation of the liver, which in turn may lead to hepatoma. Hepatoma has also been described in men following use of androgenic anabolic steroids for body building.

Pathology

The tumour grows rapidly, is usually large, arises from the liver parenchyma or a cirrhotic nodule and may be multifocal. In cut section there is bile staining, haemorrhage and necrosis. It invades through the liver capsule, along the hepatic ducts and blood vessels. Intrahepatic ducts proximal to the tumour will be obstructed and therefore dilated. The tumour is composed of hepatocytes which have lost the characteristic architecture of the portal tracts and frequently stain for α-fetoprotein (AFP).

Natural history

The tumour may remain confined to the liver, invading along the intrahepatic bile ducts and hepatic veins, or breach the liver capsule, leading to invasion of adjacent structures such as the hepatic veins, portal vein, inferior vena cava, right hemidiaphragm, right kidney, right adrenal, stomach and transverse colon. The hilar lymph nodes at the base of the liver and portal nodes are frequently involved.

The lungs are the most common site of distant metastases, although bone, skin and brain may also be involved. Spread beyond the liver capsule may lead to diffuse peritoneal involvement, which in turn may cause malignant ascites.

Symptoms

There is often a long history of increasing ill-health with hepatic pain caused by distension of the liver capsule, which contains many stretch receptors. The onset of pain may be acute and severe if precipitated by a sudden haemorrhage into the tumour which leads to its rapid enlargement. Swollen legs are a common complaint in advanced cases owing to a combination of hypoalbuminaemia and compression of the inferior vena cava. Systemic symptoms such as anorexia, nausea, weight loss, fever and malaise are frequent.

Signs

There may be evidence of an underlying cirrhosis such as clubbing, leuconychia, palmar erythema, jaundice, spider naevi, gynaecomastia, testicular atrophy, ascites, ankle oedema, dilated superficial abdominal wall veins and splenomegaly. Signs of hepatic encephalopathy are rare. The liver may be diffusely enlarged due to cirrhosis, focally enlarged due to the hepatoma or both. An arterial bruit and hepatic rub may be heard over the tumour because of its rich vascular supply and capsular invasion, respectively.

Differential diagnosis

A poorly differentiated hepatoma may cause confusion with a carcinoma of unknown primary metastasizing to the liver. A high serum AFP or positive staining for AFP within a biopsy supports the diagnosis of hepatoma.

Investigations

Liver function tests, clotting parameters

Liver function derangement is common but more likely to be caused by an underlying cirrhosis rather than the hepatoma itself. Assessment of clotting is necessary prior to liver biopsy or any invasive procedure.

Hepatitis serology

Serology for types A, B, C and D should be performed.

Serum α-fetoprotein

This is elevated in 90 per cent of cases. It is a useful diagnostic test, of value in monitoring response to therapy (especially surgery) and in predicting relapse.

Chest X-ray

This is mandatory prior to surgery to exclude pulmonary metastases, with a CT scan of the thorax if there is any suggestion of metastases from the plain radiographs.

Liver ultrasound and percutaneous biopsy

This localizes and measures the tumour, assesses the inferior vena cava and other large blood vessels for obstruction, and permits percutaneous biopsy under direct vision. A random biopsy of the contralateral lobe is desirable in patients for whom resection is planned.

Computed tomography of the liver and upper abdomen

This complements information obtained from abdominal ultrasound and facilitates percutaneous biopsy when the tumour is not adequately localized by ultrasound. Typically, it demonstrates a large necrotic filling defect in the liver (Fig. 9.4). It is also very useful for excluding invasion of the portal vein and/or hepatic veins. It is mandatory if surgery or radiotherapy is planned.

Magnetic resonance imaging of liver

This may provide additional information for the surgeon regarding the extent of the tumour within the liver and thereby determine operability.

Laparoscopic biopsy

This is indicated if multiple percutaneous biopsies have failed to give a result.

Angiography

This will define the tumour precisely in terms of its size, position and vascular supply, and is mandatory prior to surgical resection or embolization. Computed tomography or MRI angiography is desirable.

Staging

The TNM system (see Chapter 2) is widely used.

- Tis – carcinoma *in situ*.
- T0 – no evidence of primary.
- TX – primary cannot be assessed.
- T1 – solitary tumour 2 cm or less in greatest dimension, without vascular invasion.
- T2 – solitary tumour 2 cm or less in greatest dimension, with vascular invasion; or multiple tumours limited to one lobe, none >2 cm without vascular invasion; or solitary tumour >2 cm without vascular invasion.
- T3 – solitary tumour >2 cm in greatest dimension with vascular invasion; or multiple tumours limited to one lobe, none >2 cm with vascular invasion; or multiple tumours limited to one lobe, any >2 cm with or without vascular invasion.
- T4 – multiple tumours in more than one lobe; or tumour(s) involving a major branch of the portal or hepatic vein(s); or tumour(s) with direct invasion of adjacent organs other than gallbladder; or tumour(s) with perforation of visceral peritoneum.
- N0 – no regional lymphadenopathy.
- N1 – regional lymph nodes involved.
- M0 – no distant metastases.
- M1 – distant metastases.

Treatment

RADICAL TREATMENT

Surgery

Up to 90% of the liver can be resected as the remaining portion has a remarkable capacity for regeneration. Patients requiring very extensive surgery or those with cirrhosis may be considered for hepatectomy and liver transplant. Meticulous preoperative staging is required whenever such surgery is planned.

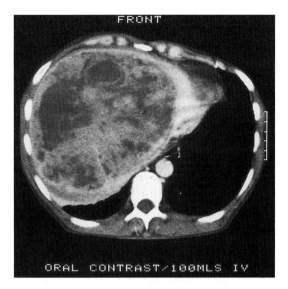

FIG 9.4 Computed tomography image of the upper abdomen showing a very large, round, necrotic tumour arising from the substance of the liver. Biopsy confirmed hepatoma.

Radiotherapy

High-dose radiotherapy with curative intent is impractical at this anatomical site and hepatoma is relatively resistant to radiation.

PALLIATIVE TREATMENT

Surgery

Hepatomas derive their blood supply from the hepatic artery and ligation of this vessel close to the liver may palliate local symptoms, particularly pain. The portal vein must be patent to prevent ischaemic necrosis of the liver and a cholecystectomy must be performed in case there is necrosis of the gallbladder. Mortality from this procedure is less than 5 per cent, but the response is short-lived because of the development of a collateral tumour circulation.

Radiotherapy

Low doses of radiation may be given with the expectation of relieving hepatic pain.

Chemotherapy

Adriamycin, 5-FU and cisplatin are the most active agents and may be considered for patients symptomatic from metastases. Response rates are low (20–30 per cent) with peripheral venous administration. Regional chemotherapy delivered via the hepatic artery is also being studied. Other possible systemic treatments include:

- somatostatin (Octreotide);
- tamoxifen.

Hepatic artery embolization

This is less invasive than ligation of the artery, and has a longer symptomatic response as the collateral circulation develops more slowly, and it is anatomically more selective. Unlike ligation, it may be repeated when symptoms recur. Responses of up to 50 per cent are seen.

Percutaneous ethanol injection (PEI)

This is an effective chemical means of inducing tumour necrosis in small tumours. It is relatively free of serious toxicity.

Tumour-related complications

A number of non-metastatic manifestations are recognized including:

- hypoglycaemia (insulin-like peptides);
- polycythaemia (erythropoietin-like peptides);
- hypercalcaemia (parathyroid hormone-like peptides);
- feminization (oestrogens);
- pyrexia of unknown origin (pyrogens);
- porphyria cutanea tarda (porphyrins).

Portal vein thrombosis will lead to splenomegaly, ascites and oesophageal varices, while hepatic vein thrombosis will lead to a Budd–Chiari syndrome with ascites, hepatomegaly and leg oedema. Inferior vena cava obstruction will lead to oedema below the umbilicus. Sudden haemorrhage may occur into the tumour causing acute right upper abdominal pain or into the abdomen causing abdominal pain and distension and may lead to death.

Treatment-related complications

Surgery

Partial hepatectomy may lead to hepatic decompensation if the function of the remaining liver is poor. Transplant patients will also have the problems of rejection and chronic immunosuppression to overcome.

Radiotherapy

Hepatic irradiation invariably causes anorexia, nausea and vomiting during treatment, and radiation hepatitis may result when a large volume of liver has been irradiated.

Hepatic artery embolization

Ectopic embolic phenomena may lead to infarction of other abdominal viscera.

Prognosis

Untreated, most patients die within 1 year. Surgery is the only potentially curative treatment and even after liver transplantation for carefully selected patients, less than 20 per cent will have long-term disease-free survival.

Prevention

Vaccination against hepatitis B, health education and improved food storage to avoid contamination with aflatoxin may decrease the incidence of hepatoma in endemic areas.

Screening

Measurements of AFP and liver ultrasound are probably the most sensitive investigations for screening and detecting hepatoma while it is operable. High-risk populations would include hepatitis B surface antigen positive individuals with cirrhosis or other conditions where the risk of hepatoma is very high (e.g. haemochromatosis).

Rare tumours

Angiosarcoma

This is very rare and associated with medical exposure to Thorotrast and industrial exposure to vinyl chloride monomer.

CHOLANGIOCARCINOMA

This is a malignant tumour arising from the epithelium lining the extrahepatic biliary tract.

Epidemiology

This is rare in developed countries. For example, in the UK there are fewer than 1000 new cases and 300 deaths recorded per annum. It is about half as common as carcinoma of the gallbladder. The peak age incidence is 50–70 years and there is a slight female predominance. It is more common is areas where liver flukes are endemic, e.g. Southeast Asia.

Aetiology

Recognized associations include:

- liver flukes (e.g. *Clonorchis sinensis*);
- primary sclerosing cholangitis (a rare complication of chronic ulcerative colitis);
- chronic infective cholangitis secondary to gallstones;
- radiation (previous use of Thorotrast contrast medium – of historical significance only);
- congenital biliary abnormalities (e.g. choledochal cyst).

Pathology

Tumours of the upper third of the extrahepatic biliary tree tend to be diffusely sclerosing leading to a malignant stricture. Tumours in the middle third tend to be nodular while those in the lower third tend to be papillary. The tumour is usually a well-differentiated mucin-secreting adenocarcinoma with about half staining for CEA.

Natural history

Tumours of the upper third may infiltrate the liver, while those of the lower third may infiltrate the duodenum and pancreas. Tumours also spread to the hilar, superior mesenteric and coeliac lymph nodes. The liver is the most common site of distant metastases, although lung and bone may also be involved.

Symptoms

The most common presentation is with obstructive jaundice, pruritus, dark urine and pale stools. Recurrent cholangitis from subacute biliary tract obstruction may also occur.

Signs

The patient will be jaundiced, the gallbladder may be palpable (positive Courvoisier's sign) and the liver may be congested and therefore smoothly enlarged.

Differential diagnosis

Other causes of obstructive jaundice include:

- gallstones;
- benign biliary tract stricture following surgical trauma;
- sclerosing cholangitis;
- carcinoma of the head of the pancreas;
- carcinoma of the ampulla of Vater;
- lymph node metastases at the porta hepatis.

Investigations

Endoscopic retrograde cholepancreaticogram

This is the investigation of choice as it will allow an accurate anatomical localization of the tumour, brushings and biliary aspirates for cytology, and therapeutic manoeuvres such as passage of a stent to relieve jaundice.

Percutaneous transhepatic cholangiogram

This is indicated when ERCP has failed to opacify the biliary tree or adequately display the tumour because of its position.

Computed tomography scan of the upper abdomen

This will show the degree of local invasion, any enlarged regional lymph nodes and exclude liver metastases.

Staging

The TNM staging (see Chapter 2) is used for tumours of the extrahepatic ducts:

- TX – primary tumour cannot be assessed.
- T0 – no evidence of primary tumour.
- Tis – carcinoma *in situ*.
- T1 – tumour invades subepithelial connective tissue or fibromuscular layer:
  1a – tumour invades subepithelial connective tissue;
  1b – tumour invades fibromuscular layer.
- T2 – tumour invades perifibromuscular connective tissue.
- T3 – tumour invades adjacent structures: liver, pancreas, duodenum, gallbladder, colon, stomach.
- NX – regional lymph nodes cannot be assessed.
- N0 – no regional lymph node metastasis.
- N1 – metastasis in cystic duct, pericholedochal and/or hilar lymph nodes (i.e. in the hepatoduodenal ligament).
- N2 – metastasis in peripancreatic (head only), periduodenal, periportal, coeliac, and/or superior mesenteric and/or posterior pancreaticoduodenal lymph nodes.
- MX – presence of distant metastasis cannot be assessed.
- M0 – no distant metastasis.
- M1 – distant metastasis.

Treatment

RADICAL TREATMENT

As this is a very rare tumour, the optimum management with surgery and/or radiotherapy is undetermined.

Surgery

This offers the best chance of cure although only 10–20 per cent will be resectable. The optimum surgical procedure for carcinoma of the extrahepatic bile duct will vary according to its location along the biliary tree, the extent of hepatic parenchymal involvement and the proximity of the tumour to major blood vessels in this region. Distal tumours are more likely to be resectable than proximal ones. Tumours of the lower third require pancreaticoduodenectomy, while those with more proximal lesions may be carefully staged and selected for hepatic lobectomy or liver transplantation.

Radiotherapy

This tumour is rarely cured by radiotherapy. The difficulties of giving high-dose irradiation to this region are lessened by the use of interstitial brachytherapy for localized strictures. A nasobiliary tube is inserted at ERCP or a percutaneous tube inserted under ultrasound control, and an iridium-192 source is passed down this conduit using either a wire straddling the tumour for 5–7 days or a high-dose rate afterloading technique fractionated over several treatments. Tumours with extraductal invasion are best treated with external beam irradiation and a brachytherapy boost.

PALLIATIVE TREATMENT

Surgery

Choledochojejunostomy will relieve obstructive jaundice in cases not amenable to endoscopic or percutaneous stenting. Cholecystectomy should be considered to prevent the possibility of an acute cholecystitis.

Radiotherapy

This is best reserved for palliating pain from local infiltration.

Chemotherapy

This can only be considered within clinical trial protocols. Cisplatin and 5-FU are the most active agents tested. Bearing in mind the success of CRT at other gastrointestinal sites, this is an option that deserves further study.

Tumour-related complications

These include:

- acute cholangitis, which presents with fever, rigors and right upper abdominal pain and usually responds to broad-spectrum antibiotics;
- secondary biliary cirrhosis, which is caused by chronic cholestasis.

Treatment-related complications

Surgery

The bile duct is a delicate structure prone to stricture after handling. Biliary fistulae are also a problem after anastomosis.

Radiotherapy

Insertion of a nasobiliary tube and the iridium wire carries a high risk of cholangitis. External beam irradiation carries the same morbidity as outlined for stomach cancer.

Prognosis

The mean survival in untreated cases is only 3 months. Palliative biliary drainage increases this to 9 months while radical radiotherapy gives 2-year survivals of 10–20 per cent.

CARCINOMA OF THE GALLBLADDER

This is the commonest biliary tract tumour but a rare tumour in developed countries. For example, 1400 new cases and 750 deaths are recorded per annum in the UK. In developed countries it has a peak age incidence of 60–80 years and a female-to-male ratio of 3:1. Aetiological factors include:

- gallstones – 0.5–1 per cent of cholecystectomies performed for cholelithiasis will yield an occult carcinoma of the gallbladder;
- typhoid carriage – there is a greatly increased risk due to carriage of the *Salmonella typhi* bacteria in the gallbladder, which in turn leads to a chronic cholecystitis;
- rubber plant workers;
- large gallbladder polyps;
- choledochal cysts and other biliary tract anatomical anomalies.

Many patients are diagnosed incidentally at cholecystectomy and are asymptomatic with no physical signs. Otherwise, the presentation resembles benign gallbladder disease with bouts of acute cholecystitis or more chronic and less severe right upper abdominal pain where a mass may be palpable. Eighty per cent arise at the fundus or neck of the gallbladder and 90 per cent are adenocarcinomas. The adjacent liver capsule and parenchyma are involved early and there may be lymphatic spread to the hilar nodes around the liver. The liver and lungs are the most common sites for blood-borne metastases. Staging investigations include liver function tests, chest X-ray, liver ultrasound and a CT/MRI scan of the upper abdomen. Treatment comprises cholecystectomy with a wide excision of the surrounding liver, excision of the extrahepatic bile duct and regional lymph node dissection. Low-dose radiotherapy may be of value in relieving pain caused by local infiltration, and a biliary drainage procedure will palliate biliary obstruction. In those with superficial involvement of the mucosa, the disease may be cured with cholecystectomy alone. Of those with liver involvement, 50 per cent die within 3 months of diagnosis and less than 5 per cent survive 1 year. As one would expect for a rare tumour, chemotherapy and radiotherapy strategies are far less well developed. 5-Fluorouracil is the most established agent with activity in this disease.

CARCINOMA OF THE COLON AND RECTUM

Epidemiology

There are 210 000 new cases of colorectal cancer and 110 000 deaths recorded in the European Union per annum. The vast majority occur in the over-50 age-group, the peak age incidence being at 60–80 years. Colonic primaries outnumber rectal primaries by almost 2 : 1. There has been a recent trend towards more right colonic tumours, which may reflect surveillance programmes which have decreased the incidence of left-sided cancers. For colon cancer, there is a female-to-male predominance of 4:3, while for rectal cancer there is a male-to-female predominance of 4:3. Colon cancer is commonest in social classes I and II. There is no social class trend for rectal cancer. It is predominantly a disease of the developed world, being most common in New Zealand, Canada, USA and UK, while rare in Africa and Asia.

Aetiology

Diet may account for the marked geographical variation in incidence. This is presumed to be due to changes in the bowel flora which produce carcinogens such as fecapentaenes and 3-ketosteroids from ingested food, the effect being exacerbated by the slower bowel transit time seen in people taking a low-fibre diet. The incidence has increased in Japan as a Western-style diet has been adopted, and Japanese migrants to the West have subsequently acquired the risk of the indigenous population. Important dietary factors include:

- increased meat consumption;
- high total fat consumption;
- high calorific intake;
- high alcohol intake.

Familial adenomatous polyposis (FAP) is a rare, dominantly inherited condition (i.e. there is a 50 per cent chance of inheriting the gene from an affected parent). The mutated gene is located on chromosome 5. It has a prevalence of 1 in 10 000 births. There are characteristic physical signs to indicate a gene carrier, such as congenital hypertrophy of the retinal pigment epithelium (CHRPE), osteomas of the jaw and pre-puberty epidermoid cysts. Affected individuals develop multiple benign polyps from a very young age (puberty). Inevitably, over the subsequent years, one or more of these polyps will transform into a cancer, usually during the third and fourth decades, 20–30 years before the general population. Prophylactic surgical excision of the colon and rectum is advised in young adults. Upper gastrointestinal malignancy will also develop in 5 per cent and benign desmoid tumours in 10 per cent. The latter may arise within the abdomen and may prove fatal because of relentless local spread. Gardener's syndrome is similar to familial polyposis coli but characterized by skeletal and cutaneous abnormalities (e.g. osteomas of the mandible and skull, sebaceous cysts and dermoid cysts).

Hereditary non-polyposis colon cancer (HNPCC) accounts for 20 per cent of cases. This is a dominantly inherited condition. Such families often have three or more cases of colon cancer. Unlike FAP, there are no characteristic extracolonic physical signs and there is not a propensity to develop a multitude of polyps. Colon cancer develops, on average, at 40 years of age. Cancers other than just colonic ones are associated. Families can be divided into syndromes I and II. In Lynch syndrome I, the cancers are mainly gastrointestinal. In Lynch syndrome II, endometrial and ovarian cancers may arise at a young age.

Peutz–Jeghers syndrome is characterized by the development of multiple bowel hamartomas and an increased risk of colon cancer. Turcot's syndrome is associated with the development of multiple benign adenomas but to a lesser degree than FAP. It presents during childhood with brain tumours, usually astrocytomas. Such patients have a high incidence of leukaemia after radiotherapy. Chronic inflammation of the bowel is a rare cause. In the case of ulcerative colitis, the increased risk is related to both the extent and duration of the colitis. Those with disease extending beyond the splenic flexure and/or of more than 10 years' duration are at greatest risk. Chronic Crohn's colitis also confers an increased risk of colorectal cancer.

Pathology

One-third arise in the rectum or rectosigmoid, and one-quarter in the sigmoid colon and one-tenth at the caecum. The rest are evenly distributed along the large bowel, two-thirds arising on the left side. Most cancers represent malignant change in a benign adenomatous polyp (e.g. tubular, tubulovillous or villous), the highest risk being from villous adenomas, especially those greater than 2 cm. The tumour may be nodular, ulcerating or diffusely infiltrating, and multiple primaries are found in approximately 5 per cent. The vast majority are adenocarcinomas (85 per cent glandular, 15 per cent mucinous, 2 per cent signet ring), usually well differentiated and may show evidence of a preceding benign adenomatous polyp. The tumour cells frequently stain for CEA.

Natural history

The tumour spreads longitudinally and circumferentially along the mucosa, in some cases leading to obstruction of the bowel lumen, and invades deep to the mucosa to infiltrate the muscular wall of the bowel and serosa. Penetration of the serosa leads to direct infiltration of the surrounding abdominal and pelvic viscera, while submucosal spread in the lamina propria may lead to skip lesions well away from the primary tumour. Tumour cells have a propensity

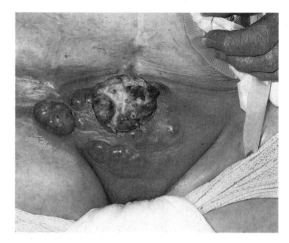

FIG 9.5 Perineal spread from rectal cancer.

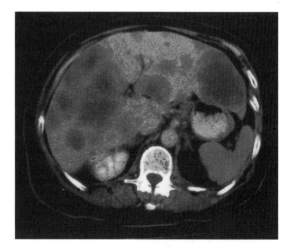

FIG 9.6 Computed tomography image of the upper abdomen in a patient with colon cancer showing multiple, well-circumscribed, hypodense lesions consistent with metastases.

to seed in abdominal scars, perineal skin (Fig. 9.5), stomas and even anal fissures. Transcoelomic spread may lead to diffuse peritoneal involvement resulting in ascites and spread to the ovaries. The regional (mesenteric) lymph nodes may be involved, and the likelihood of lymph node metastases increases with the depth of bowel wall invasion. The tumour spreads to the liver (Fig. 9.6) via the portal circulation, and from there to the lungs, bone, brain and skin. Rectal cancer has a particular propensity for local recurrence and often this leads to a presacral mass (Fig. 9.7).

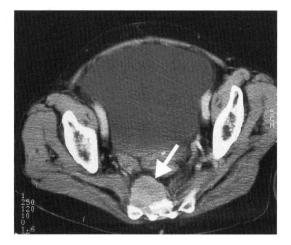

FIG 9.7 Transverse pelvic computed tomography image showing a presacral recurrence of a rectal cancer.

Symptoms

The tumour most commonly presents with symptoms referable to the large bowel, 20 per cent presenting as a surgical emergency with acute bowel obstruction or peritonitis due to perforation. In the remainder there is usually a history of one or more of the following:

- change in bowel habit;
- blood per rectum;
- mucus per rectum;
- tenesmus;
- obstructive symptoms;
- iron-deficiency anaemia.

A change in bowel habit is often the presenting symptom with an increase or decrease in frequency of defecation or a change in stool consistency. Alternating diarrhoea and constipation is highly suspicious of cancer. Blood per rectum is another symptom that leads patients to seek medical advice. It varies in quantity depending on degree of tumour ulceration and/or vascularity. The blood will be bright red and more likely streaked on the outside of the stool if the tumour arises in the rectum or sigmoid, or dark red and mixed in with the stool if the tumour arises more proximally in the colon. Mucus per rectum is more likely to be noticed with distal lesions, particularly those of a mucinous variety. Tenesmus is a frequent urge to defecate but leading to the passage of a little stool on each occasion and

a feeling of incomplete rectal emptying. This is usually seen in rectal tumours, particularly if bulky or invading deeply. Obstructive symptoms may manifest as intermittent colicky abdominal pain. They are more common in tumours of the descending colon where the faeces are more solid compared with right colon tumours where the stool is more liquid. Chronic bleeding leads to iron deficiency and in turn anaemia. It is a particular feature of right-sided colonic tumours which have few associated gastrointestinal symptoms.

Signs

The primary tumour may be palpable by digital examination of the rectum as a circumscribed area of mucosal induration, often with irregular heaped-up margins and a friable ulcer base that bleeds on contact. Proximal tumours may be palpable in the pouch of Douglas per vaginam, and caecal tumours may be palpable by abdominal examination. Signs indicative of spread outside the pelvis include:

- Troisier's sign owing to enlargement of Virchow's lymph node in the left supraclavicular fossa;
- ascites indicating peritoneal involvement;
- hepatomegaly suggesting possible liver metastases;
- Rarely, locally advanced disease in the pelvis may lead to formation of a fistula between the adjacent bladder (colo-vesical, suggested by faecal debris in the urine or pneumaturia) or vagina (colo-vaginal, suggested by leakage of faeces per vaginam).

Investigations

Digital examination of the rectum/vagina

This permits evaluation of the site, size and extent of local invasion of tumours of the rectum.

Proctoscopy and sigmoidoscopy

This is mandatory for tumours of the distal 25 cm of the large bowel, as it allows an accurate assessment of the tumour size, extent and distance from the anal verge and permits biopsy to obtain a tissue diagnosis.

Double-contrast barium enema

This is a very sensitive and specific investigation which can detect tumours 1 cm or more and should be performed in all cases. It allows rapid assessment of the large bowel from the rectum to the caecum and can detect synchronous primaries or benign polyps elsewhere. Circumferential tumours give rise to a characteristic 'apple core' stricture.

Flexible sigmoidoscopy

This visualizes tumours of the distal 50–60 cm of the large bowel and is better tolerated than colonoscopy for biopsy of such lesions.

Colonoscopy

This facilitates a detailed survey of the whole large bowel, is more sensitive than a barium enema and is useful for biopsy of tumours of the transverse and ascending colon. It is the best way of excluding a synchronous primary cancer or polyp elsewhere in the large bowel.

Computed tomography

A CT scan of the thorax/abdomen/pelvis is mandatory to delineate the locoregional extent of tumour and exclude hepatic and/or pulmonary metastases.

Endorectal ultrasound or magnetic resonance imaging

These may be particularly useful for delineating the extent of a low rectal tumour in relation to the sphincters (Fig. 9.8) and aid surgical planning.

Staging

The clinicopathological staging according to Dukes is the best known staging system.

- A – confined to the bowel wall and has not penetrated its full thickness.
- B – tumour has breached the bowel wall.
- C – regional lymph node involvement.
- D – distant metastases.

There are a number of variants in clinical use. An alternative is the TNM system (see Chapter 2).

- Tis – carcinoma *in situ*.
- T0 – no evidence of primary.
- TX – primary cannot be assessed.
- T1 – involving submucosa.
- T2 – involving muscularis propria.
- T3 – involving subserosa, non-peritonealized pericolic/perirectal tissues.
- T4 – other organs/structures/visceral peritoneum.
- N0 – no regional lymphadenopathy.
- N1 – three or fewer pericolic/perirectal lymph nodes.
- N2 – >3 pericolic/perirectal lymph nodes.
- N3 – nodes on named vascular trunk/apical node(s).
- M0 – no distant metastases.
- M1 – distant metastases.

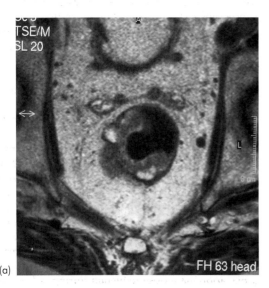 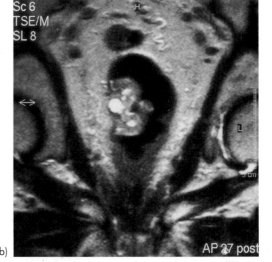

FIG 9.8 Magnetic resonance image of a rectal carcinoma. (a) Transverse view; (b) coronal view.

Treatment

RADICAL TREATMENT

Surgery

This is the only curative treatment modality. Eighty per cent of all tumours are resectable. Prior to resection of the primary tumour, a detailed inspection and palpation of the open abdomen and pelvis is performed to document the exact extent of disease, with special reference to the liver, and suspicious tissues should be biopsied if not part of the main resection. The ovaries should be checked in women as there they represent a potential site of spread.

Tumours of the colon are treated by hemicolectomy with either immediate reanastomosis (usual) or formation of a temporary colostomy which can be closed at a later date. Some surgeons ligate the vascular pedicle prior to mobilization of the tumour to try to prevent vascular dissemination of tumour.

Rectal cancer surgery is difficult and technically challenging because of the relative inaccessibility of the rectum. The usual operation is an anterior resection. This may be associated with a high risk of local recurrence of up to 30% in some series, mainly due to the problems involved in balancing morbidity from surgery against the need to attain an adequate cuff of normal tissue around the tumour-bearing tissue, and to some extent variations in surgical skill. In recent years, there has been much interest in total mesorectal excision (TME). This involves a meticulous circumferential surgical excision down the avascular plane between the mesorectum and the pelvic side wall. In those patients where a clear circumferential resection margin (CRM) is attained following TME, the risk of local recurrence is far lower than when the CRM is involved:

- Dukes' B CRM − : <5 per cent local recurrence at 5 years;
- Dukes' B CRM + : 60 per cent local recurrence at 5 years;
- Dukes' C CRM − : 25 per cent local recurrence at 5 years;
- Dukes' C CRM + : 85 per cent local recurrence at 5 years.

Abdominoperineal resection may be required for the lowest rectal tumours, but in many cases can be avoided with current surgical techniques. In each case, the mesentery containing the regional lymph nodes is also resected.

Radiotherapy

Radiotherapy has little role in the curative treatment of colon cancer. This is because:

- local recurrence is not a major cause of relapse;
- it is difficult to determine accurately the volume to be irradiated;
- the proximity of a number of organs at risk limit the dose of radiation that can be delivered.

Conversely, rectal cancer has a higher risk of recurrence due to the technical difficulties and anatomical challenges faced by the surgeon. The volume to be irradiated is also far easier to define and there are fewer dose-limiting organs at risk in the lower pelvis.

Preoperative radiotherapy may be of use in rectal cancer for converting an inoperable or partly fixed tumour to one that is operable, and thereby offers a chance of a curative approach to treatment. Despite the use of only moderate doses of radiation (e.g. 25 Gy in five fractions on consecutive days), and surgery within a short time after completing radiotherapy, there is a surprisingly large reduction in the odds of recurrence of rectal cancer (approximately 60 per cent), reducing the absolute risk of recurrence from 20 per cent to less than 10 per cent. A meta-analysis of individual studies suggests a significant survival advantage with a reduction in the odds of dying of rectal cancer of approximately 20 per cent, equivalent to approximately a 7 per cent in absolute survival benefit. Preoperative short-course radiotherapy is thus considered by many to be the standard of care for all stages of disease. However, some of this benefit is offset by an increase in mortality from non-cancer causes within 1 year of receiving radiotherapy. It should also be noted that many of the trials of preoperative radiotherapy were conducted in an era before TME surgery was widely performed.

Postoperative radiotherapy to the region of the primary tumour decreases the odds of local recurrence in carcinoma of the rectum by approximately 40%, reducing the absolute risk of recurrence by 5 per cent from 15–20 per cent to 10–15 per cent. There is, however, in contrast to preoperative radiotherapy, no statistically significant benefit in terms of a survival advantage. In practice, postoperative radiotherapy may be reserved for those deemed to be at high risk for local recurrence (e.g. T4 cancers with invasion of adjacent pelvic viscera, involved CRM). Evidence is emerging that synchronous CRT may be of value in high-risk rectal cancers. Typically, radiotherapy is used synchronously with 5-FU, applying a dose reduction during radiotherapy to limit additive toxicity.

Radiation given with curative intent in inoperable cases is limited by the close proximity to radiosensitive normal tissues which makes it very difficult to give a tumoricidal dose and the fact that colorectal cancer is not particularly radiosensitive. There is also a high incidence of occult metastases in this group which limits the treatment outcome.

Chemotherapy

Despite an 80 per cent resection rate, almost half of such patients will have a relapse of their disease in the liver, usually within 2 years of surgery. Much effort has therefore been put into assessing the role of adjuvant chemotherapy to eradicate the micrometastases which have been shed from the tumour prior to, or during its resection. Chemotherapy has a role in the adjuvant therapy of both colonic and rectal cancers.

The most active chemotherapy agent in colorectal cancer is 5-FU, with response rates of 15–25 per cent in metastatic disease. Improved response rates can be seen when 5-FU is 'modulated' by combining it with calcium leucovorin (folinic acid) which enhances the inhibition of the enzyme thymidylate synthetase required by the cancer cells to produce DNA.

Patients that have had surgery for Dukes' C tumours benefit from 6 months' adjuvant therapy with 5-FU/folinic acid chemotherapy. This strategy will yield an absolute reduction in mortality of approximately 6 per cent at 5 years. Not surprisingly, for such a common cause of cancer-related death, this strategy is now standard practice. The issue of adjuvant chemotherapy for Dukes' B disease is still unresolved. Most oncologists believe that there is a significant survival benefit for these patients but that it is smaller in magnitude than for Dukes' C patients, perhaps amounting to a 2–3 per cent absolute survival benefit at 5 years. It is likely that recent trials have been underpowered to detect such an advantage because of the small numbers of Dukes' B patients included in clinical trials. It is reasonable to offer adjuvant chemotherapy to patients with Dukes' C tumours and those with selected Dukes' B tumours (e.g. those with venous invasion, T4 cancers, etc.).

Possible strategies include:

- bolus 5-FU;
- protracted venous infusion 5-FU;
- perioperative portal vein infusion of 5-FU.

Bolus 5-FU and folinic acid is a simple regime. Delivered weekly or 4-weekly for 6 months, it produces relatively little toxicity. The main side-effects are stomatitis, diarrhoea and myelosuppression. There is no evidence that high-dose folinic acid confers any advantage over low-dose, which is far more cost-effective.

Meta-analysis of trials of protracted venous infusion (PVI) of 5-FU versus bolus 5-FU has shown a significant advantage for the former approach in the context of metastatic disease. It is therefore reasonable to assert that PVI will be at least as effective as bolus 5-FU in the adjuvant setting. Protracted venous infusion is delivered at a dose of $300 \text{ mg/m}^2/\text{day}$ through an indwelling venous catheter, which has the advantage of continuous and reliable venous access but the potential disadvantages of the risk of infection and/or venous thrombosis. Toxicity mirrors bolus 5-FU, and occasionally necessitates a reduction in daily 5-FU dose. There is a much higher incidence of palmar–plantar erythema (PPE) which is apparent as redness, dryness and tenderness of the skin of the palms of the hands and soles of the feet. This responds to prescription of the vitamin pyridoxine 50 mg t.d.s. There is, however, much less haematological toxicity.

It is recognized that most patients dying of colorectal cancer will develop hepatic metastases as a result of the nature of blood flow via the portal circulation. Perioperative portal vein infusion of 5-FU allows a relatively high concentration of 5-FU to be delivered directly into the portal circulation via an indwelling catheter inserted at the time of definitive bowel surgery. This technique remains investigative although there is evidence of prolonged disease-free survival and overall survival with this approach.

PALLIATIVE TREATMENT

Meta-analysis of the randomized trials addressing active treatment versus best supportive care shows an unequivocal advantage to a proactive approach. Active treatment yields a 35 per cent mortality reduction, equivalent to a 16 per cent 1-year absolute improvement in survival, and improvement in median survival from 8 months for best supportive care to 12 months for active treatment. These benefits are independent of the age of the patient.

Surgery

If the tumour is inoperable, a bypass procedure or defunctioning colostomy may be of value in alleviating symptoms. In the case of those with liver metastases, it is well worth undertaking further investigations to assess the patient with respect to their suitability for partial hepatic resection. A CT scan should be undertaken to assess the liver and exclude local recurrence at the site of the original primary tumour. The hepatic disease can be assessed further by MRI ± angiography. Of those patients undergoing potentially curative excisions of all tumour-bearing liver, 25 per cent will survive 10 years.

Radiotherapy

This is of benefit in inoperable disease, local recurrence after surgery and symptomatic metastases. It is very effective in relieving bleeding, mucorrhoea and local pain, with response rates of about 75 per cent. Symptomatic pre-sacral recurrence is a particular problem after surgery and can be helped greatly by radiotherapy. In an era where more patients will have received preoperative radiotherapy, retreatment of the pelvis poses a dilemma for the oncologist.

Chemotherapy

For the palliation of metastatic disease, PVI 5-FU produces superior response rates to bolus doses (23 per cent versus 11 per cent). The addition of leucovorin to bolus 5-FU also improves the response rate (23 per cent versus 13 per cent). Addition of mitomycin C delivered 6-weekly also improves response rates of PVI 5-FU. Another strategy is to 'chronomodulate' 5-FU to exploit circadian variations in its metabolism. This entails infusing 5-FU for 12 hours overnight. Meta-analysis of trials of hepatic arterial infusion (HAI) of 5-FU versus bolus 5-FU delivered into a peripheral vein indicates superior response rates for HAI (42 per cent versus 14 per cent).

Despite these many strategies, one of the most favoured is the de Gramont regimen, which is a hybrid of infused and bolus 5-FU with high-dose folinic acid modulation, which combines all of these approaches and is highly active in metastatic disease:

- $200 \, \text{mg}/\text{m}^2$ folinic acid as a 2-hour infusion on days 1 and 2;
- 5-FU $400 \, \text{mg}/\text{m}^2$ as i.v. bolus on days 1 and 2;
- 5-FU infusion $600 \, \text{mg}/\text{m}^2$ over 22 hours on days 1 and 2;
- repeated every 2 weeks.

In recent years, a number of new, effective drugs have been marketed. Including oxaliplatin, irinotecan, capecitabine and oral 5-FU analogues. Current clinical trials are concentrating on how best to blend these drugs to yield the optimum trade-off between efficacy and toxicity.

Oxaliplatin is a water-soluble platinum derivative, which is highly active in colorectal cancer. Combined with de Gramont 5-FU, when compared with the de Gramont regime alone, oxaliplatin produces a doubling on response rate to 50 per cent and a superior progression-free survival (9 months versus 6 months) with relatively little penalty in terms of additional toxicity.

Irinotecan (CPT 11) is also an active agent. It is usually reserved for metastatic disease that has become refractory to 5-FU. There is good evidence that second-line CPT 11 is superior to best supportive care and PVI 5-FU in terms of symptom control and 1-year survival without a quality of life disadvantage. Evidence is also emerging of improved objective response rates when irinotecan/5-FU is compared with 5-FU alone.

Capecitabine is an oral formulation of a 5-FU-like prodrug that is converted into the active cytotoxic agent by an enzyme – thymidine phosphorylase (TP) – found at high concentration within malignant cells. It is given at a dose of $2500 \, \text{mg}/\text{m}^2$ daily in two divided doses for 14 days followed by a 1-week period of rest before the next cycle begins. Apart from some potential therapeutic gain in sparing normal cells and being preferentially activated within tumour tissue, it has the convenience of being easy to administer. Preliminary data suggest superiority to standard 5-FU (26 per cent response rate versus 17 per cent for 5-FU) with lower rates of stomatitis and myelosuppression, the latter in turn leading to lower rates of neutropenic fever and sepsis. Other oral formulations of 5-FU are now available. As experience of their use accrues, it is likely that their greater convenience and perhaps greater efficacy will lead to them superseding intravenous 5-FU for the treatment of metastatic colorectal cancer.

Prognosis

Dukes' staging and operability are the most important prognostic factors. The 5-year survivals are 90 per cent, 70 per cent and 40 per cent for Dukes' A, B and C tumours, respectively.

Unfavourable histopathological features include:

- increasing anatomical extent of tumour – depth of local invasion, lymph gland involvement (increasing number and proximal location are poor features) and distant metastases;
- incomplete surgical excision of tumour (e.g. CRM positivity following TME);
- infiltrative tumour margins rather than expansile;

- no peritumoral lymphoid reaction at deepest point of invasion and absence of lymphoid aggregates in the surrounding tissue;
- increasing tumour grade (decreasing differentiation);
- venous invasion;
- lymphatic invasion;
- perineural invasion;
- signet-ring and small cell types;
- preoperative CEA >5 mg/l.

Screening

For asymptomatic individuals, screening was previously thought to be expensive and unrewarding. However, it has been shown to allow diagnosis of colorectal cancer at an early stage, as shown by an increase in the proportion of Dukes' A and B tumours in the screened population. This in turn leads to an apparent survival advantage for the screened population. The most cost-effective and socially acceptable method of screening is faecal occult blood testing (FOBT). A tiny sample of stool is obtained non-invasively and chemically tested for the presence of blood. The specimen collection can be undertaken in the patient's own home and mailed back to the laboratory. Ninety-five per cent will be negative at the first screen, while 3–4 per cent will be weakly positive. Most of these will

Case history: colon cancer

A 60-year-old man presents to his general practitioner with a 6-week history of intermittent bright red blood per rectum, noticed as smearing on the lavatory paper associated with some perianal irritation. His bowels are regular and he has no other symptoms of note. Visual inspection of the anal orifice shows a prolapsed haemorrhoid and digital examination of the rectum is declined as he has had similar symptoms over the preceding 5 years. A diagnosis of haemorrhoids is made and the symptoms settle by the time he returns for a prescription of antihypertensive medicines 2 weeks later.

Eight weeks later, he returns with a 4-week history of more frequent and profuse passage of fresh blood per rectum. This is associated with mucoid discharge per rectum and a feeling of incomplete rectal evacuation. Rectal examination is strongly suggested and this reveals an ulcerating tumour of the mid-rectum. He is referred to a colorectal surgeon for further investigation. Digital examination confirms a tumour distinct from the prostate, with an impression of tethering laterally. Rigid sigmoidoscopy shows no other mucosal abnormality and biopsies confirm a moderately differentiated adenocarcinoma. Barium enema confirms no other mucosal abnormality elsewhere in the large bowel. Chest X-ray is normal. Computed tomography (CT) scan of the abdomen and pelvis shows no evidence of liver metastases, no pelvic lymphadenopathy and no evidence of direct invasion of the adjacent pelvic viscera. The serum carcinoembryonic antigen (CEA) is twice the upper limit of normal (normal range <4 μg/l) and the liver function tests normal. After discussion at the multidisciplinary team meeting, he is referred to a clinical oncologist and receives five fractions of preoperative radiotherapy using fields encompassing the rectum and immediate lymphatic drainage. One week later, he undergoes a total mesorectal excision with immediate reanastomosis. Histopathological review confirms a moderate/poorly differentiated adenocarcinoma that penetrates through the full thickness of the rectal wall but has a clear circumferential resection margin and clear margins of excision proximally and distally. There is no involvement of the perirectal or other pelvic lymph nodes but prominent venous invasion is noted. The CEA returns to normal during the immediate postoperative period. His tumour is therefore designated as Dukes' B and he receives 6 months of adjuvant 5-fluorouracil (5-FU)/folinic acid chemotherapy because of the vascular invasion and poorly differentiated elements of the tumour.

He remains entirely well on routine follow-up until 18 months later when a routine preclinic CEA estimation is found to be 12 times the upper limit of normal at 48 μg/l. There are no adverse physical signs. This triggers restaging investigations. A CT scan reveals two metastases in the left lobe of the liver and no evidence of loco-regional recurrence of the original primary tumour. The chest is clear. There is no radiological abnormality elsewhere. Magnetic resonance imaging (MRI) of the liver confirms a smaller third metastasis in the left lobe close to the other two and no involvement of the major hepatic vessels. He is referred to a hepato-biliary surgeon and is deemed medically fit for salvage surgery. A segmental resection of the left lobe of the liver is performed. The CEA returns to normal postoperatively. He remains well and disease-free 4 years later.

retest as negative after dietary restriction (no vitamin C, no iron supplements, no non-steroidal anti-inflammatory drugs (NSAIDs), no red meat, no fresh fruit). This leaves approximately 2 per cent with a positive FOBT who will require further investigation (e.g. colonoscopy, sigmoidoscopy/double-contrast barium enema). Less than 10 per cent of these individuals will be found to have a bowel cancer. As with any screening method, a very small proportion of patients will have a false-negative result. One European cost-effectiveness analysis of FOBT suggested a cost of approximately €20 000 per cancer detected and approximately €10 000 per life year gained.

High-risk groups require regular colonoscopy, in particular those with familial polyposis coli, those with strong family histories of colon cancer or a longstanding history of extensive ulcerative colitis.

Prevention

Dietary interventions such as increasing fibre and reducing animal fats may be a useful strategy. This approach is vindicated by observations that the descendants of Japanese migrants to Hawaii acquire the higher risk of cancer seen in indigenous Hawaiians as they adopt their dietary habits. There is evidence that NSAIDs reduce the odds of developing colorectal cancer by approximately half, particularly in women. Prompt diagnosis and excision of large bowel benign polyps will prevent subsequent transformation into a cancer.

CARCINOMA OF THE ANUS

Epidemiology

This is a rare tumour. For example, in England and Wales, there are only 300 new cases and 200 deaths recorded per annum. It comprises about 4 per cent of large bowel tumours with a peak incidence at 50–70 years and a slight female predominance overall. Anal margin tumours are more common in men, while anal canal tumours are more common in women.

Aetiology

Homosexual activity, in particular ano-receptive intercourse, is associated with anal cancer, and there is evidence that this is due to transmission of the human papilloma virus types 16 and 18 (50 per cent of cancer sufferers test positive for these); it is analogous with carcinoma of the cervix. There is also evidence among attendees of sexually transmitted disease (STD) clinics that up to 60 per cent of homosexuals will have asymptomatic anal intra-epithelial neoplasia (AIN), which is comparable to cervical intra-epithelial neoplasia (CIN).

Pathology

The tumour may arise from skin at the anal margin or from the anal canal, appearing as a nodule, polyp or ulcer with everted edges. Ninety per cent are squamous carcinomas; most of the remainder are adenocarcinomas arising from mucous glands. Anal margin tumours are well differentiated as they are akin to squamous carcinomas of the skin, whereas 75 per cent of anal canal tumours are poorly differentiated. There may be *in situ* carcinoma in the surrounding epithelium.

Natural history

The tumour will spread circumferentially and longitudinally within the anus and may invade the lower rectum or perianal skin. Deeper infiltration leads to involvement of the sphincters, ischiorectal fossae, vagina and urethra. Lymphatic spread occurs in 10 per cent and is more common with anal canal tumours. The first station lymph nodes are the inguinal groups, from which there may be spread to the iliac nodes. Involvement of the distal rectum may lead to spread to the inferior mesenteric nodes. Haematogenous spread is very uncommon at presentation. Sites of distant metastases include the liver, lungs and skeleton.

Symptoms

Patients present with anal symptoms such as:

- discharge;
- irritation/discomfort;
- bleeding;
- tenesmus.

Minor symptoms are frequently neglected by both patients and physicians alike as they resemble those from haemorrhoids, which are far more prevalent.

Signs

Tumours of the anal verge or most distal part of the anal canal should be easily seen on parting the

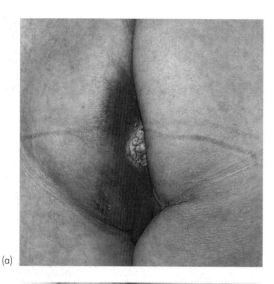

(a)

(b)

FIG 9.9 Anal margin carcinoma. Papilliform tumour arising from skin at anal verge. (a) Distant view; (b) close view with buttocks parted.

buttocks (Fig. 9.9). The tumour should be palpable as an indurated ulcer or nodule on digital examination. Enlarged inguinal nodes should be sought,

although a proportion of enlarged nodes will be secondary to infection.

Differential diagnosis

This includes:

- genital warts – these may be confused with a papilliform, well-differentiated carcinoma;
- Crohn's disease of the anus;
- syphilis;
- basal cell carcinoma/melanoma.

Investigations

Proctoscopy

This is an essential investigation, permitting the tumour to be visualized directly and biopsied, and complements the findings of a digital rectal examination.

Examination under anaesthetic (EUA)

This is the best staging investigation in an anxious or uncooperative patient. In a woman, a full bimanual examination is mandatory to assess the extent of local spread. An EUA will also permit the taking of a generous biopsy with minimal distress and discomfort.

Fine-needle aspiration (FNA) of any enlarged inguinal lymph nodes

This will help to distinguish reactive lymph nodes from malignant ones which is important in planning treatment.

Chest X-ray

This should be performed to exclude lung metastases.

Computed tomography of the pelvis

This permits an assessment of the degree of deep invasion of the tumour and is of value in excluding impalpable pelvic lymphadenopathy when the inguinal nodes are involved. It also surveys the liver.

Endo-anal ultrasound/magnetic resonance imaging

This may offer more precise information on the local extent of the tumour.

Staging

The TNM staging system (see Chapter 2) is used:

- TX – primary tumour cannot be assessed.
- T0 – no evidence of primary tumour.
- Tis – carcinoma *in situ*.
- T1 – tumour 2 cm or less in greatest dimension.
- T2 – tumour more than 2 cm but not more than 5 cm in greatest dimension.
- T3 – tumour more than 5 cm in greatest dimension.
- T4 – tumour of any size that invades adjacent organ(s), e.g., vagina, urethra, bladder (involvement of the sphincter muscle[s] alone is not classified as T4).
- NX – regional lymph nodes cannot be assessed.
- N0 – no regional lymph node metastasis.
- N1 – metastasis in perirectal lymph node(s).
- N2 – metastasis in unilateral internal iliac and/or inguinal lymph node(s).
- N3 – metastasis in perirectal and inguinal lymph nodes and/or bilateral internal iliac and/or inguinal lymph nodes.
- MX – distant metastasis cannot be assessed.
- M0 – no distant metastasis.
- M1 – distant metastasis.

Treatment

RADICAL TREATMENT

Surgery

Anal margin tumours may be treated by wide local excision alone, with more extensive surgery reserved for salvage of local relapse. In anal canal tumours, an abdominoperineal resection (APR) is necessary, which will result in the patient having a permanent colostomy. Preoperative counselling by a stomatherapist should be arranged in all patients in whom an APR is planned. Patients with cytologically positive inguinal nodes should undergo a block dissection of the groins.

Chemoradiotherapy (CRT)

Non-surgical treatment has the advantage of allowing sphincter preservation. Most local recurrences occur within 1 year of completing treatment and can still be salvaged by an APR. Radiotherapy alone is associated with a 60 per cent local recurrence rate, compared with 40 per cent for CRT. Chemoradiotherapy has therefore become the standard of

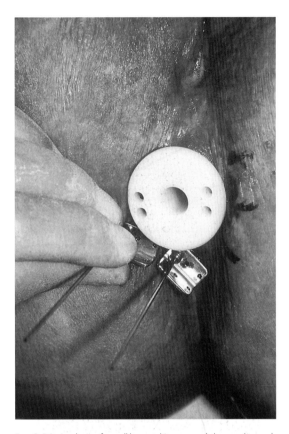

FIG 9.10 Implant of small-bore tubes around the anal canal, which will be loaded with radioactive iridium wire.

care for this disease. With CRT, 5-FU is delivered continuously during weeks 1 and 5 of radiotherapy with bolus mitomycin C on the first day of radiotherapy. Radiotherapy is delivered to the pelvis and inguinal nodes bilaterally at a dose of 45 Gy in 25 fractions over 5 weeks. This is followed, after a short break, by a boost dose of 15–20 Gy to the anal tumour alone, either by external beam radiation over 1.5 weeks or by interstitial brachytherapy (Fig. 9.10). A poor objective response after the initial phase of CRT is an indication to proceed immediately to APR. CRT is associated with an increased severity of acute treatment reactions, particularly with respect to perineal skin reactions and diarrhoea. Five-year survival is approximately 70 per cent.

PALLIATIVE TREATMENT

Surgery

In the exceptional case of a very advanced inoperable tumour leading to anal occlusion, a defunctioning colostomy may be justified.

Radiotherapy

Pelvic/perineal radiotherapy may be used to palliate symptomatic local recurrence after radical surgery.

Tumour-related complications

An advanced tumour may lead to an aberrant connection between the anal canal and the perineum, vagina or urethra, leading to faecal incontinence. The ischiorectal fossae are anatomically close to the anus and particularly prone to secondary infection and abscess formation.

Treatment-related complications

Radiotherapy

The perianal region does not tolerate radiotherapy well as the skin is constantly subjected to friction when sitting or walking, trauma when patients are having to defecate frequently, moisture from sweating and perhaps discharge from the anus. During radiotherapy the patient can be expected to experience diarrhoea, tenesmus and perianal irritation/soreness. These symptoms will begin 1–2 weeks after starting radiotherapy and persist for 4–8 weeks after it has finished. In the longer term, chronic proctocolitis may manifest as diarrhoea, tenesmus, bleeding and mucus per rectum, which can be treated conservatively with topical steroids. Small bowel stricture, intestinal obstruction and bladder contracture may occur in 10–20 per cent of cases. Infertility is inevitable for both males and females. High doses of radiation to the groins may lead to occlusion of the lymphatics and to chronic lymphoedema, which is best managed with pressure garments.

Surgery

The main morbidity in the short term is from dehiscence of the perineal wound and pelvic infection. Extensive pelvic surgery such as an APR may damage autonomic nerves leading to urinary incontinence and impotence in men. The psychosexual trauma and effect on body image may be considerable.

Chemotherapy

In addition to the usual complications from these chemotherapy drugs, CRT leads to severe gastrointestinal toxicity causing anorexia, nausea, vomiting, diarrhoea and intense cutaneous inflammation.

Prognosis

The overall 5-year survival is 70 per cent. Adverse features include anal canal v. anal margin tumours, increasing TNM stage at presentation and poorly differentiated tumours.

Screening/prevention

The high incidence of AIN in STD clinics may make screening a worthwhile exercise in this small group, particularly in male homosexuals. 'Safe sex' practices among homosexual males may also help prevent papilloma virus transmission. A greater awareness of the disease may lead to earlier diagnosis rather than *ad hoc* prescription or purchase of proprietary haemorrhoid remedies.

10 UROLOGICAL CANCER

RENAL CELL CARCINOMA (HYPERNEPHROMA)

Epidemiology

This accounts for 2 per cent of all malignancies with over 4000 cases each year in the UK. It is slightly more common in males than females. The incidence is high in Europe, particularly Denmark, and lowest in Japan.

Aetiology

There are several aetiological factors:

- smoking tobacco increases the risk of renal cell carcinoma;
- cadmium exposure may also be a factor;
- rarely, it occurs in a familial pattern and has been associated with *HLA-BW44* and *HLA-DR8*;
- there is increased incidence in von Hippel–Lindau disease, horseshoe kidneys and adult polycystic kidneys.

Pathology

Tumours may arise from any part of the renal tissue: one-quarter involve the whole kidney, one-third the upper pole, and one-third the lower pole. Macroscopically, the tumour is usually solid, expanding the renal tissue with a central area of necrosis or cystic degeneration and other haemorrhagic areas. Occasionally, a tumour may arise within the wall of a cyst. Renal cell tumours are thought to arise from the lining cells of the proximal convoluted tubule.

Microscopically, they are adenocarcinomas composed of characteristic clear cells, although the degree of differentiation can vary from a well-differentiated tumour to a highly anaplastic appearance.

Natural history

The tumour invades the surrounding kidney and may grow into the renal vein and thence into the inferior vena cava (IVC).

Lymph node spread involves the renal hilar nodes and progresses to the para-aortic chain. Blood–bone metastases characteristically go to the lung and bone, although many other sites including skin, central nervous system and liver are also recognized. Approximately 25 per cent of patients will present with metastatic disease and of the remainder a further 30–40 per cent will eventually express distant metastases.

Spontaneous regression of metastases, typically lung deposits monitored on chest X-ray, is often referred to in the context of renal cell cancer. While such events undoubtedly occur, the true incidence is extremely low, the verified incidence being around 7 per cent of patients with metastatic disease. Spontaneous regression of the primary tumour is virtually unknown.

Symptoms

Haematuria, which is typically painless, is the most common presenting symptom. Loin pain may occur acutely owing to haemorrhage within the tumour or chronically as the tumour enlarges.

Symptoms of metastases may be present, in particular bone pain or even pathological fracture (bone metastases) and cough with or without haemoptysis (lung metastases).

Symptoms of paraneoplastic conditions associated with renal cell cancer may be present, these include hypercalcaemia and polycythaemia. There may also be general symptoms of malignancy such as malaise, anorexia and weight loss.

Signs

The primary tumour may be palpable as a mass in the loin, and in 10–20 per cent of patients there is associated fever.

Differential diagnosis

Other causes of haematuria should be considered, in particular benign renal adenomas, tumours of the renal pelvis, renal tract stones and bladder tumours. Other causes of loin pain which should be taken into account include renal stones or hydronephrosis.

Investigations

Blood tests

A full blood count may show anaemia due to chronic haematuria or polycythaemia due to tumour production of erythyropoietin-like substances. Serum calcium may be raised.

Radiography

Chest X-ray may show typical 'cannon-ball' metastases.

Computed tomography scan

The renal tumour will be imaged on both ultrasound or computed tomography (CT) scan. The latter will also give information on renal vein/IVC invasion and involvement of surrounding structures. The role of intravenous urography (IVU) where CT is widely available is debatable. Figure 10.1 shows the appearance of a renal carcinoma on CT scan.

Fine-needle aspirate or biopsy

Tissue diagnosis may be obtained by fine-needle aspirate cytology or biopsy.

Isotope bone scan

Isotope bone scans are not routinely recommended but X-ray skeletal survey may be of value. The

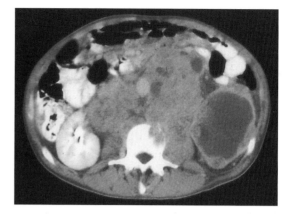

FIG 10.1 Computed tomography scan demonstrating a large renal carcinoma rising from the right kidney.

typical lytic bone lesions of renal cell carcinoma may give false negative bone scan images.

Staging

Full TNM staging (see Chapter 2) is not often used in the clinical assessment of renal cell cancers. Important features are the size of the primary tumour and involvement of surrounding structures, including the renal vein, which will determine operability of the primary, and the presence of distant metastases.

Treatment

SURGERY

Radical nephrectomy in which the perirenal fat, perirenal fascia, adrenal gland and regional nodes are removed *en bloc* is the operation of choice with superior local control rates to simple nephrectomy. Tumour invading the renal vein can be successfully removed and this is therefore not an absolute contraindication to radical treatment.

PALLIATIVE TREATMENT

Local irradiation of painful bone metastases may be required. Brain metastases may benefit from cranial irradiation, or if solitary, without extensive disease elsewhere, surgical excision may be considered.

Lung metastases may also be amenable to surgical excision in the occasional patient that presents some years after treatment of the primary tumour with a solitary lung metastasis.

SYSTEMIC TREATMENT

Renal cancer is responsive to biological therapies such as interferon and interleukin 2 (IL2). Response rates of around 15 per cent are seen with interferon and 20–30 per cent with IL2. There is no effective chemotherapy for renal cell cancer but the addition of 5-fluorouracil (5-FU) to interferon and IL2 has been shown to enhance activity.

Hormone responses occur with progestogens, although the true response rate is probably quite low, perhaps less than 10 per cent.

Treatment with either biological agents or progestogens is at best palliative in the setting of widespread metastatic disease – a recent trial comparing interferon with medroxyprogesterone reported a 1-year survival of 12 per cent and overall a 1-month advantage in progression-free survival for interferon. More toxic regimes including interferon, interleukin and 5-FU are currently under evaluation.

Tumour-related complications

Complications of renal cell carcinoma include hypercalcaemia and polycythaemia. Renal function is usually unaffected provided that the contralateral kidney is normal.

Prognosis

The prognosis for tumour localized to the kidney is good, with 5-year survival after radical nephrectomy of around 50 per cent. Even in the presence of metastases, renal cell cancer often has a long and indolent course so that 5–10 per cent of patients with lung metastases will survive for 5 years or more.

Screening and future prospects

Simple urinalysis for microscopic haematuria and cytology are readily available. However, while sensitive, it is non-specific and results in unacceptably high false-positive rates for routine application.

It is of interest that this tumour is one of the few to show responses to the biological response modifying agents and future developments in this area may well lead to further new treatments. Thalidomide is currently under investigation as a systemic agent for renal cell cancer.

PROSTATE CANCER

Epidemiology

The incidence of prostate cancer is rising. This may reflect an increasing proportion of the population aged over 70 years, a greater diagnostic rate and possibly a true increase in incidence in younger men.

There are around 14 000 cases in the UK each year with an incidence of 50 in 100 000, compared with 91 in 100 000 black men and 51 in 100 000 in white men in the USA, and 6 in 100 000 in Japan. In the UK it ranks third behind lung and large bowel cancer for deaths from cancer.

Aetiology

It is rare under 45 years but increases with age, being almost universal at post-mortem in men aged over 80 years. It is more common in married men, and is related to the number of sexual partners, frequency of sexual activity and a history of sexually transmitted disease. A positive correlation with circulating testosterone levels and a negative correlation with oestrogen levels has been claimed.

When seen in young men under 45 years there may be a familial pattern with first-degree relatives affected. An association with breast cancer in female relatives has also been described linked to the BRCA gene. Benign prostatic hypertrophy is often also present, but no direct causal relationship has been demonstrated.

It is more common in city dwellers than rural communities, and is associated with a high fat and meat diet, and an occupational exposure to cadmium.

Pathology

Cancer of the prostate develops most commonly in the peripheral part of the gland; this accounts for 70 per cent, while only 10 per cent arise centrally. The remainder arise in the transitional zone. Eighty-five per cent are diffuse multifocal tumours. *In situ* cancer (prostate intraepithelial neoplasia, PIN) is now a recognized precursor to invasive disease and may be seen in adjacent parts of a gland containing invasive cancer.

Microscopically, prostate cancer is typically an adenocarcinoma of varying differentiation. Various grading systems based on morphological appearances have been described, all of which correlate with outcome. The commonly used system is the Gleason score, which is based on the pattern of

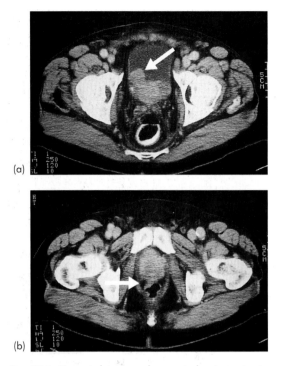

(a)

(b)

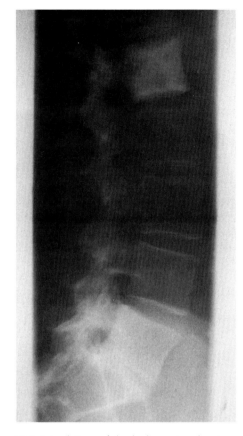

Fig 10.2 Computed tomography scans showing extensive local infiltration of prostate carcinoma into (a) the bladder and (b) posteriorly into the rectum.

growth of the tumour and is recorded as the sum of a primary and secondary grade, giving a summed score from 2 to 10. A Gleason score of 7 or above correlates with a relatively poor outcome. Another poor prognostic feature is perineural invasion.

Where there is doubt as to the primary origin of a tumour deposit, a prostatic primary will be characterized by staining for acid phosphatase and prostate-specific antigen. Androgen and progestogen receptors have been demonstrated on the surface of prostate cancer cells although the value of this in routine clinical use remains uncertain.

Natural history

Local growth results in infiltration of the prostate gland and surrounding tissues, particularly into the seminal vesicles, bladder and rectum as shown in Fig. 10.2.

Lymph node metastases are recognized with initial involvement of pelvic nodes but this is less frequent than the predominant picture of blood-borne dissemination.

Distant spread is usually blood-borne, typically by retrograde venous spread through the vertebral plexus of veins, so that bone metastases to the spine

Fig 10.3 Lateral X-ray of the lumbar spine showing metastases in L1 causing extensive sclerotic changes compared with surrounding normal vertebrae.

are common although all parts of the skeleton may be affected (Fig. 10.3).

Soft tissue metastases (e.g. lung or liver) although well recognized are uncommon in prostatic cancer.

Symptoms

Prostate cancer is often asymptomatic and found either at post-mortem or incidentally during the investigation of another condition. The following symptoms may be present:

- prostatic outflow obstructive symptoms, with frequency, hesitancy, poor stream, nocturia and terminal dribble;
- haematospermia;
- bone pain or, less often, spinal cord compression, due to bone metastases;
- hypercalcaemia;
- general symptoms of malignancy, including malaise, anorexia and weight loss.

Signs

The tumour may be palpable per rectum as a hard nodule or diffusely infiltrating abnormality, which in more advanced cases may be found to invade surrounding pelvic tissues. Typically, there is loss of the midline sulcus of the gland, which is present in the normal or hypertrophied prostate.

Bone metastases may be clinically apparent when complicated by pain, pathological fracture or neurological signs.

Differential diagnosis

Benign prostatic hypertrophy may produce the same symptoms of bladder outflow obstruction and indeed may coexist with prostatic cancer.

Investigations

Routine blood tests

A full blood count may show a reduction of haemoglobin, white cells or platelets with widespread bone metastases. Hypercalcaemia and uraemia should be excluded on routine biochemistry.

Intravenous urography

Intravenous urography will demonstrate the enlarged gland indenting the bladder and any associated hydronephrosis.

Computed tomography scan

This gives more detail of surrounding soft tissue, in particular lymph node enlargement.

Ultrasound

Transrectal ultrasound is the most sensitive means of assessing the prostate gland and may be used to direct needle biopsy towards suspicious areas of the gland. Doppler flow studies may give even greater detail of the internal structure of the gland and highlight abnormal areas.

Magnetic resonance imaging

Excellent views of the prostate gland and its relation to surrounding normal soft tissue structures such as bladder and rectum can be obtained by magnetic resonance imaging (MRI). The best definition is obtained using specific rectal coils. It is probably the investigation of choice for staging prostate cancer; an example is shown in Fig. 10.4.

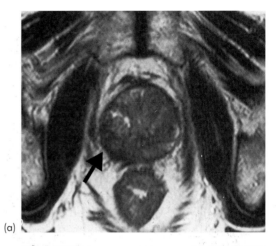

(a)

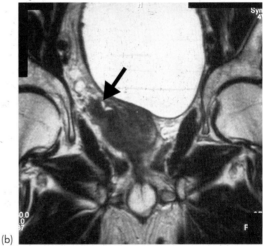

(b)

FIG 10.4 Magnetic resonance imaging scan of prostate demonstrating (a) early extracapsular invasion and (b) seminal vesicle invasion.

Prostate-specific antigen

Prostate-specific antigen (PSA) is measured in the blood and is more specific than acid phosphatase for diagnosis and monitoring of the disease although it may be slightly elevated (up to 10 ng/ml) in benign prostatic hypertrophy. It has largely replaced measurement of serum acid phosphatase which, while raised in the presence of bone metastases, is far less sensitive.

Isotope bone scan

Isotope bone scan is the most useful screening test for bone metastases. A positive scan is shown in Fig. 10.5.

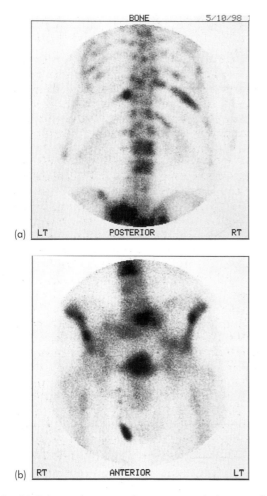

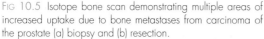

Fɪɢ 10.5 Isotope bone scan demonstrating multiple areas of increased uptake due to bone metastases from carcinoma of the prostate (a) biopsy and (b) resection.

Histological confirmation is made either at transurethral resection of the prostate (TURP) or on transrectal ultrasound-guided needle biopsy per rectum. Previous fears that TURP may cause dissemination of cancer cells are unfounded, but in the absence of major bladder outflow symptoms a needle biopsy is to be preferred.

Staging

Staging of cancer of the prostate is a little confused because of the existence of two different systems, the TNM system (see Chapter 2) and the Jewitt system (widely adopted in the USA). The two systems are shown in Table 10.1. The important principles are to distinguish early localized carcinoma of the prostate from locally extensive disease from that which has already metastasized.

TABLE 10.1 Staging of prostatic cancer

TNM	Jewitt	
TO, T1	A1, A2	Asymptomatic incidental finding
T2	B1, B2	Confined within capsule of gland
T3, T4	C1, C2	Extension beyond capsule of gland
N1, N2, N3	D1	Involvement of regional nodes
M1	D2	Distant metastases

Treatment

Radical treatment is indicated for prostatic cancer which is localized to the prostate gland with no evidence on the basis of isotope bone scan or serum prostate-specific antigen of distant metastases. A PSA level of under 20 ng/ml virtually excludes the possibility of bone metastases, while a level of >50 ng/ml carries a very high probability of distant spread even if the bone scan is 'normal'.

RADICAL PROSTATECTOMY

This is indicated for disease that is localized to the gland (i.e. stages T1 and T2). The operation involves removal of the entire prostate and adjacent bladder neck, both seminal vesicles, the vasa deferentia and surrounding fascia. It requires considerable surgical expertise. Complications include erectile impotence and occasional urinary incontinence. 'Nerve sparing' techniques to preserve the neurovascular bundle responsible for penile erection are used but may not be possible where there is tumour infiltration close to these critical structures.

Postoperative radiotherapy may have a role where excision margins are close to or involved with tumour or when pelvic lymph nodes are involved. A rising PSA level, which should be undetectable after prostatectomy, suggests residual prostatic tissue and is an indication for postoperative radiotherapy.

RADICAL RADIOTHERAPY

This is indicated for all patients with disease localized to the pelvis. There is no evidence that prophylactic treatment of pelvic lymph nodes is of value and a small treatment volume encompassing known disease in the prostate and seminal vesicles is adequate. Localization with CT scanning greatly increases the accuracy of treatment. Prostate

Case history: prostate cancer

MJ, a 68-year-old man had been noticing for some weeks a nagging pain in the back with some local tenderness over the lumbar spine. The pain was worse on standing and walking but never went away completely. He had done no recent heavy work to provoke it. For several years he had noted that he passed water more frequently and had started having to get up at night two or three times to pass water also. He consulted his general practitioner who confirmed some local tenderness in the lumbar spine and in view of his urinary symptoms performed a rectal examination. This revealed an enlarged hard irregular prostate gland.

His GP arranged for X-rays of the spine and some blood tests including a serum prostate-specific antigen (PSA). This returned with an elevated level at 385 ng/ml and the X-rays showed scattered sclerotic changes compatible with metastatic disease. He was referred to a specialist oncology clinic where it was confirmed that the above findings were compatible with a diagnosis of metastatic prostate cancer. The raised PSA level was considered sufficient to confirm the diagnosis and no biopsy of the prostate gland was recommended. Treatment was started with cyproterone acetate tablets for 2 weeks and a goserelin subcutaneous implant was given. When reviewed 6 weeks later MJ reported a considerable improvement in his back pain but was complaining of intermittent hot flushes. It was explained that these were a common side-effect of the goserelin injections. A repeat PSA had fallen to 26 ng/ml and he was recommended to continue with the goserelin at 3-monthly intervals.

MJ remained well for the next 2 years, the hot flushes regressing and his pain remaining well controlled. He then noted over a period of a few days increasing difficulty in climbing stairs accompanied by a return of his backache. The following day he was unable to pass water and reported a loss of feeling in his legs. His GP referred him for an urgent assessment to his local casualty department. There he was found to be in urinary retention, with a grade 3–4 weakness of the lower limbs and a reduction in pin-prick and light-touch sensation to the level of the umbilicus. A urinary catheter was inserted and an urgent magnetic resonance scan was performed. This showed extensive spinal metastases with involvement of the spinal canal at T10. Urgent transfer to the local cancer centre was arranged. He was started on dexamethasone and immediate local radiotherapy to the lower thoracic spine was given over the next week. A repeat PSA level was found to be 376 ng/ml. Following completion of radiotherapy his pain settled once more. The power in his lower limbs improved and he was able to walk independently with the aid of a stick. He also regained control of his bladder function.

Three months later he returned to his GP complaining of a poor appetite, scattered aches and pains in his ribs and spine, and severe constipation. His wife who accompanied him reported also that he had become increasingly confused. His GP performed some further blood tests and his serum calcium was found to be elevated at 3.7 nmol/l. Urgent admission to his local hospital was arranged and he was treated with intravenous saline and an infusion of pamidronate. Over the next few days his symptoms improved and his calcium fell to 2.9 nmol/l. He was discharged home a week later and remained well for 3 weeks when his earlier symptoms started to return and a further blood calcium level showed that this has risen again to 3.9 nmol/l. Admission to hospital was arranged again and treatment with pamidronate and intravenous fluids was repeated. On this occasion the response was slower and the calcium level remained at 3.2 nmol/l. MJ became increasingly confused and immobile. Ten days after admission his calcium was noted to be rising once more and he had a fever. Chest X-ray showed patchy consolidation and his condition continued to deteriorate as he developed bronchopneumonia from which he died 3 days later.

radiotherapy is an area where conformal radiotherapy and intensity modulated beams are increasingly used, with doses of over 90 Gy now technically feasible with these new techniques.

Brachytherapy techniques with permanent implants of radioactive iodine-125 or palladium-103 offer an alternative approach to external beam radiotherapy in patients with early localized disease. A permanent iodine seed implant is shown in Fig. 10.6. Combined treatments using external beam with a brachytherapy boost, usually by a temporary implant using an iridium afterloading technique, are also advocated as a means of increasing radiation dose without additional side-effects.

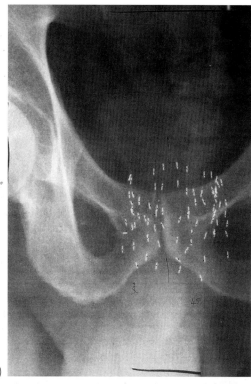

(a)

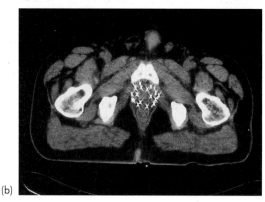

(b)

FIG 10.6 Plain X-ray showing iodine seeds (a) after implantation into prostate gland and (b) computed tomography scan showing position taken 1 month after the implant procedure.

The principal side-effects include bowel and bladder irritation, but in the majority of patients potency is preserved. Brachytherapy is associated with very few bowel effects and a low level of impotence, although acute urethritis immediately following the procedure may be more pronounced than with external beam treatment.

HORMONE THERAPY

Hormone therapy by androgen deprivation or blockade is effective in most patients (see Chapter 6 and below). It is usually reserved for relapse or those presenting with metastatic disease. It may, however, have a role in primary treatment for locally advanced tumours prior to definitive radiotherapy by allowing initial reduction of tumour bulk and early control of local symptoms. Current evidence shows an advantage in disease-free but not overall survival for at least 6 months neo-adjuvant anti-androgen treatment prior to definitive local treatment, the greatest advantage being seen in those with high-grade tumours. It is also of value in patients with severe coexisting medical or surgical conditions that preclude more radical local treatment, particularly where the prognosis from such a condition is short.

PALLIATIVE TREATMENT

For metastatic disease hormone therapy will achieve a response in most patients. Hormone therapy may be given in a number of forms, as shown in Table 10.2. All of these are equally effective and the choice will in general be based on patient acceptability and availability.

Anti-androgen drugs include cyproterone acetate, flutamide and bicalutamide. Stilboestrol has been used in the past but is limited by excessive cardiovascular side effects. Gonadotrophin-releasing hormone (GnRH) analogue drugs include goserelin and leuprorelin.

TABLE 10.2 Hormone therapy for prostate cancer: relative clinical merits

Bilateral orchidectomy	Anti-androgen drugs	Gonadotrophin-releasing hormone analogue
Surgical procedure	Oral medication	Monthly injection
Permanent	Reversible	Reversible
Compliance guaranteed	Tablets may be missed	Compliance guaranteed
Patient acceptance variable	Readily accepted	Readily accepted

First-line treatment for a patient presenting with metastatic prostate cancer will generally be either a GnRH analogue or an oral anti-androgen such as flutamide or bicalutamide. Around 80 per cent of patients will respond to this manoeuvre. When initiating treatment with a GnRH analogue drug the initial exposure should be covered by a period of 10–14 days oral anti-androgen administration to cover the initial flare seen with these agents. There is no evidence that continuing combination therapy, sometimes referred to as MAB (maximal androgen blockade) has major advantages over single-agent therapy. Permanent androgen deprivation by orchidectomy may then be offered to responders with the alternative of continuing with medical treatment.

Patients will inevitably relapse despite an initial response, the median duration of response being around 18 months. Unfortunately response to a second hormone manoeuvre is usually disappointing and further treatment will be based on control of specific symptoms.

Chemotherapy may be considered for selected patients with relapse after hormone treatment. Mitozantrone is the only drug for which there is good evidence of a palliative effect when given with prednisolone.

Other palliative treatments which will be of value in these patients include the appropriate use of analgesics and coanalgesics together with palliative radiotherapy using either external beam therapy or the radio-isotope strontium-89 for bone pain. Palliative radiotherapy may also be indicated for neurological complications.

Hypercalcaemia will require active management when symptomatic (see Chapter 22).

Tumour-related complications

Complications include:

- obstructive hydronephrosis;
- hypercalcaemia;
- spinal cord compression.

Treatment-related complications

SURGERY

Surgery may lead to impotence and urinary incontinence.

RADIOTHERAPY

Bowel and bladder damage may result from external beam radiotherapy. Impotence may also occur but less often than after surgery.

Brachytherapy is only rarely associated with long-term bowel or bladder problems but can be followed by an immediate period of post-implant acute urethritis.

HORMONE THERAPY

Androgen blockade is commonly associated with hot flushes, lethargy, reduced libido and varying degrees of impotence. Oral anti-androgens may cause nausea and, rarely, hepatic dysfunction.

Prognosis

While aggressive forms of prostatic cancer are recognized, particularly in young men, in the majority of cases the natural history of the disease will span several years. Because of this it is difficult to judge the results of treatment on short-term survival figures.

Untreated, localized carcinoma of the prostate will still give a 5-year survival of 80 per cent, although many will have locally progressive disease. After radical treatment, surgical or radiotherapeutic, 10-year survivals in excess of 80 per cent are to be expected, falling to around 50 per cent for disease extending outside the capsule of the gland.

Patients presenting with metastastic disease have a median survival of 18–24 months.

Screening and future prospects

Digital rectal examination, serum prostate-specific antigen and transrectal ultrasound offer a high chance of detecting preclinical prostate cancer. Extensive studies are currently underway in Europe to evaluate the effect of screening healthy men. This is already common practice in the USA, where 50 per cent of prostate cancers are detected while still localized to the gland, compared with only 10 per cent in the UK. However the impact of such approaches on overall survival remains uncertain.

Vaccines and monoclonal antibodies to tumour-specific antigens are currently under investigation as an alternative means of therapy.

Rarer tumours

Transitional cell tumours of the prostate arising from the urethra usually present and are managed in the same way as other urothelial tumours.

BLADDER CANCER

Epidemiology

There are around 12 500 cases of bladder cancer in the UK each year. It is twice as common in men as in women and is unusual under the age of 50 years, being most common in the 70s and 80s age-groups.

Aetiology

- Chemical carcinogens – these include aniline dyes; rubber industry byproducts such as β-naphthylamine and benzidine, and drugs, (e.g. exposure to excessive amounts of phenacetin or cyclophosphamide).
- Smoking.
- Chronic irritation – this is related to bladder diverticulae and infection with schistosomiasis is also important in those areas where this is common, being associated with squamous carcinomas in younger age groups.

Pathology

Macroscopically, bladder cancer can appear as papillary or solid lesions and may be solitary or more usually multiple. The usual area of the bladder affected is the lateral wall and involvement of the bladder base is also common.

Microscopically, the majority of cancers are transitional cell tumours of varying differentiation graded from well to poorly differentiated using a numerical scale G1–G3. These account for 90 per cent of all bladder cancers. Of the remainder, 7 per cent are squamous carcinomas and 3 per cent are adenocarcinomas.

Natural history

Most bladder cancers probably arise as fairly indolent papillomas which, left untreated, progress both in terms of dedifferentiation and local invasion. The primary tumour invades locally into the bladder muscle wall and thence into perivesical fat. More advanced disease may involve prostate, anterior vaginal wall or rectum.

Lymphatic spread involves pelvic lymph nodes and then para-aortic nodes. Blood-borne metastases arise particularly in lungs and bone.

In many, if not all patients, there is a generalized instability of the urothelium and a risk of further tumours developing not only elsewhere in the bladder but also throughout the ureters and renal pelvises. Biopsies of adjacent sites frequently demonstrate dysplasia and a clinical picture of multiple recurrent transitional cell tumours throughout the tract is well recognized.

Symptoms

These may include:

- painless haematuria and other urinary symptoms such as frequency, urgency and dysuria;
- cough, haemoptysis or bone pain caused by metastases are less frequent presentations of bladder cancer;
- general symptoms of malaise, anorexia and weight loss.

Signs

In most patients there will be no clinical signs of bladder cancer. Bladder tumours are rarely palpable per rectum or per vaginam and only in advanced cases will a suprapubic mass be palpable.

Differential diagnosis

Other causes of haematuria should be considered, including urinary tract infection, stones and renal tumours.

Investigations

Blood tests

Routine blood investigations may reveal anaemia due to chronic haematuria and renal impairment if there is obstructive hydronephrosis.

Radiography

Chest X-ray will demonstrate metastases, if present.

Urine tests

Urine cytology may reveal malignant cells and is a useful screening test. Negative urinalysis, however, should not exclude further investigations.

Intravenous urography

This may demonstrate a filling defect in the bladder and renal tract obstruction if present. It is also important to exclude tumours in other parts of the urinary tract since a generalized instability of the urothelium is often present with multiple tumours developing between the renal pelvis and the urethra.

Cystoscopy

Cystoscopy is the definitive investigation at which mucosal abnormalities can be carefully documented and biopsies taken. Transurethral resection of bladder tumour (TURBT) can also be performed during the course of this.

Computed tomography scan

This will demonstrate extravesical extension of tumour and lymph node enlargement if present. Typical appearances of a large bladder cancer are shown in Fig. 10.7.

Staging

The TNM staging system (see Chapter 2) is commonly used.

- Tis – carcinoma *in situ*.
- T1 – superficial invasive carcinoma confined to subepithelial connective tissue.
- T2 – invasion of bladder muscle:
  2a – invasion of superficial muscle;
  2b – invasion of deep muscle.
- T3 – invasion through muscle wall of bladder.
- T4 – disease beyond the bladder:
  4a – invasion of surrounding pelvic structures;
  4b – distant metastases.

The important features in deciding on appropriate therapy are the extent of local invasion into the bladder wall, tumour differentiation and distant spread.

Treatment

LOCAL RESECTION

Transurethral resection is performed for superficial (T1) bladder tumours followed by careful cystoscopic surveillance. Recurrence will occur in around 50 per cent and progression to a higher stage or worse grade will occur in around 15 per cent. This is

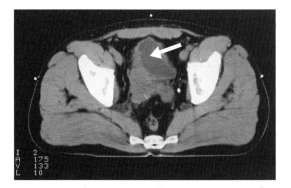

FIG 10.7 Computed tomography scan showing extensive bladder cancer with extravesical extension.

particularly the case in large tumours, high-grade tumours and those with multiple areas of mucosal dysplasia or frank malignancy. In patients that fail initial resection further local resection may be attempted. Where there are multiple recurrences and when there is progression to a high-grade tumour then alternative therapies may be required.

INTRAVESICAL CHEMOTHERAPY

This will improve local control of superficial bladder cancer. Various agents have been used, including Adriamycin, thiotepa and mitomycin C. More recently, BCG has been used and may give better results, although a higher incidence of local complications may occur and, although rare, pulmonary infection has been reported. Typically, an initial course of weekly instillations for 6 weeks is given; there is some evidence that maintenance treatment thereafter may reduce the incidence of relapse.

RADICAL RADIOTHERAPY

This may take the form of an interstitial implant for localized superficial bladder tumours or more usually external beam treatment. This is indicated for progressive high-grade T1 tumours and as initial treatment for T2 and T3 tumours.

Preoperative radiotherapy may be selected for patients undergoing primary surgery for invasive bladder cancer.

CYSTECTOMY

This may be considered for progressive superficial bladder cancer and locally advanced muscle-invading tumours. There is some evidence that elective preoperative radiotherapy improves results compared with surgery alone as a primary treatment for invasive bladder cancer. It is also used to salvage recurrence after radical radiotherapy and involves removal of the bladder and perivesical tissues together with pelvic lymphadenectomy.

For multifocal lesions, urethrectomy is also recommended. Urine is diverted via an ileal conduit to the abdominal wall.

Partial cystectomy is occasionally used for a localized superficial tumour or where there is only minimal muscle invasion.

There are two prevailing philosophies in the treatment of invasive bladder cancer. Many centres offer all patients radical radiotherapy and reserve surgery for salvage. This approach results in initial bladder preservation and complete regression of the bladder tumour in around 60 per cent but local recurrence requiring salvage surgery may occur in over half of these. The alternative approach is to offer selected patients, particularly those under 65 years, elective cystectomy with which 5-year survivals of around 35 per cent are to be expected, with or without bladder preservation. No survival advantage between these two approaches has become apparent.

PALLIATIVE TREATMENT

This may be required for locally advanced tumours or in the frail and elderly who cannot tolerate radical treatment. Local radiotherapy will help haematuria and local pain, given in short, low-dose schedules over 1 or 2 weeks.

Bladder cancer is sensitive to chemotherapy. Currently drug combinations such as CMV (cisplatin, methotrexate and vinblastine) or gemcitabine with cisplatin are used and response rates of 50–60 per cent can be achieved, some of which are complete responses. There is no role for chemotherapy in the routine primary management of bladder cancer but useful palliation may be obtained in selected patients with symptoms related to uncontrolled local tumour or soft tissue metastases.

Tumour-related complications

Complications include haematuria, leading to clot retention and clot colic, and ureteric obstruction, leading to hydronephrosis and renal failure.

Treatment-related complications

SURGERY

Cystectomy has an operative mortality particularly in the elderly. Stoma problems (e.g. prolapse, bleeding or stricture) may arise and impotence occurs.

RADIOTHERAPY

This may result in both bowel and bladder damage.

Prognosis

The 10-year cause-specific survival ranges from around 70 per cent for T1 bladder cancer to 20 per cent for T3 and less than 5 per cent for T4 tumours.

Screening and future developments

Urine cytology is currently in use for patients at high risk by virtue of industrial exposure to known bladder carcinogens.

Chemoradiation combinations are under investigation to improve the results of local treatment and surgical developments in reconstructive surgery enable increasing numbers of patients to consider bladder reconstruction after cystectomy.

Rarer tumours

The squamous and adenocarcinomas of the bladder are in general treated in the same way as the transitional cell tumours. Generally, their prognosis is worse and they respond less well to non-surgical treatments.

CANCER OF THE TESTIS

Epidemiology

Testicular tumours occur most commonly in men aged between 20 years and 40 years. In the UK, there are almost 1500 cases per year with an incidence of 57 per million, which is five times the incidence in Japan. In the USA it is more common in white people than in black people.

Aetiology

Many testicular tumours are thought to arise as a developmental abnormality in those with mal-descent, which increases the likelihood of a testicular tumour by up to 40-fold. Other factors are a contralateral testicular tumour (the incidence of second malignancy in the other testis being around 3 per cent) and possibly previous orchitis, although this remains speculative.

Pathology

There are two main types of testicular tumour: seminoma and teratoma. Around 40 per cent are seminomas and 32 per cent teratomas, with a further 14 per cent which contain components of both seminoma and teratoma.

Macroscopically, seminomas are solid tumours, well circumscribed, often lobulated and pale in appearance. In contrast, teratomas are often haemorrhagic and contain cystic areas.

Microscopically, seminoma is composed of sheets of uniform rounded cells and may contain granulomata. Particularly well-differentiated variants are recognized (spermatocytic seminoma) as are more aggressive types (anaplastic seminoma). In contrast, teratoma may contain a range of cell types with varying differentiation. Undifferentiated teratoma contains no recognizable mature elements. Trophoblastic elements may predominate and there may be recognizable yolk sac elements.

Natural history

Testicular tumours invade locally into the tunica vaginalis and along the spermatic cord. Lymph node spread occurs relatively early to para-aortic nodes and thence to mediastinal nodes. Blood-borne spread is most commonly to the lungs and liver.

Symptoms

These include:

- testicular swelling or discomfort, particularly with a past history of maldescent;
- gynaecomastia due to excess β-human chorionic gonadotrophin (HCG) secretion from the tumour;
- backache from enlarged para-aortic nodes;
- cough, haemoptysis or dyspnoea from lung metastases.

Signs

These may include:

- testicular swelling, which may have an associated hydrocele;
- central abdominal mass due to palpable para-aortic nodes;
- pleural effusion;
- gynaecomastia due to stimulation by high levels of HCG.

Differential diagnosis

The following conditions will need to be ruled out:

- benign hydrocele;
- testicular torsion;
- other causes of backache, such as degenerative spinal disease;
- other causes of lymphadenopathy (e.g. lymphoma).

Investigations

Routine investigations may demonstrate renal impairment due to ureteric obstruction by enlarged para-aortic nodes. Abnormal liver function tests may reflect liver metastases. Chest X-ray may demonstrate metastases as either lung deposits or pleural effusion.

Ultrasound

Testicular ultrasound will demonstrate a solid mass, sometimes with cystic elements in the testis.

Serum markers

There are specific serum markers for germ cell tumours. These are serum α-fetoprotein (AFP) and HCG and should be measured both prior to any surgical intervention and serially thereafter. Their value in monitoring response to treatment is shown in Fig. 10.8. Placental alkaline phosphatase is of value for seminoma but is also affected by cigarette smoking and may therefore be misleading in smokers, and lactate dehydrogenase (LDH) is a further marker of use in seminoma.

Around 90 per cent of patients with teratoma will have elevated AFP or HCG and 40–50 per cent will have both markers raised. The absolute level and rate of fall after treatment are useful prognostic features.

Computed tomography scan

A CT scan of the pelvis and abdomen is essential to evaluate pelvic nodes and liver and a CT scan of the lungs will give accurate assessment of lung metastases. Figure 10.9 demonstrates the appearances of para-aortic lymph involvement and lung metastases on CT scan.

Staging

The TNM staging system (see Chapter 2) is sometimes used to describe the extent of the primary tumour but for the overall disease the Royal Marsden Hospital staging system is more widely applied (Table 10.3).

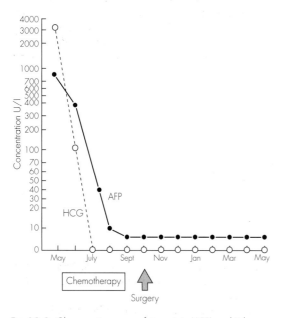

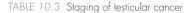

Fig 10.8 Changes in serum α-fetoprotein (AFP) and β-human chorionic gonadotrophin (HCG) from diagnosis through treatment with chemotherapy and later surgical removal of a residual tumour mass in a patient presenting with advanced testicular germ cell tumour.

TABLE 10.3 *Staging of testicular cancer*

T stage	
Tl	Limited to testis
T2	Involving tunica albuginea or epididymis
T3	Invading spermatic cord
T4	Invading scrotum
N1	Single node <2 cm max diameter
N2	Single node 2–5 cm max diameter or multiple nodes <5 cm max diameter
N3	Any node >5 cm max diameter
M1	Distant metastases
Royal Marsden stage	
I	Limited to testis
II	Involving nodes below diaphragm
III	Involving nodes both sides of diaphragm
IV	Distant metastases
IVL	Lungs
IVH	Liver

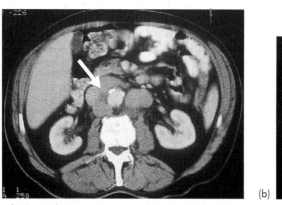

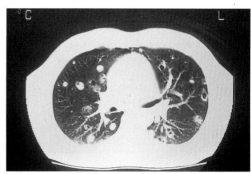

Fig 10.9 Computed tomography scans demonstrating (a) enlarged para-aortic lymph nodes and (b) lung metastases from testicular teratoma.

Treatment

All patients will proceed to inguinal orchidectomy with removal of the affected testis. Scrotal interference should be avoided at all costs because of the risk of tumour implantation in the scrotal wound and subsequent relapse.

STAGE 1 TUMOURS

If there is no evidence of residual tumour after surgery then the prognosis is extremely good and around 85 per cent of patients will be cured with no further treatment.

Seminomas proceed to a course of radiotherapy to the para-aortic nodes. A low dose of only 20 Gy is required. As an alternative to this, a single course of carboplatin is under evaluation.

Teratomas are entered into a programme of intensive surveillance with monthly measurement of serum markers and regular abdominal and chest CT scans. Those with adverse features such as anaplastic tumour and vascular invasion will receive a short course of chemotherapy.

STAGE 2, 3 OR 4 TUMOURS

Seminomas will proceed to chemotherapy for all but those with very small para-aortic nodes. The drugs used are usually cisplatin or carboplatin with the possible addition of etoposide. Small-volume disease may be treated by radiotherapy alone to the para-aortic and pelvic nodes and radiotherapy may be given following chemotherapy in other patients.

Teratomas will proceed to chemotherapy. For good prognosis tumours, standard chemotherapy will be 3-weekly cycles of BEP (bleomycin, etoposide and cisplatin). High-risk patients with extensive disease or very high markers (AFP >1000 U/l, HCG >10 000 U/l) will receive more intensive regimes using weekly administration of alternating drug schedules containing bleomycin, vincristine, cisplatin, methotrexate and etoposide (BOP or POMBACE).

In recurrent or resistant cases there is increasing use of high-dose chemotherapy with peripheral blood progenitor cell or autologous bone marrow support.

PELVIC SURGERY

Pelvic lymphadenectomy is advocated as part of the primary treatment of germ cell tumours in some centres, particularly in the USA. In the UK and Europe, it is more usual to give initial treatment with chemotherapy and use surgery electively for those patients with primary teratomas and having residual tumour masses after full chemotherapy. This occurs in around 20 per cent of patients and excision of these masses is important to remove not only residual malignant teratoma but also benign differentiated teratoma, since this retains the potential to develop into a malignant form at a later date. At surgery, approximately 20 per cent are malignant teratoma, 50 per cent differentiated teratoma and the remainder are necrotic with no viable tumour.

Tumour-related complications

Gynaecomastia sometimes occurs owing to high levels of HCG.

Treatment-related complications

Unilateral orchidectomy has no physiological effect on potency but this may be affected after pelvic lymphadenectomy.

Abdominal radiotherapy may be related to subsequent peptic ulceration.

Chemotherapy causes alopecia, which is reversible. Cisplatin may cause peripheral neuropathy and ototoxicity. Renal impairment, which is usually reversible may also occur. Bleomycin may cause skin changes and pneumonitis in high doses.

Fertility is impaired after chemotherapy but recovery usually occurs after standard BEP chemotherapy and there are increasing reports of success in fathering children after treatment for testicular cancer. Despite this, semen storage is routinely advised for patients undergoing this type of chemotherapy. Potency is not affected.

Prognosis

Few patients now die from testicular cancer. Cure is virtually guaranteed for stage 1 tumours and is expected in around 85 per cent of those with more advanced stages. However relapse after primary chemotherapy heralds a poor outlook, with only 20–30 per cent of patients surviving long term with salvage treatment.

Screening

Health education programmes aimed at self examination are the main form of population screening.

Rarer tumours

The remaining tumours that occur in the testis are lymphomas (7 per cent) and the rare pure yolk sac tumours, Sertoli cell tumours and interstitial cell tumours. Mesotheliomas arising from the tunica vaginalis are also described. Lymphomas are managed as for any extranodal lymphoma while other rare tumours are managed by surgical excision.

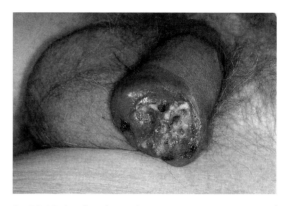

FIG 10.10 Locally advanced primary squamous carcinoma of the penis with destruction of the glans.

CANCER OF THE PENIS

Epidemiology

Penile cancer is rare in the UK with only 300 cases reported per year, and it accounts for less than 1 per cent of deaths from cancer in men. It is more common in other parts of the world, particularly in Africa and China where it accounts for around 15 per cent of male cancers.

Aetiology

It is virtually unknown in populations that practise circumcision. A relationship with papilloma virus has been proposed.

Pathology

Macroscopically, it may be a papilliferous or solid growth on the shaft or glans of the penis. Ulceration may occur. It may develop insidiously beneath the foreskin.

Microscopically, penile cancer is a squamous carcinoma, often well or moderately differentiated.

Natural history

The tumour will invade the shaft of the penis as shown in Fig. 10.10 and spread to inguinal lymph nodes, as shown in Fig. 10.11. Blood-borne spread occurs relatively late to lungs and liver.

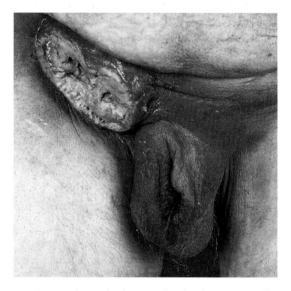

FIG 10.11 Advanced right inguinal nodes disease caused by metastases from a carcinoma of the penis. The primary tumour was treated some months earlier when no metastases were apparent by amputation.

Symptoms

Tumours are usually asymptomatic but there may be local discharge and odour.

Signs

The primary tumour is usually obvious on clinical examination. Palpable inguinal nodes are present in up to half of patients.

Differential diagnosis

Other penile skin lesions should be considered, including lymphogranuloma venereum, condylomata acuminata, chancroid, traumatic ulceration, leucoplakia, Bowen's disease, erythroplasia of Queyrat and giant penile condylomata (Buschke–Lowenstein tumour).

Other causes of inguinal lymphadenopathy need to be taken into account, in particular chronic infection, which accounts for around 50 per cent of the associated lymphadenopathy.

Investigations

Routine investigations are rarely helpful, although a chest X-ray will be necessary to exclude lung metastases.

Biopsy

A biopsy or cytological scrapings will confirm the diagnosis.

Fine-needle aspiration

Fine-needle aspiration (FNA) of enlarged nodes should be used to distinguish metastatic nodes from infected and inflammatory nodes.

Computed tomography scan

Where inguinal nodes are involved, a pelvic CT scan is of value to assess further lymphatic spread.

Staging

The commonly used staging system is the Jackson staging which is shown alongside the formal TNM staging (see Chapter 2) in Table 10.4.

Treatment

RADICAL TREATMENT

This will be appropriate even where there is inguinal node involvement.

Surgery

This will usually involve partial or complete amputation, as shown in Fig. 10.11, unless the tumour is small and confined to the prepuce when local excision by circumcision may be adequate. Penile reconstruction may be considered.

Radiotherapy

This can be delivered by either external beam treatment or the use of brachytherapy with an interstitial implant or penile mould. The penis is preserved reserving surgery for salvage.

Treatment of involved nodes should be by block dissection of the groin. In the case of fixed inoperable nodes, local irradiation can be performed. Advanced fixed fungating nodes are shown in Fig. 10.10.

PALLIATIVE TREATMENT

This may be indicated for locally advanced disease or where there are distant metastases. Usually, a short palliative course of radiotherapy to the primary site, nodes or local recurrence will help prevent local pain and fungation.

There is no recognized chemotherapy for penile cancer, although responses are seen in advanced disease using schedules containing drugs such as cisplatin, methotrexate, 5-FU and mitomycin C.

Tumour-related complications

Interference with micturition and potency is seen.

TABLE 10.4 Staging for cancer of the penis

T Stage		Jackson stage	
T1	Superficial subepithelial	I	Limited to glans or prepuce
T2	Invading corpus cavernosa	II	Invading shaft; no nodes
T3	Invading urethra or prostate	III	Invading shaft; node positive
T4	Invading adjacent structures	IV	Fixed inoperable nodes or distant metastases

Treatment-related complications

Radiotherapy may result in urethral stricture in about 10 per cent of cases.

Prognosis

Survival with stage 1 disease is over 85 per cent at 5 years falling to 35 per cent for stage 3 tumours. Long-term survival with stage 4 disease is unusual.

11 GYNAECOLOGICAL CANCER

CERVICAL CANCER

Epidemiology

Carcinoma of the cervix accounts for around 20 per cent of cancers in women, being third in order of incidence after breast and lung cancer, with over 4500 cases each year in the UK and an annual incidence of 17 per 100 000. It is predominantly a disease of women in their 40s and 50s but is showing an increase in younger age groups. It is common in lower socio-economic groups and there is a wide geographical variation, the highest levels of the disease being in South America with incidence figures of up to 80 in 100 000.

Aetiology

It is associated with sexual activity, particularly in women starting intercourse at an early age and having multiple partners. It is more common in women that are or that have been married than in single women. There is some evidence that the male partner is implicated, being associated with partners of lower socio-economic groups and the identification of high-risk males who have more than one partner that develops cervical cancer.

A common factor uniting the above risk factors may be viral infection, with both herpes simplex type 2 infection and human papilloma virus types 16 and 18 being implicated in cervical carcinogenesis.

Pathology

Macroscopically, there are two common presentations:

- proliferative growth at the cervix with surface ulceration;
- diffusely infiltrating tumour with the mucosa intact due to tumour arising in the endocervical canal (the latter is sometimes described as a 'barrel-cervix').

Microscopically, 95 per cent of cervical cancers are squamous carcinomas of varying differentiation. The remaining 5 per cent are adenocarcinomas arising from the external os or endocervix.

Natural history

Local spread in all directions occurs as shown in Fig. 11.1. Lymph node spread occurs relatively early, being identified in around 15 per cent of stage 1 tumours.

From paracervical nodes there is spread to internal and external iliac nodes, presacral and obturator nodes. Subsequent spread is then up the para-aortic node chain. Blood-borne metastases occur, affecting in particular the lungs, liver and bone.

Symptoms

Presentation is frequently asymptomatic as a result of an abnormal cervical smear test. Local pain is

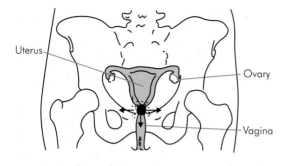

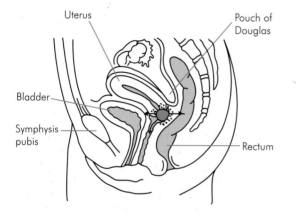

FIG 11.1 Patterns of local spread from cervical carcinoma.

unusual unless there is extensive pelvic infiltration. If symptoms are present they may include:

- vaginal bleeding, particularly after intercourse;
- vaginal discharge;
- renal failure owing to bilateral ureteric obstruction;
- haematuria or rectal bleeding owing to local spread;
- low back and sacral pain owing to pelvic and para-aortic lymphadenopathy;
- general symptoms of malignancy, including anorexia, malaise and weight loss.

Signs

Pelvic examination is mandatory, at which the tumour will usually be apparent at the cervix as a proliferative or ulcerative growth or a diffuse infiltration. It is important to note extension onto the vaginal mucosa, and on rectal examination any evidence of spread into the parametrium or rectal mucosa.

Differential diagnosis

Other cervical lesions should be considered, such as a cervical erosion.

Where bladder or rectal involvement is diagnosed it may be difficult to distinguish clinically between primary tumours of these sites invading the cervix, although this is usually apparent on histology.

Investigations

Routine investigations may reveal anaemia due to bleeding and a raised white cell count where there has been chronic infection. Renal failure will be apparent on routine biochemical tests and a chest X-ray will be needed to exclude metastases.

Cervical cytology

This may have been performed to diagnose malignancy and vaginal swabs taken at the same time may demonstrate the nature of an infective discharge.

Biopsy

A full examination under anaesthetic including a cystoscopy should be performed in all cases, at which time biopsies can also be taken.

Computed tomography scan

A computed tomography (CT) scan of the abdomen and pelvis will help assess local extension and enlargement of pelvic and para-aortic lymph nodes.

Intravenous urography

Intravenous urography (IVU) will assess ureteric obstruction, although this can now usually be seen clearly on CT.

Magnetic resonance imaging

For definition of soft tissue changes around the cervix and assessment of the primary tumour magnetic resonance (magnetic resonance imaging, MRI) is superior to CT, as shown in Fig. 11.2

Staging

The FIGO staging system is generally accepted in clinical assessment of cervical cancer.

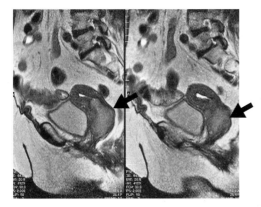

Fɪɢ 11.2 Magnetic resonance imaging scan demonstrating locally advanced carcinoma of the cervix.

- Stage 1 – A, microinvasive disease limited to the cervix;
  B, confined to the cervix with invasion >5 mm depth from surface or >7 mm spread in a horizontal direction.
- Stage 2 – A, extension to vaginal mucosa but not into lower third of vagina;
  B, extension to parametrium but not reaching pelvic side wall.
- Stage 3 – A, extension to lower third of vagina;
  B, extension to pelvic side wall.
- Stage 4 – A, involvement of bladder and rectal mucosa;
  B, distant metastases.

Case history: cancer of the cervix

A 38-year-old woman presents with a 3-month history of post-coital bleeding. One year previously she had a normal cervical smear report when she saw her general practitioner (GP) for family planning advice. The GP has referred her to a consultant gynaecologist, having performed a pelvic examination at which he found a hard irregular cervix and considered the likely cause of bleeding to be a cervical carcinoma. The gynaecologist confirmed the clinical history and on examination found a hard ulcerating tumour at the cervix with no obvious extension beyond this site. He subsequently performed examination under anaesthetic confirming a stage 1B carcinoma of the cervix with no parametrial or vaginal extension. A biopsy showed poorly differentiated squamous carcinoma. A cystoscopy was normal.

Further investigations included a normal full blood count and chest X-ray, a magnetic resonance imaging (MRI) scan confirmed a 3 cm mass at the cervix but no extension beyond that and an intravenous urography (IVU) was normal. Treatment was recommended with radical hysterectomy at which the uterus and cervix with an upper cuff of vagina and parametrial tissue were removed together with a pelvic lymph node dissection. Histological examination of the specimen confirmed a moderately differentiated carcinoma of the cervix but three out of five left pelvic lymph nodes were positive and two out of eight right-sided pelvic lymph nodes were positive. As a result of this finding, postoperative radiotherapy was recommended. The patient received a standard 5-week course of postoperative radiotherapy to the pelvis. During this time she experienced some diarrhoea and urinary frequency.

Three months later she was well but complaining of some bowel frequency attributed to the radiotherapy. When seen 6 months later she complained of some persistent low back pain. Clinical examination was normal but a computed tomography (CT) scan showed large lymph nodes in the para-aortic region. The chest X-ray showed three small volume metastases in the left lung field and five metastases in the right lung.

Chemotherapy was recommended. The patient received a course of cisplatin, methotrexate and bleomycin. During treatment she suffered nausea and vomiting, and for the following week had some nausea but otherwise tolerated the treatment well. She returned 3 weeks later for a second course of treatment, which had similar side-effects. Two weeks later she returned to the hospital earlier than planned with persistent nausea and vomiting. She was drowsy and slightly confused. Urgent investigations revealed a serum creatinine of 800 and abdominal ultrasound showed bilateral hydronephrosis. Bilateral nephrostomies were inserted and over the subsequent three days as urine drainage was re-established her creatinine fell to 260. At this point she developed a high fever and her full blood count had fallen with a profound neutropenia, total neutrophil count 0.3. She was treated with intravenous antibiotics using ceftazidime but continued to have a high fever. The culture from her urine draining through the nephrostomy showed a staphylococcal infection. Flucloxacillin was added to an antibiotic regimen and her fever settled. Two days later she complained of acute chest pain and shortness of breath. She became acutely hypotensive and despite active resuscitation died from a presumed pulmonary embolus.

Treatment

Radical treatment will be considered for all patients except those with widespread metastatic disease or bladder or rectal involvement. Presentation with renal failure is not an absolute contraindication to radical treatment and in selected cases percutaneous nephrostomies to re-establish renal drainage may be performed prior to treatment as shown in Fig. 11.3.

LOCALIZED TO THE CERVIX (STAGE 1)

Surgery

Radical surgery is the treatment of choice in the form of a radical hysterectomy (Wertheim's hysterectomy) during which, in addition to the removal of the uterus, tubes and ovaries, the upper vagina, parametrium and pelvic lymph nodes are also included in the resection.

Radiotherapy

Radical radiotherapy may be given for early stage cancer of the cervix and the results in terms of survival are no worse than those after radical surgery, although there may be a greater incidence of long-term morbidity. It is usually therefore reserved for elderly patients and those medically unfit for surgery but is an acceptable option for younger women that refuse surgery, and those with bulky (>4 cm) tumours.

Postoperative radiotherapy may be indicated following Wertheim's hysterectomy where the excision margins are not clear of tumour and where there is involvement of the removed pelvic lymph nodes in the resection.

Preoperative radiotherapy has been advocated in the past but it has no proven value and using the above criteria only 20 per cent of women will require irradiation in addition to surgery.

TUMOUR BEYOND CERVIX (STAGES 2 AND 3)

Radiotherapy

Radical radiotherapy will be the treatment of choice, increasingly given along with chemotherapy (see

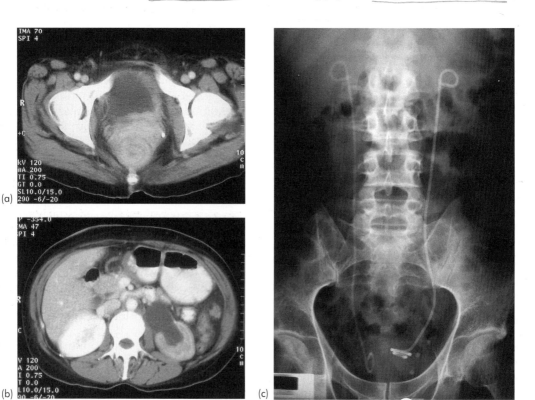

FIG 11.3 Computed tomography scan demonstrating (a) extensive local infiltration from cervical cancer into the bladder base (b) with associated hydronephrosis. Insertion of ureteric stents is necessary in this situation if renal function is to be preserved, as shown in the plain X-ray (c).

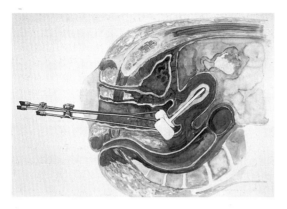

FIG 11.4 Intrauterine tube and vaginal sources in position for treatment of carcinoma of the cervix demonstrating their position relative to surrounding anatomical structures.

below). This will involve a course of external beam treatment to the whole pelvis covering the major node chains up to the bifurcation of the aorta, delivering a dose of 40–50 Gy over 4–5 weeks. Intracavitary treatment to the cervix will follow this, using an intrauterine tube and vaginal source to give a further 25–30 Gy to the cervix and surrounding tissues. A typical arrangement of intracavitary applicators is shown in Fig. 11.4.

Chemotherapy

There is now evidence to suggest that the results of radical radiotherapy for cervical cancer are improved if chemotherapy is given during radiotherapy. The optimum drugs and timing of chemotherapy is currently under investigation but cisplatin is probably an important component of any chemoradiation schedule given once or twice weekly during the 5 weeks of external beam treatment.

In contrast, the use of adjuvant chemotherapy, usually given prior to radiotherapy in locally advanced disease, has been disappointing and to date no proven advantage has emerged in clinical trials.

PALLIATIVE TREATMENT

Where there are distant metastases or locally advanced pelvic disease then radical local treatment is inappropriate. Chemotherapy for advanced and recurrent disease has only limited activity and complete response is extremely rare. The most effective drug schedules are combinations of cisplatin, methotrexate and ifosfamide, and there may be considerable associated toxicity.

Palliative radiotherapy for advanced local disease may be worthwhile and is particularly indicated for the control of local bleeding and pelvic pain. Other procedures such as a palliative colostomy may be required where there is rectal involvement or fistulae develop.

HORMONE REPLACEMENT

Cervical cancer is not hormone dependent. This means that hormone manipulation is not a useful approach to treatment but also that following radical treatment, in young women in particular, hormone replacement therapy should be considered.

Tumour-related complications

These include:

- renal failure owing to bilateral ureteric obstruction;
- acute haemorrhage from the tumour may occasionally result in hypovolaemic shock;
- fistulae between bladder or rectum and vagina;
- pyometra owing to obstruction of the cervical canal by tumour.

Treatment-related complications

Radical surgery may result in urinary urgency and urge or stress incontinence. Lower limb lymphoedema following pelvic node dissection may also be seen.

Radical radiotherapy may result acutely in bowel and bladder toxicity with radiation cystitis and diarrhoea. Chemoradiation schedules may enhance the toxicities of radiotherapy and, in addition, cause pancytopenia with the risk of neutropenic sepsis. Long-term sequelae from radiotherapy may include reduced bladder volume, telangiectasia causing haematuria or rectal bleeding, chronic diarrhoea and vaginal stenosis. Rarely, bowel or bladder fistulae may occur, although subsequent investigations often reveal recurrent disease in this setting.

Prognosis

Outcome is closely related to stage at presentation, with a 5-year survival of around 80 per cent for stage 1 and 2A tumours, falling to only 20–30 per cent for stage 3 and less than 5 per cent for stage 4. Within stage 1 tumours, prognosis is related to tumour bulk and differentiation.

For microinvasive and *in situ* carcinoma of the cervix surgery is almost always curative, emphasizing the importance of early diagnosis in this condition, where curative treatment is readily available for early stage disease.

Screening

Screening for cervical neoplasia by cervical smear testing is widespread and there is good evidence that in the USA and Scandinavia the rate of decline in cervical cancer can be related to intensity of screening.

Around 3 million cervical smears are performed in the UK each year and it has been estimated that this has reduced the incidence of invasive cancers by around 30 per cent. Current recommendations are for all sexually active women below the age of 50 years to have cervical smears at 3- to 5-yearly intervals. A major problem with this, as with any screening programme is to achieve good rates of compliance, particularly in those groups at high risk. It is also important to recognize the limitation of smear screening since a number of women will still be diagnosed despite having a recent normal smear. Overall, the accuracy of cervical smear cytology is only around 80 per cent despite technically good smears and accurate interpretation.

Future prospects

The greatest impact is likely to be made by extending the current screening programmes to reach all those women at risk with high rates of compliance in order to detect early curable disease.

Current developments in treatment are looking at optimizing the use of chemoradiation in advanced disease.

Rarer tumours

Five per cent of cervical cancers are adenocarcinomas. These are generally treated in the same way as the more common squamous cancers and, stage for stage, they have a similar prognosis.

ENDOMETRIAL CANCER

Epidemiology

Compared with cancer of the cervix, cancer of the endometrium affects the older, predominantly postmenopausal age group, the median age at presentation being 61 years. The incidence in the UK is 14 per 100 000, similar to that of cervical cancer, with around 4000 cases each year, although the mortality is lower, which reflects its natural history. There is far less geographical variation than cervical cancer, although it is relatively rare in Japan where the incidence is about one-tenth of that in Europe and the USA.

Aetiology

Endometrial carcinoma occurs typically in obese nulliparous women who have a tendency to diabetes and cardiovascular disease.

High levels of circulating oestrogens are a known cause and it is a recognized complication of an oestrogen-secreting granulosa cell tumour of the ovary. There is no proven association with therapeutic use of oestrogens in hormone replacement therapy but there is increasing evidence linking endometrial cancer with prolonged tamoxifen use for breast cancer.

Pathology

Macroscopically, the tumour arises within the uterine cavity and may be polypoid or a more diffuse, even, multifocal growth arising from the endometrium.

Microscopically, the tumour is an adenocarcinoma which may be of varying grade, usually designated from G1 (well differentiated) to G3 (poorly differentiated). A serous papillary type is recognized which has a particularly poor prognosis.

Natural history

There is local invasion into the myometrium and cervix. The tubes and ovaries may also be involved and the tumour occasionally extends into parametrial tissues or involves the bladder or rectum. This is far less common than in cancer of the cervix.

Lymph node spread may occur, involving pelvic lymph nodes, and submucosal lymphatic permeation along the vaginal walls is well recognized. Distant metastases by blood-borne spread most frequently involve lungs and bone.

Symptoms

The classic presentation of endometrial cancer is with postmenopausal bleeding. In the premenopausal woman heavy and/or irregular periods may be the only symptom. There may be an associated vaginal discharge.

General symptoms of malaise, anorexia and weight loss are usually mild and symptoms from metastatic disease are unusual at presentation.

Signs

On pelvic examination the uterus may feel bulky and a vaginal discharge or bleeding from the os may be apparent. Often, no physical signs can be detected.

Differential diagnosis

Other causes of postmenopausal bleeding should be considered, such as atrophic vaginitis and, in premenopausal women, other causes of irregular menstrual bleeding such as fibroids.

Investigations

Routine investigations may reveal anaemia due to chronic blood loss. Other abnormalities are unusual.

Biopsy

While positive cytology may be obtained from cervical smears or sampling of the endometrial cavity this cannot be relied upon and the diagnosis is confirmed by examination of endometrial biopsies. These may be obtained by examination under anaesthetic, at which time the cervical canal and uterine cavity are dilated in turn and fractional curettage performed to obtain endometrial samples. However, increasingly this is being replaced by outpatient sampling using a pipelle and hysteroscopy with endometrial biopsy under direct vision.

Radiology

A chest X-ray will be performed to exclude distant metastases. Further imaging of the pelvis is usually reserved for more advanced cases (stages 2, 3 or 4) when a CT scan will be used to assess local spread and lymph node status.

Staging

Carcinoma of the endometrium is staged using the FIGO system.

- Stage 1 – A, confined to the endometrium, no myometrial invasion;
  B, confined to the endometrium, invasion <50 per cent of myometrium;
  C, confined to the endometrium, invasion >50 per cent of myometrium.
- Stage 2 – invasion of cervix.
- Stage 3 – spread to pelvic tissues.
- Stage 4 – A, spread to bladder or rectum;
  B, distant metastases.

Treatment

A major feature of endometrial cancer is the predominance of stage 1 tumours at presentation, accounting for 70–80 per cent of patients.

SURGERY

Total abdominal hysterectomy and bilateral salpingo-oophorectomy is the treatment of choice for disease localized to the endometrium.

A Wertheim's hysterectomy (see above) is indicated when there is cervical involvement (stage 2).

RADIOTHERAPY

Postoperative radiotherapy is considered for patients following hysterectomy for stage 1 disease, depending on the risk factors for local and distant dissemination. Well-differentiated tumours with myometrial invasion may receive vaginal irradiation only. Moderately or poorly differentiated tumours and those invading into outer third of the myometrium are considered to have a greater risk of lymph node spread and therefore receive both external beam radiotherapy to the pelvic nodes and intravaginal treatment.

Radical radiotherapy may, on occasions, be given for elderly unfit patients with stage 1 disease and is the treatment of choice for those with bulky stage 2 and stage 3 tumours. This will take the form of external beam treatment to the pelvis followed by intracavitary treatment to the uterine cavity and upper vagina.

PALLIATIVE TREATMENT

Palliative radiotherapy may be given for locally advanced tumours and for painful bone metastases.

Endometrial cancer is a hormone-dependent tumour and metastatic disease will respond to progestogens such as medroxyprogesterone acetate or megestrol. Response rates are between 20 per cent and 30 per cent, and useful palliation of symptomatic metastases may be achieved. Responses to gonadotrophin-releasing hormone analogues such as leuprorelin are also recognized. There is no good evidence to support the use of these agents as adjuvant treatment.

Occasionally, chemotherapy using cisplatin and Adriamycin may be offered to younger fit patients with advanced disease; objective tumour responses are seen in 20–30 per cent of patients.

Tumour-related complications

Pyometra or haematometra may occur owing to obstruction of the uterine cavity.

Treatment-related complications

Hysterectomy may result in urinary urgency and urge or stress incontinence. Pelvic radiotherapy may be associated with late bowel and bladder toxicity, causing frequency, haematuria, rectal bleeding and rectal or vaginal stenosis.

Prognosis

The prognosis for endometrial carcinoma is good since the majority of patients present with stage 1 disease for which there are cure rates in excess of 85 per cent. Prognosis for more advanced stages falls as would be anticipated, with 5-year survival rates of around 65 per cent for stage 2 and 35 per cent for stage 3. Survival stage for stage is worse for women over 60 years than younger women and also for those with the papillary serous type of cancer.

Prevention

The early diagnosis of endometrial cancer is aided by its early presentation with postmenopausal bleeding. It is therefore vital that all women with this symptom are investigated appropriately to exclude endometrial cancer.

Rarer tumours

Sarcomas of the endometrium may arise, presenting in the same way as endometrial cancer. They may be pure sarcomas, such as a leiomyosarcoma arising from a fibroid, or mixed tumours, such as the mixed mesodermal tumour which contains both epithelial and stromal components, the latter in the form of malignant sarcomatous cells.

The prognosis for endometrial sarcomas is poor. Treatment is surgical removal at hysterectomy and postoperative radiotherapy is usually given to reduce the likelihood of local relapse. There is no proven role for chemotherapy, although distant metastases are a common problem with these tumours.

OVARIAN CANCER

Epidemiology

There are almost 6000 cases of carcinoma of the ovary in the UK each year, accounting for around 5 per cent of cancer in women and over 4000 deaths per year. There is a similar incidence in the USA but a low incidence in Japan, which approaches that of American women in immigrants to the USA.

Aetiology

Ovarian cancer tends to occur in women over the age of 40 years that are nulliparous and of higher socio-economic groups. There is increasing evidence that genetic factors are important in the development of ovarian cancer, and a link with the breast cancer-associated gene *BRCA1* as well as with blood group A has been demonstrated.

No specific environmental agents have been identified as directly contributing to the development of ovarian cancer.

A familial pattern is seen in some cases.

Pathology

The common appearance of ovarian cancer is that of a cystic enlargement of the ovary. Two common types are recognized macroscopically:

- the pseudomucinous cyst, characteristically a large, multiloculated tumour mass containing mucinous material;
- the serous cyst, containing clear fluid within a thin-walled cyst containing papillary structures.

Other tumours may form solid masses (typical of a Brenner tumour) or characteristic teratomas.

The microscopic appearances of ovarian cancer are variable and the classification often complex.

Epithelial adenocarcinomas are the commonest ovarian cancers with several variants recognized, such as clear cell carcinomas and endometrioid carcinomas. Germ cell tumours are the other major group of tumours of the ovary but, in contrast, to the testis the majority are benign teratomas.

Rarer tumours include those derived from gonadal stroma, such as the granulosa cell and Sertoli cell tumours, which are, respectively, oestrogen- and androgen-secreting mixed mesodermal tumours analogous to those that grow in the uterus and lymphomas.

Metastases may also present in the ovary, typically from carcinoma of the breast or stomach (Krukenberg tumours).

Natural history

Local growth occurs within the ovary, spreading through the cyst wall onto the surface. Transcoelomic spread across the peritoneal cavity results in the classic appearance of multiple seedlings visible throughout the pelvic and abdominal cavities studding the peritoneal surfaces. Involvement of the omentum is also common and ascites is frequently found at operation.

Lymph node spread occurs to para-aortic nodes in the first instance. Blood-borne metastases to liver and lungs are seen in more advanced disease. Meig's syndrome is the presence of a pleural effusion accompanying an ovarian tumour which has the features of a transudate and is cytologically negative for carcinoma cells.

Symptoms

Ovarian cancer may remain asymptomatic for some time and often presents with vague symptoms of abdominal discomfort and pelvic pain. In more advanced cases this may be associated with abdominal swelling due to either tumour or ascites and urinary and bowel disturbance due to local pressure.

General symptoms of malignancy including malaise, anorexia and weight loss may also be present and metastases may cause dyspnoea or bone pain.

Signs

Abdominal swelling and distension with a palpable mass or clinical signs of free fluid (shifting dullness to percussion and a fluid thrill) may be present. An ovarian mass may be palpable per vaginam or per rectum and a pleural effusion may be detectable clinically by dullness to percussion and absent breath sounds. A left supraclavicular node may be palpable in advanced cases.

Differential diagnosis

Other causes of abdominal swelling should be considered, including ascites from other causes, hepatomegaly or splenomegaly, benign ovarian masses and intestinal obstruction.

Investigations

Routine investigations will often be unremarkable, although in advanced cases there may be electrolyte disturbance from intestinal obstruction or ureteric obstruction causing renal failure.

Radiography

Chest X-ray may demonstrate metastases or a pleural effusion.

Ultrasound

This will image the ovaries and give information regarding the nature of ovarian cysts. Liver ultrasound will evaluate the presence or absence of liver metastases.

Computed tomography scan

A CT scan of the abdomen and pelvis will demonstrate the primary tumour and also pelvic and para-aortic lymph node enlargement, together with liver metastases if present. An example of a massive intra-abdominal tumour mass from carcinoma of the ovary is shown in Fig. 11.5.

Serum markers

Serum CA125 is a valuable blood marker for ovarian cancer and is a useful monitor of response to treatment, as demonstrated in Fig. 11.6.

Creatinine or ethylenediamine tetra-acetic acid clearance

Creatinine clearance or ethylenediamine tetra-acetic acid (EDTA) clearance may be necessary to measure renal function for those patients requiring chemotherapy.

Staging

The FIGO staging system for ovarian cancer is in common use.

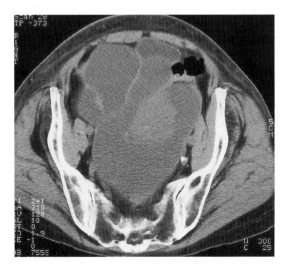

FIG 11.5 Computed tomography scan demonstrating extensive intra-abdominal tumour from carcinoma of the ovary.

- Stage 1 – confined to the ovary:
     (a) one ovary involved;
     (b) both ovaries involved.
- Stage 2 – Spread to the pelvis.
- Stage 3 – Spread to the abdominal cavity.
- Stage 4 – Blood-borne metastases.

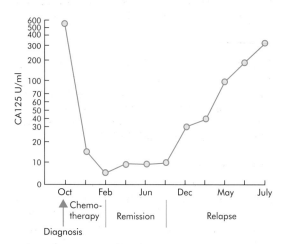

FIG 11.6 Changes in serum CA125 from high levels at diagnosis, falling through chemotherapy and later rising at relapse.

Treatment

SURGERY

All patients with operable disease will proceed to laparotomy at which total abdominal hysterectomy, bilateral salpingo-oophorectomy and omentectomy are performed, together with careful examination of the para-aortic nodes, liver and peritoneal surfaces including the subdiaphragmatic regions and biopsy of any suspicious areas. Prognosis is directly related to the residual bulk of tumour and so maximum tumour debulking should be attempted in all patients, even where complete clearance is not possible.

CHEMOTHERAPY

For patients with stage 1 disease adjuvant chemotherapy with six cycles of cerboplatin or cisplatin is recommended.

For more advanced disease localized to the abdominopelvic cavity (i.e. stages 2 and 3), chemotherapy is also indicated. The drugs of choice are currently cisplatin or its analogue carboplatin, given for six cycles at monthly intervals together with paclitaxel.

Case history: cancer of the ovary

A 48-year-old woman presents with a 1-year history of intermittent abdominal discomfort and a 1-month history of progressive abdominal distension. An abdominal ultrasound has shown a complex mass in the left ovary. Her CA125 is measured at 3562. Other investigations including a full blood count, renal function and chest X-ray are normal. She proceeds to laparotomy at which a large clinically malignant tumour is seen in the right ovary, with multiple seedlings found throughout the abdominal cavity. Five litres of ascites are drained from the abdominal cavity. A total abdominal hysterectomy, bilateral salpingo-oophorectomy is performed leaving behind multiple small nodules on the peritoneum. Postoperatively, a course of chemotherapy is recommended. She proceeds to receive a five course treatment of carboplatin and paclitaxel. During treatment she suffers alopecia and complains at the end of her course of tingling in the fingers, particularly when attempting to use them for fine movements. Her CA125 at completion of chemotherapy has fallen to 23.

Following chemotherapy she makes a good recovery and returns to a normal lifestyle.

Two years later she presents to her casualty department with a 3-day history of nausea, vomiting and constipation. On clinical examination she is found to be in intestinal obstruction. An emergency laparotomy is performed which reveals widespread multiple areas of obstruction of the small bowel secondary to scattered nodules of tumour. Biopsy confirms recurrence of her ovarian cancer. No attempt at resection is made and postoperatively she makes a slow but steady recovery with gradual resolution of her obstructive symptoms. Second-line chemotherapy is offered but she declines. Within 2-weeks she has a further episode of abdominal obstruction which is managed conservatively with intravenous fluids and subcutaneous diamorphine and cyclizine. The symptoms are well-controlled but her general condition deteriorates and she dies peacefully 10 days later.

For stage 4 disease with soft tissue metastases the outlook is poor and treatment may not influence the outcome. For patients with good general status, chemotherapy may be considered as for earlier stage disease. This group of patients may be considered for developmental chemotherapy, and the role of high-dose chemotherapy with bone marrow support is also being evaluated in this setting.

PALLIATIVE TREATMENT

Chemotherapy may be of value where relapse occurs after a long period of remission (>1 year). Relapse within the first year responds less well to further chemotherapy and heralds a particularly poor prognosis.

Radiotherapy may be of value for symptomatic pelvic masses, vaginal bleeding from disease invading the vagina and bone metastases.

Tumour-related complications

Ascites and pleural effusions may occur. Intestinal obstruction is common in the advanced phases of the disease.

Treatment-related complications

Cisplatin may cause neurotoxicity with peripheral neuropathy or less frequently spinal cord damage. Ototoxicity may result in tinnitus and high-tone deafness. Reduced renal function is common but overt renal failure should not occur provided that the patient is well hydrated and renal function is properly monitored.

Both paclitaxel and carboplatin may cause significant bone marrow depression. Paclitaxel will in addition cause alopecia and may be associated with peripheral neuropathy.

Prognosis

The outlook for stage 1 ovarian cancer is good, with 10-year survival figures of over 80 per cent. For more advanced disease the results of current chemotherapy give 5-year survival figures of 35–50 per cent. The survival of patients with stage 4 disease is usually only a few months.

Screening

Screening programmes for ovarian cancer have been proposed using serum CA125 measurements and abdominal ultrasound. At present they are recommended for those with a strong positive family history but routine population screening is not justified.

Rare tumours

Brenner tumours

These are fibromas of the ovary and are usually benign in nature. Treatment is surgical removal.

Teratomas

Arising in the ovary, these are usually benign although malignant teratomas analogous to those arising in the testis are recognized. Treatment should include adjuvant chemotherapy following surgical removal using drug combinations such as BEP (bleomycin, etoposide and cisplatin).

Dysgerminomas

These are germ cell tumours arising in the ovary analogous to seminomas arising in the testis. For stage 1 tumours, surgery is often curative. More advanced tumours are usually very radio-sensitive and postoperative pelvic radiotherapy is recommended. Chemotherapy using drugs such as VAC (vincristine, actinomycin D and cyclophosphamide) may be used for more widespread disease.

Granulosa cell tumours

These are usually low grade and generally cured by surgery although local recurrence some years later is recognized. Characteristically, they secrete oestrogens and may be associated with the synchronous development of an endometrial cancer.

Sertoli–Leydig cell tumours

These are usually of low malignant potential and cured by oophorectomy.

Sarcomas

These are rare and typically mixed mesodermal tumours having both sarcomatous and epithelial elements. Their prognosis is poor unless localized within the ovary at the time of surgery.

Lymphomas

These may arise within the ovary and are typically high-grade non-Hodgkin's lymphomas treated as extranodal lymphomas at any other site with adjuvant chemotherapy with or without pelvic radiotherapy.

Metastases

These may present in the ovary, usually from stomach or breast cancer. The classic bilateral ovarian metastases from carcinoma of the stomach are sometimes referred to as Krukenberg tumours.

CANCER OF THE VAGINA

Epidemiology

Carcinoma of the vagina is rare, accounting for only 1 per cent of all gynaecological cancer and around 130 deaths each year in the UK. It is a disease predominantly of elderly women unless associated with maternal use of stilboestrol.

Aetiology

Chronic irritation of the vaginal mucosa is typically seen following long-term use of a vaginal ring pessary for vaginal prolapse.

Maternal use of stilboestrol during pregnancy is associated with the development of clear cell adenocarcinoma of the vagina during adolescence.

Vaginal intraepithelial neoplasia (VAIN) is a recognized epithelial change analogous to cervical intra-epithelial neoplasia (CIN) at the cervix and may progress to frank carcinoma.

Pathology

Macroscopically, the tumour may present as an ulcer, papilliferous growth or diffuse infiltration of the vaginal mucosa. Microscopically, the usual picture is of a squamous carcinoma. Rarely, adenocarcinomas may arise and there is a clear cell variant related to maternal stilboestrol use.

Natural history

Direct extension results in invasion of the parametrium, bladder or rectum. Lymph node spread is to internal iliac and pelvic nodes (from the upper two thirds of the vagina) and to inguinal and femoral nodes (from the lower third). Blood-borne spread to liver and lungs may also occur in advanced disease.

Symptoms

These include vaginal discharge and bleeding; local pain is unusual unless there has been extensive pelvic infiltration.

Signs

Tumour will usually be visible and palpable on speculum and digital vaginal examination. Inguinal nodes may be palpable with tumours of the lower vagina.

Differential diagnosis

This includes atrophic vaginitis, metastases from the cervix or endometrium and a tumour of the urethra or Bartholin's gland.

Investigations

The diagnosis will be confirmed at examination under anaesthetic when biopsies can be taken. Routine investigations may show chronic anaemia from blood loss and, rarely, renal failure owing to ureteric obstruction from pelvic infiltration or lung metastases on chest X-ray.

Fine-needle aspiration

Palpable inguinal nodes should be investigated further by fine-needle aspiration (FNA) to distinguish inflammatory nodes from metastases.

Computed tomography scan

Staging should include a CT scan of the pelvis to assess pelvic lymph nodes.

Staging

Vaginal carcinoma is staged using the FIGO classification.

- Stage 1 – limited to the vaginal mucosa.
- Stage 2 – extension to submucosa and parametrium but not to pelvic side walls.
- Stage 3 – extension to pelvic side wall.
- Stage 4 – bladder, rectum or distant metastases.

Treatment

SURGERY

Early disease may be treated by radical hysterectomy and total vaginectomy with pelvic lymphadenectomy. Inguinal node dissection may also be required for tumours in the lower third of the vagina. Vaginal reconstruction should be offered to women undergoing this procedure.

RADIOTHERAPY

Radiotherapy may also be considered for those with early tumours who are unwilling to accept vaginectomy, reserving surgery to salvage patients who recur, for those unfit for surgery and stage 2 and 3 disease. It will take the form of external beam irradiation to the pelvis including the inguinal nodes for lower third tumours followed by intracavitary or interstitial treatment to give a high dose of radiation directly to the vaginal mucosa and adjacent tissues.

PALLIATIVE TREATMENT

Radiotherapy is helpful for locally advanced or recurrent disease. This may take the form of external beam treatment where there is a major pelvic component or intracavitary treatment for bleeding or ulcerated disease locally in the vagina.

There is no recognized effective chemotherapy for vaginal carcinoma.

Tumour-related complications

These may include vaginal haemorrhage and sepsis, and renal failure owing to urethral obstruction.

Treatment-related complications

Recognized acute complications of pelvic radiotherapy include radiation cystitis and diarrhoea. Late complications may include vaginal stenosis and fistulae into bladder or rectum, particularly where there has been local infiltration by tumour.

Prognosis

Over 80 per cent of stage 1 patients can expect cure; 50 per cent of patients with stage 2 and 30 per cent of those with stage 3 tumours will survive 5 years.

Screening

Female offspring of mothers that received stilboestrol during pregnancy are at recognized high risk and will benefit from regular screening by clinical examination and vaginal smears.

Vaginal intraepithelial neoplasia seems to be related to earlier cervical malignancy and therefore these patients should also receive regular vaginal smears following treatment of a cervical cancer.

Rarer tumours

Adenocarcinoma and clear cell carcinoma are usually treated surgically, and radiotherapy reserved for palliation of advanced tumours.

CANCER OF THE VULVA

Epidemiology

Cancer of the vulva accounts for only 5 per cent of all gynaecological cancers and around 600 cases occur in the UK each year. It is usually seen in older, postmenopausal women.

Aetiology

Chemical carcinogenesis was seen historically in the 'mulespinners' exposed to mineral oils. There are also dystrophic conditions of the vulval skin, including leucoplakia, lichen sclerosus et atrophicus and Paget's disease of the vulva. True carcinoma *in situ* is also seen in the vulval skin.

Pathology

Macroscopically, the tumour is typically a papilliferous growth or an ulcer arising from the medial side of the labium majorum (Fig. 11.7). Bilateral tumours may be seen – the so-called 'kissing cancer'.

Microscopically, vulval carcinomas are squamous carcinomas. Other rare tumours which can arise in the vulva include basal cell carcinomas, melanomas, sarcomas and tumours of the female urethra and Bartholin's gland.

Natural history

Local invasion of surrounding soft tissue occurs early and in advanced cases pubic bone may become involved. Lymphatic spread is to the inguinal nodes before progressing along the pelvic node chain. Blood-borne spread to lungs may occur but is a late event.

Symptoms

There may be long-standing symptoms of skin dystrophy with local irritation. A lump may be obvious to the patient. Swelling of the legs may occur due to inguinal nodes or femoral vein involvement.

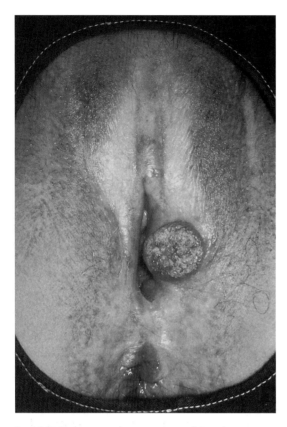

Fig 11.7 Primary squamous carcinoma of the vulva.

Pain is usually a late symptom caused by bone invasion.

Signs

The local tumour will be apparent as an ulcer or papilliferous growth. Inguinal nodes may be palpable, with associated leg oedema.

Differential diagnosis

Vulval dystrophies may be a forerunner of invasive cancer, as discussed above. Infective conditions such as condylomata, lymphogranuloma inguinale or lymphogranuloma venereum should be considered. In the past, tuberculous or syphilitic lesions have also been described in the differential diagnosis but are rarely seen today.

Investigations

The tumour is usually apparent clinically and diagnosis is confirmed by a full examination under anaesthetic and biopsy.

Fine-needle aspiration

Palpable nodes should be investigated with FNA for cytological confirmation of malignancy as many will be only inflammatory.

Computed tomography scan

In the presence of palpable nodes, CT scan of the pelvis will assess proximal spread into the iliac node chain.

Radiography

Chest X-ray will exclude the presence of lung metastases.

Staging

Staging uses the TNM classification (see Chapter 2).

- T1 – confined to the vulva, 2 cm, or less in diameter.
- T2 – confined to the vulva, > 2 cm in diameter.
- T3 – involving the urethra, vagina, perineum or anus.
- T4 – invading the rectal or bladder mucosa, urethral mucosa or underlying bone.
- N0 – no nodes palpable.
- N1 – mobile nodes in either groin, not clinically suspicious of malignancy.
- N2 – mobile nodes in either groin, clinically suspicious of malignancy.
- N3 – fixed or ulcerated nodes.

Treatment

SURGERY

Wide excision of the vulva (vulvectomy) with bilateral femoral and inguinal node dissection is usually recommended.

RADIOTHERAPY

For inoperable disease, radical radiotherapy can be given using both external beam treatment and interstitial implantation of the tumour. A radical dose may be given but acute reactions in this area can be severe and are often dose limiting. Reactions are particularly severe in patients receiving combined chemoradiotherapy schedules delivering 5-fluorouracil (5-FU) and mitomycin C with radiation; at present it is uncertain whether this approach gives better local control than radiotherapy alone.

PALLIATIVE TREATMENT

Local toilet surgery may be required or, where there is extensive posterior infiltration, a defunctioning colostomy. Radiotherapy is of value for local pain, discharge and bleeding.

There is no recognized chemotherapy for vulval carcinoma, although responses are described following combinations effective against squamous carcinomas such as mitomycin C and 5-FU or methotrexate and 5-FU.

Tumour-related complications

These may include:

- local haemorrhage and discharge;
- oedema of either or both legs may develop owing to venous or lymphatic obstruction;
- urethral invasion may cause difficulty with micturition and anal invasion may result in faecal incontinence.

Treatment-related complications

Radical surgery may be complicated by delayed wound healing. Leg oedema may occur where there has been extensive dissection of the groin.

Prognosis

Survival is related to the extent of disease at presentation and general condition, which in the frail and elderly may preclude radical surgery.

Following radical surgery for localized disease over 80 per cent of patients will survive 5 years. The presence of lymph nodes is a poor prognostic sign, reducing 5-year survival to around 40 per cent.

Rare tumours

Basal cell carcinomas

They are usually cured by local surgery unless they have invaded deeper structures. They may also be treated by radiotherapy.

Melanomas

These are best treated with wide surgical excision. For more advanced local lesions or patients with distant metastases palliative radiotherapy may be of value in obtaining local control.

Sarcomas

These are also best treated by wide surgical excision.

CHORIOCARCINOMA

Epidemiology

Choriocarcinoma is a malignant tumour arising from the placental tissues. It is a rare tumour which occasionally may arise in association with a normal pregnancy but is far more common as a complication of a hydatidiform mole.

The incidence of hydatidiform mole is around 1 in 1000 pregnancies in the UK of which 3 per cent will develop into choriocarcinoma. The incidence of choriocarcinoma following term delivery where there is no mole is around 1 in 50 000 pregnancies. There is no recognized geographical variation.

Aetiology

Hydatidiform mole is more common in pregnancies in women under 20 years and over 40 years. Past history of a mole predisposes to subsequent mole pregnancies.

Pathology

Macroscopically, choriocarcinoma arises within the uterus following normal pregnancy, ectopic pregnancy, spontaneous abortion or hydatidiform mole. It is characteristically a haemorrhagic tumour with no detectable placental remnant.

Microscopically, the distinction between a benign mole and choriocarcinoma is made by the absence of villi in the choriocarcinoma, with areas of necrosis and haemorrhage. The cells of the trophoblast have malignant features with many mitoses and pleomorphic cells with multiple nucleoli.

Natural history

Local invasion involves the uterine wall at an early stage. Lymph node metastases are rare. Early blood-borne dissemination occurs to lungs, liver and the central nervous system. Other common distant sites involved are skin, bowel and spleen. Bone metastases are rare.

Symptoms

These include vaginal bleeding within 1 year of pregnancy and abdominal or pelvic discomfort.

Up to one-third of patients may present with symptoms of metastatic disease, such as cough, haemoptysis, weight loss, headache or fits.

Signs

The uterus may be enlarged and tender on pelvic examination or a pelvic mass may be palpable. Chest signs secondary to lung collapse or effusion may be present, the liver may be enlarged and palpable and there may be focal neurological signs associated with brain metastases.

Differential diagnosis

Choriocarcinoma must be distinguished from hydatidiform mole. Other causes of uterine bleeding such as fibroids and cervical or endometrial carcinoma should be considered.

Investigations

Blood tests

Blood levels of human chorionic gonadotrophin (HCG) are important. This is raised in normal pregnancy but also with hydatidiform mole and choriocarcinoma. It is an important indicator of tumour bulk in choriocarcinoma and an invaluable tumour marker for monitoring treatment.

Ultrasound

Ultrasound of the uterus gives a characteristic picture in hydatidiform mole and choriocarcinoma. It can also be used to assess the extent of local invasion through the uterine wall and fallopian tube and ovarian involvement.

Computed tomography scan

A CT scan of the chest is used to exclude pulmonary metastases below the size detectable on plain chest X-ray. A scan of the brain may be indicated where there are neurological symptoms or signs.

Histology

The diagnosis of choriocarcinoma will be confirmed histologically on examination of the uterine contents removed at examination under anaesthetic and suction evacuation.

Staging

There is no recognized staging system for choriocarcinoma. However, a prognostic score has been described by which patients can be divided into those with a good, intermediate and poor prognosis. This uses a number of parameters including age, parity, preceding pregnancies, HCG level, number, site and size of metastases.

Treatment

Because of its rarity and the complex nature of its treatment, all patients should be referred to a major centre experienced in the management of choriocarcinoma.

SURGERY

Suction evacuation of the uterus is the initial treatment in all cases.

CHEMOTHERAPY

Subsequent chemotherapy is based on close monitoring of serum HCG levels. Indications for treatment include:

- very high levels persisting after evacuation (>20 000 IU);
- rising levels of HCG;
- continued uterine bleeding;
- metastatic disease.

All the above are signs of active choriocarcinoma.

Low-risk patients

Low-risk patients who are young with disease restricted to the uterus and vagina or those with lung metastases are treated with methotrexate as a single agent.

Intermediate-risk patients

Intermediate-risk patients who are over 39 years with localized disease or have spleen or liver metastases receive chemotherapy with actinomycin D, vincristine and etoposide.

High-risk patients

Those with metastases in the gastrointestinal tract or liver receive more intensive chemotherapy using etoposide, actinomycin D, methotrexate, vincristine and cyclophosphamide. Multiple drugs are used in this context to prevent resistance emerging in surviving cells.

Because of the high risk of central nervous system (CNS) metastases, prophylactic treatment with intrathecal methotrexate is also recommended for high-risk patients and all those with lung metastases.

Established CNS metastases are treated with dexamethasone and multiple-drug chemotherapy as for the high-risk group.

Tumour-related complications

Bleeding from the uterus or metastatic sites resulting in gastrointestinal, intracerebral or intrapulmonary haemorrhage may be seen. Respiratory failure may complicate multiple pulmonary metastases or may be precipitated by their treatment owing to rapid tumour lysis.

Treatment-related complications

Rapid tumour destruction with chemotherapy of widespread metastases may cause not only respiratory failure but also extensive metabolic disturbance (tumour lysis syndrome; see Chapter 22).

Many patients have proceeded after successful treatment to have further pregnancies without complications. There is, however, some concern that oral contraceptive treatment in the immediate period after chemotherapy may provoke further relapse; therefore, oral contraception should be avoided for 6 months following completion of chemotherapy.

Prognosis

The outlook for patients with choriocarcinoma is extremely good. It is only those that have high-risk disease, including those over 40 years with bulky (>5 cm) metastases, multiple sites or more than a total of eight metastases, brain metastases and very high HCG levels (>10 000 IU) in whom survival of less than 100 per cent can be anticipated and even in this group over 80 per cent will be cured.

Screening

Routine screening of pregnant women is not indicated but high-risk patients that have had previous trophoblastic disease (mole or choriocarcinoma) should have careful monitoring of HCG following delivery.

12 CNS TUMOURS

A discussion of the general principles will be followed by specific examples.

Epidemiology

These are uncommon tumours with 29 000 new cases and 21 000 deaths registered in the European Union per annum. One to two per cent of autopsies performed after death from other causes reveal occult brain primary tumours. There is a bimodal age incidence with peaks at 5–9 years and 50–55 years, varying with the type of tumour (e.g. medulloblastomas are very rare beyond adolescence; glioblastomas are very rare in adolescents and children). There is a slight male predominance in all types except meningioma.

Aetiology

In the vast majority of cases no aetiological factors can be identified. Several associations have been identified but these conditions are themselves very rare. Genetic predisposition to CNS tumours has been identified in the following rare syndromes.

- Neurofibromatosis – neurofibroma, and neurofibrosarcoma, optic nerve glioma, ependymoma, meningioma.
- Tuberose sclerosis – glioma and hamartoma.
- von Hippel–Lindau syndrome – cerebellar haemangioblastoma.
- Li Fraumeni syndrome – gliomas.
- Gorlin's syndrome – medulloblastoma.

Industrial exposure to vinylchloride has been associated with the development of gliomas. The controversy regarding a cause and effect relationship between electromagnetic radiation and CNS tumours continues. In human immunodeficiency virus (HIV)-positive cases, primary cerebral lymphoma is associated with infection by the Epstein–Barr virus.

Pathology

The classification of tumours according to their cell of origin is outlined in Table 12.1. Eighty per cent

TABLE 12.1 Classification of primary CNS tumours according to the tissue of origin

Tissue of origin	Tumour
Glial (50%)	Astrocytoma, oligodendroglioma, ependymoma
Meninges (25%)	Meningioma, meningiosarcoma
Pituitary (20%)	Craniopharyngioma, adenoma
Vascular (2%)	Angioma, haemangioblastoma
Pineal (<1%)	Pinealoma, pineoblastoma
Germ cells (<1%)	Teratoma, dysgerminoma
Miscellaneous	Chordoma, medulloblastoma, lymphoma

are intracranial and 20 per cent are spinal; childhood tumours tend to be located in the cerebellum, whereas adult tumours tend to be located in the cerebral hemispheres. Highly malignant tumours will have necrosis and haemorrhage on cut section, oedema of the surrounding cerebral tissue, and may not be well circumscribed. Multifocal high-grade gliomas and lymphomas are recognized. Calcification is seen in craniopharyngiomas, oligodendrogliomas and some meningiomas, making them visible on a plain skull X-ray.

Spinal tumours may be classified further according to their origin in relation to the dural/spinal cord anatomy into three groups:

- extradural (e.g. metastases, chordoma);
- intradural extramedullary (e.g. meningiomas, neurofibromas);
- intramedullary (e.g. astrocytomas, ependymomas, haemangioblastomas, lipomas, dermoids).

Tumours may be subclassified into grades according to the degree of differentiation. This grading reflects the expected behaviour of the tumour and takes into account factors such as the degree of tumour cellularity, the number and appearance of mitotic figures and the presence of necrosis.

Natural history

Direct infiltration is the main mode of spread and the cause of death of the majority of patients dying from CNS tumours. All CNS tumours, even if benign, enlarge by infiltrating and/or compressing the adjacent neural tissue, and in turn the increasing peritumoral oedema around the tumour leads to raised intracranial pressure. Raised intracranial pressure may also be caused by hydrocephalus arising from compression of the ventricular system, leading to impaired drainage of cerebrospinal fluid (CSF) and ventricular dilatation proximal to the block. Local infiltration will also lead to focal brain damage manifested as focal neurological signs, and some tumours cross the corpus callosum in the midline to involve the contralateral hemisphere (Fig. 12.1). Tumours prone to CSF seeding include medulloblastoma, ependymoma, pineoblastoma, germ cell tumours and lymphoma. This results in meningeal deposits anywhere from the foramen magnum down to the mid sacrum (Fig. 12.2). Insertion of a shunt to relieve hydrocephalus may rarely lead to distant dissemination of tumour. Lymphatic spread is not seen as the neural tissue does not have

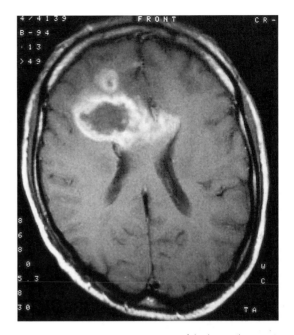

FIG 12.1 Magnetic resonance image of the brain, showing a high-grade glioma infiltrating across the corpus callosum.

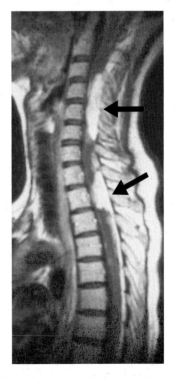

FIG 12.2 Sagittal magnetic resonance image of the cervico-thoracic spine and spinal cord. This patient has multiple meningeal tumour deposits.

a true lymphatic drainage system. Distant metastases are extremely rare, but are described in patients with very aggressive tumours such as glioblastomas which have invaded the dural venous sinus system and in medulloblastomas.

Symptoms and signs

CEREBRAL TUMOURS

Patients with cerebral tumours usually present with one or more of the following:

- epilepsy;
- raised intracranial pressure;
- focal neurological deficit.

The patient may present with an epileptic fit, which may be generalized, affecting the whole body or focal, affecting a region or single part of the body which is related to the anatomical origin within the brain. A cerebral tumour should be considered in any patient presenting *de novo* in this manner, particularly with focal epilepsy. Raised intracranial pressure may lead to headaches with an early morning predominance, nausea, vomiting, somnolence, apathy, poor concentration, memory impairment and personality change. Clinically, there may be papilloedema, upgoing plantar responses, evidence of impaired higher mental functions and impairment of consciousness. Local pressure from a tumour will lead to dysfunction of the affected tissue due to ischaemia, which will be manifested clinically by focal neurological signs corresponding to the affected portion of the brain. These will be upper motor neurone in type, for example spasticity, hyperreflexia and upgoing plantar reflexes in the case of a hemiparesis.

SPINAL TUMOURS

These may present with one of the following:

- spinal cord compression;
- cauda equina compression.

Spinal cord compression may arise when the lesion lies between the foramen magnum and the lower limit of the cord at the junction of the first and second lumbar vertebrae. There will be a pattern of upper motor neurone loss of function below the level of the block, associated with a sensory level and sphincter disturbance.

Cauda equina compression may arise if the lesion is somewhere below the lower limit of the spinal cord affecting only nerve roots and therefore the signs are those of a lower motor neurone lesion affecting the lower limbs (i.e. hypotonia, weakness, wasting, fasciculation, hyporeflexia, downgoing plantar reflexes and a dermatomal sensory loss). The urethral and anal sphincters may also be impaired.

Investigations

Contrast enhanced computed tomography

This will give information regarding the location, size and degree of local invasion of the tumour. The advent of spiral computed tomography (CT) heralded an era of improved image reconstruction in planes other than the usual axial images. It is particularly good for delineating the skeletal anatomy but poor at surveying the posterior fossa because of the thickness of the bone in this region and proximity of mastoid air cells, both of which can lead to streak artefacts. Artefacts from surgical clips and dental amalgam can also produce problems.

Magnetic resonance imaging

Magnetic resonance imaging (MRI) should be considered the investigation of choice for imaging of CNS tumours. The high lipid content of neural tissue leads to high contrast and in turn a high spatial resolution. The ability to image directly in non-axial planes (rather than reconstruct non-axial planes as in CT) lends itself to high-quality images of the brain and spinal cord. These are ideal for neurosurgical planning and radiotherapy treatment planning. It is also vastly superior to CT in demonstrating the subtle changes of meningeal disease. However, MRI is not as useful as CT in showing the skeletal anatomy.

Magnetic resonance angiography

Magnetic resonance angiography (MRA) is a useful tool for delineating the arterial blood supply to a tumour, allowing optimal planning of management.

Positron emission tomography

Cerebral tissue avidly takes up glucose as a metabolic substrate. Systemic administration of the positron-emitting isotope of fluorodeoxyglucose permits imaging of the brain. Tumours, particularly high-grade gliomas, will concentrate the tracer and therefore form an image against the background of the surrounding normal brain. Other metabolic substrates such as amino-acids (e.g. methionine) may also be exploited for positron emission tomography (PET). Functional imaging from PET can provide useful information on tumour activity and extent complementary to that obtained from CT and MRI.

Stereotactic needle biopsy or open biopsy

This is essential to obtain a specimen for histological diagnosis. When surgical resection is not feasible, for example with a tumour located at a critical site such as the brainstem, a needle biopsy will be the least traumatic means of sampling a tumour. Otherwise, open biopsy and tumorectomy are performed, and have the advantages of providing a larger specimen for histological analysis and potentially being of therapeutic benefit by allowing complete excision or debulking of the tumour.

Lumbar puncture

This may be of value in providing further information to assist in diagnosis and treatment, for example in providing CSF for cytology in carcinomatous meningitis and high-risk non-Hodgkin's lymphoma and, in the case of germ cell tumours, allowing assay of CSF α-fetoprotein (AFP) and β-human chorionic gonadotrophin (HCG). However, a lumbar puncture should not be routinely performed in patients with brain tumours due to the risk of coning (compression and herniation of the brainstem through the foramen magnum), which may be fatal. Lumbar puncture should always be preceded by fundoscopy and a CT or MRI scan of the brain to exclude raised intracranial pressure.

Myelography

This is now an obsolete investigation, having been superseded by CT and MRI. It entails the instillation of radio-opaque contrast into the subarachnoid space by either lumbar puncture or cisternal puncture.

Treatment

The skill and advice of a neurosurgeon should always be sought when planning investigation and treatment of such patients. Ideally, this should be in the context of a multidisciplinary team comprising an oncologist, neurosurgeon and neuroradiologist.

SURGERY

This is the treatment of choice for all brain and spinal tumours as most are relatively radioresistant, making them incurable by radiotherapy alone. Complete excision should be the goal of the neurosurgeon both to clear the tumour and to obtain adequate tissue for diagnosis. However, CNS tissue is not tolerant of trauma, is critical to normal body functioning and has no powers of regeneration, and frequently the best that can be expected is surgical debulking. Tumours of the brainstem and pineal region are notoriously difficult to resect and are associated with high operative morbidity and mortality.

RADIOTHERAPY

The CNS is not tolerant of high doses of radiation and therefore curative doses carry the risk of permanent neurological impairment. Radiotherapy has a complementary role to surgery, being ideal for eradicating small-volume disease left behind after attempted surgical clearance, but may also be used to treat radiosensitive tumours arising in critical areas of the brain, with a high expectation of cure (e.g. a dysgerminoma arising in the pineal region). Focused radiotherapy techniques such as stereotactic arc therapy, gamma-knife treatments and intensity-modulated radiotherapy (IMRT) permit high-dose treatment to small volumes of brain with relatively little irradiation of the surrounding normal brain. They are therefore ideally suited to the 'curative' treatment of small tumours (e.g. solitary brain metastases), boost treatments following whole-brain radiotherapy or retreatment of recurrences after radiotherapy.

CHEMOTHERAPY

Only germ cell tumours are potentially curable by chemotherapy alone. The role of chemotherapy in other CNS tumours is mainly palliative in intent. The blood–brain barrier acts as an obstacle to the free passage of chemotherapy drugs. Lipid-soluble drugs such as the nitrosoureas BCNU and CCNU, procarbazine, vincristine, cisplatin and very high doses of methotrexate enter the brain in sufficiently high concentrations. More recently, the oral agent temozolamide has been shown to be of benefit in the management of gliomas. Methotrexate and cytosine arabinoside given intrathecally by lumbar puncture or intraventricularly via an indwelling Ommaya reservoir are of value as regional chemotherapy in the management of meningeal deposits from lymphoma, leukaemia and solid tumours.

SUPPORTIVE THERAPY

Dexamethasone, 4–16 mg daily, is very effective at relieving raised intracranial pressure. Prolonged usage does, however, lead to symptoms and signs of Cushing's syndrome, oral candidiasis and proximal myopathy, which may exacerbate neurological deficits. Mannitol given intravenously is useful as an adjunct in an acute exacerbation of raised intracranial pressure. Anticonvulsants should only be given for documented fits, and patients with epilepsy or recent craniotomy should be advised not to drive until fit-free according to national guidelines. Many patients will have problems with the activities of daily living owing to neurological deficit and referral to a neurophysiotherapist, occupational therapist and social worker is very important.

ASTROCYTOMA

These arise from astrocytes in the brain or spinal cord, and are most common in adults but may arise during childhood. They are divided histologically into low grade (grades 1 and 2) and high grade (grades 3 and 4) which correlate with prognosis. Grade 4 tumours are termed glioblastoma multiforme. These constitute 50 per cent of astrocytomas, arising in adults with a peak incidence of 50 years. They are usually found in cerebral hemispheres, especially the frontal and temporal lobes, are extensively necrotic (Fig. 12.3) and haemorrhagic and are often associated with oedema of the adjacent brain. Tumours close to the midline may spread to the contralateral hemisphere via the corpus callosum or basal ganglia. Glioblastomas are occasionally multifocal (Fig. 12.4). Spinal cord astrocytomas are very rare (Fig. 12.5).

Surgery should be performed with the aim of complete macroscopic and microscopic resection,

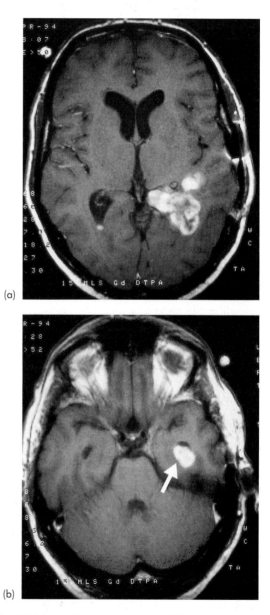

(a)

(b)

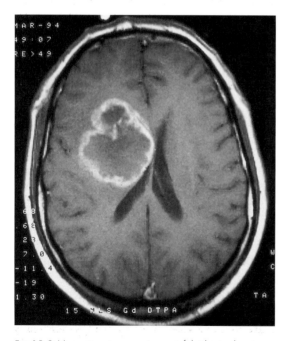

Fig 12.3 Magnetic resonance image of the brain showing a large high grade glioma. Note the necrotic centre and compression of the adjacent ventricle.

Fig 12.4 Magnetic resonance image of the brain showing a multifocal high grade glioma. (a) Several foci are seen in the parieto-occipital lobe; (b) further focus in the temporal lobe.

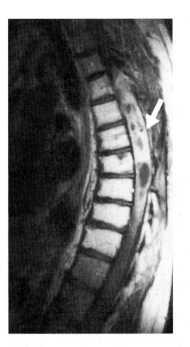

Fig 12.5 Sagittal magnetic resonance image of the thoracic spine. There is a part-solid, part-cystic mass arising from the spinal cord suggestive of an astrocytoma.

although this goal is not often attained due to the diffusely infiltrative nature of the tumour and its position within the brain. Postoperative radiotherapy will not be necessary for grade 1 tumours that have been completely resected. All other grades and incompletely resected grade 1 tumours (in practice, the vast majority) should receive postoperative radiotherapy to maximize local control and in turn prolong survival.

Poor prognostic factors include high-grade tumours, advanced age, poor neurological performance status, limited surgical resection and a presentation other than epilepsy. Five-year survival for grade 1 tumours is about 60 per cent, but high-grade tumours have an extremely poor prognosis, with a median survival of 3 months when biopsy alone is performed, 8 months when treated with radiotherapy and a 1-year survival of 30 per cent. In addition to demonstrating innate radioresistance, gliomas are relatively resistant to chemotherapy. This is not helped by the sanctuary effect conferred by the blood–brain barrier. Meta-analysis of individual randomized trials demonstrates a 5 per cent absolute survival advantage at 2 years for chemotherapy, equating to an increase in 2-year survival from 15 to 20 per cent. Patients with a good performance status should be considered for chemotherapy

to prolong symptom-free survival and overall survival. Active drugs include the nitrosoureas BCNU and CCNU, *Vinca* alkaloids, procarbazine and cisplatin. The combination PCV (procarbazine–CCNU–vincristine) is widely used, has been shown to be superior to single-agent BCNU and has been particularly active in anaplastic astrocytomas. More recently, temozolamide has been demonstrated to be moderately active, and has the advantage of being an oral agent. The anti-angiogenic drug thalidomide is being tested in clinical trials.

OLIGODENDROGLIOMA

These constitute only 5 per cent of gliomas, arising exclusively in adults with a mean age of 40 years. They are usually found in the cerebral hemispheres, particularly in the frontal lobes (50 per cent) and adjacent to the ventricles, and 20 per cent are bilateral. They are slow-growing, well-circumscribed tumours; 40 per cent have foci of calcification and, unlike gliomas, there is little associated oedema for their size. Patients often have a history of epilepsy or gradual deterioration in higher mental functions. Low-grade tumours are compatible with a long survival after surgery alone which may be curative. The principles of management mirror those for astrocytomas.

MENINGIOMA

These constitute 15 per cent of intracranial tumours, are most common in adults and are the only CNS tumours which are more common in females. They arise from the arachnoid mater, adjacent to the major venous sinuses, the most common sites being the parasagittal region, olfactory groove, sphenoidal ridge and suprasellar region and may arise as an intradural extramedullary spinal tumour. They are usually benign, slow-growing, well circumscribed, may erode overlying skull and 20 per cent are partly calcified. More locally invasive malignant variants are occasionally seen. Primary treatment is surgery, although their proximity to the venous sinuses can lead to perioperative problems and careful case selection is important. Radiotherapy is considered after incomplete surgical excision without which approximately 50 per cent of patients will sustain a recurrence. Radiotherapy will reduce the risk of recurrence by half in this context. Radiotherapy is also used for inoperable cases or recurrence after surgery. Focused radiotherapy techniques such as multiple arc rotations, gamma-knife or IMRT are ideal for treating well-circumscribed, spheroidal, benign tumours of this nature. The prognosis is very good as the natural history is measurable in years and decades. Chemotherapy has no defined role in this disease.

PITUITARY ADENOMA

Pituitary adenomas may be classified according to the staining characteristics of the cell of origin into three groups:

- chromophobe adenomas (50 per cent) are often large, forming the bulk of non-secretory tumours but may secrete prolactin;
- eosinophil adenomas (40 per cent) are much smaller than chromophobe adenomas and may secrete growth hormone or prolactin;
- basophil adenomas (10 per cent) are usually small, and may secrete adrenocorticotropic hormone (ACTH), rarely thyroid-stimulating hormone (TSH), luteinizing hormone (LH) or follicle-stimulating hormone (FSH).

Adenomas may present with headache or with more specific abnormalities. The optic chiasma is a close anatomical relation of the pituitary fossa below and therefore suprasellar extension may lead to chiasmal compression and visual disturbance. Testing of the visual fields to confrontation and perimetry typically reveals a bitemporal hemianopia, although occasionally lateral extension may involve the cavernous sinuses resulting in a palsy of the 3rd, 4th and 6th cranial nerves. Examination of the fundi may reveal a pale disc consistent with optic atrophy. Hypopituitarism may occur as a result of compression of the pituitary gland adjacent to the tumour or pressure on the hypothalamus. Growth hormone secretion is the first to be impaired followed by the gonadotrophins. Diabetes insipidus indicates superior extension into the supraoptic nuclei. Hypothalamic pressure may also lead to a loss of hypothalamic regulation and, in turn, disturbances in homeostasis such as loss of temperature regulation, disturbance of appetite and sleep. Eighty per cent of pituitary adenomas are hormonally active. Prolactin may be elevated in half the cases owing to loss of the

inhibitory hormone produced by the hypothalamus or direct secretion by the eosinophilic or chromphobe adenoma cells. Eosinophilic adenoma may also produce growth hormone and basophilic adenomas may secrete ACTH; less than 1 per cent secrete TSH.

Investigations

Referral to an endocrinologist

An expert baseline endocrine assessment is mandatory before surgery and after treatment the patient will require lifelong follow-up and hormone replacement therapy.

Visual field perimetry

This is the most objective means of documenting visual field defects, and gives a hard copy which can be stored in the patient's notes for comparison at a later date.

Plain radiographs

An antero-posterior (AP) and lateral skull X-ray will document any bony expansion of the pituitary fossa.

Computed tomography and magnetic resonance imaging

Computed tomography and MRI of the pituitary fossa provide a detailed assessment of the bony walls of the pituitary fossa, the pituitary itself and potential sites of local tumour spread. They are an indispensable part of planning surgery and/or radiotherapy (Fig. 12.6).

Treatment

SURGERY

Hypophysectomy provides a tissue diagnosis, instant decompression of the optic chiasma and other adjacent structures, and a cessation of hormone hypersecretion. Complete resection of the pituitary tumour and its extensions will provide optimum long-term local control for macro-adenomas but partial removal of the pituitary may suffice for a micro-adenoma. A trans-sphenoidal approach is preferred whenever possible, but if there is much suprasellar or lateral extension a frontal (transcranial) approach will give greater access.

RADIOTHERAPY

There is a high recurrence rate after surgery alone for macro-adenomas, but the addition of radiotherapy

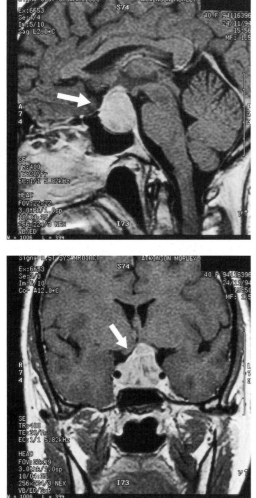

(a)

(b)

FIG 12.6 Pituitary adenoma. (a) Sagittal magnetic resonance image of the brain showing an enhancing tumour, which occupies the pituitary fossa and extends into the suprasellar region. (b) Coronal magnetic resonance image from the same patient. Note the proximity of the tumour to the cavernous sinuses.

increases 10-year disease-free survival from 10 per cent to over 80 per cent. Radiotherapy alone is successful in the long-term control of hormone hypersecretion, although the maximum benefit is expressed after some years. In acromegalics, there is a 20 per cent per annum decline in growth hormone levels, but normalization may never occur, particularly if pretreatment levels were very high. Similar results are seen in prolactin- and ACTH-secreting tumours. Focused radiotherapy techniques (see the meningioma section above) may have an important role in pituitary tumours in the future.

BROMOCRIPTINE

This is a dopamine agonist which mimics the prolactin inhibitory hormone produced by the hypothalamus, and is of value in the treatment of prolactinoma, when it may induce dramatic tumour regression.

CRANIOPHARYNGIOMA

This is very rare, usually arising in children, and constitutes 10 per cent of all childhood intracranial tumours. It is most common in Japan but rare in the USA and Western Europe. It is a suprasellar tumour arising from nests of epidermoid cells in the pars tuberalis (Rathke's pouch). It is slow-growing and benign, with three-quarters being partly cystic and calcified (Fig. 12.7).

Presentation is as for pituitary adenomas and surgery is the treatment of choice, with radiotherapy having the same role as for pituitary tumours: i.e. after incomplete excision or for inoperable cases. Historically, the cystic nature of these tumours made them amenable to instillation of radioisotopes such as ^{90}Yttrium and ^{32}Phosphorus. Prognosis is very good with an 80 per cent 5-year survival and 70 per cent 5-year disease-free survival.

PINEAL TUMOURS

These are rare. Characteristically they present with obstructive hydrocephalus because of their proximity to the CSF ventricular outflow pathway or ocular palsies, especially paralysis of upward gaze (Parinaud's syndrome). Surgery is particularly difficult and hazardous in this region. A ventriculoperitoneal shunt may be required. Germinomas and astrocytomas are the commonest tumours in the pineal region. Rarer, intrinsic tumours of the pineal gland include:

- pinealoma;
- pineoblastoma.

Pinealoma is very rare, but is the most common pineal tumour with a peak incidence of 15–25 years; it is slow-growing, well-circumscribed, non-invasive and treated by surgical excision. Pineoblastoma is even rarer and much more aggressive than pinealoma; CSF dissemination is a frequent complication.

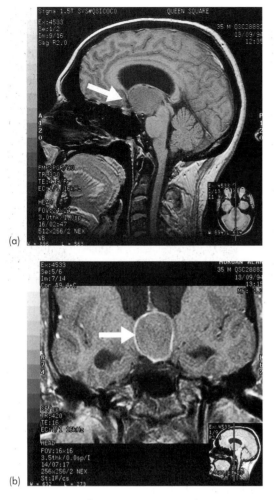

(a)

(b)

FIG 12.7 Craniopharyngioma. (a) Sagittal magnetic resonance image of the brain showing a solitary, well-circumscribed, cystic mass in the suprasellar region. (b) Coronal magnetic resonance image from the same patient.

GERM CELL TUMOURS

Teratomas and dysgerminomas (analogous to seminoma) may arise from islands of ectopic germ cells in the suprasellar region (Fig. 12.8) or pineal. Patients with confirmed CNS disease should be referred to a regional centre specializing in the treatment of germ cell tumours. The tumours are radiosensitive and chemosensitive but the prognosis is not as good as for their testicular counterparts. Serum and CSF AFP and HCG measurements are useful to confirm diagnosis and monitor response to treatment.

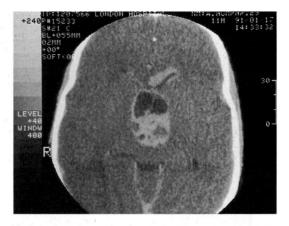

FIG 12.8 Transverse computed tomography image of the brain of a young child showing a complex cystic lesion arising in the suprasellar region. The appearances in this age suggest a suprasellar teratoma.

EPENDYMOMA

These constitute 10 per cent of childhood intracranial tumours with a peak incidence during the first decade of life. They arise throughout the CNS from cells lining ventricles, central canal of the spinal cord and choroid plexus, although the vast majority arise near the 4th ventricle; 40 per cent are supratentorial and 60 per cent infratentorial. They are well circumscribed, usually well differentiated, slow-growing and may be calcified (Fig. 12.9). Spread via CSF is well-recognized, particularly if high grade and infratentorial.

Combined surgery and radiotherapy give the greatest chance of local control. Selected patients at high risk of CSF dissemination receive radiotherapy to the craniospinal axis. The prognosis is a 5-year survival of about 50 per cent, falling to 40 per cent at 10 years.

MEDULLOBLASTOMA

This is the most common intracranial tumour in children (see chapter 18), accounting for 20 per cent of intracranial tumours in the under-16s with 80 per cent arising in those under 15 years of age, most during the first decade. The cells of origin are fetal elements of the external granular layer of the cerebellum, and the tumour is found centrally in the vermis in children and more laterally in the hemispheres in young adults. There is a high risk of

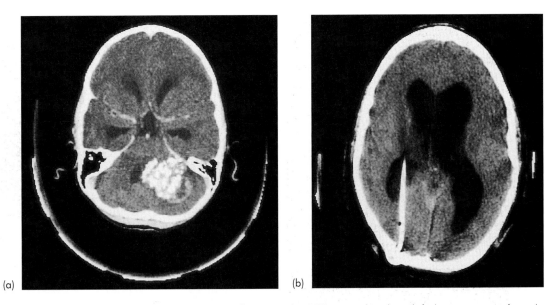

FIG 12.9 Ependymoma. (a) As seen on computed tomography (CT) as a heavily calcified mass arising from the posterior fossa of a child dilatation. (b) A CT image from the same child, showing obstructive hydrocephalus leading to massive ventricular dilatation. A shunt has been inserted to relieve this.

spread via CSF (one-third of cases) and it occasionally metastasises outside the CNS, usually to bone. It presents with cerebellar ataxia and/or obstructive hydrocephalus.

Patients require a posterior fossa craniotomy and tumorectomy, a shunt being inserted to relieve raised intracranial pressure. Medulloblastoma is one of the most radiation-sensitive CNS tumours. Radiotherapy to the craniospinal axis is invariably indicated and the 5-year survival is approximately 50 per cent. Trials comparing chemotherapy (vincristine and CCNU) and radiotherapy with radiotherapy alone have not shown a substantial advantage for the combined modality treatment. A major issue is the impaired growth development and neuropsychiatric consequences of CNS irradiation in infants and young children.

CHORDOMA

This is a very rare tumour which presents in adult life, arising from notochord remnants in the axial skeleton anywhere from the sella turcica to the sacrum. In adults, these remnants persist in the nucleus pulposus of the intervertebral disc. Fifty per cent are sacrococcygeal, 35 per cent arise in the spheno-occipital region and 15 per cent in the vertebral column. They are slow-growing, wellcircumscribed, gelatinous, extradural tumours with areas of haemorrhage and necrosis, often reaching large size and causing compressive symptoms. A characteristic histological finding is the so-called 'physaliferous' cells. They are locally invasive and may be confused with metastatic adenocarcinoma or chondrosarcoma, with less than 10 per cent metastasizing to distant sites.

Radical excision should be attempted although it is rarely possible, and postoperative radiotherapy is necessary in the majority, giving a 50 per cent 5-year survival, falling to 20 per cent at 10 years. There is little published data on the use of chemotherapy. A sarcoma protocol may be appropriate for palliation of symptoms refractory to radiotherapy or to control distant metastatic disease.

HAEMANGIOBLASTOMA

Haemangioblastomas are more common in children and form part of the von Hippel–Lindau syndrome. They are usually cerebellar in origin, with the hemispheres affected more than the vermis. The tumour is slow-growing, well circumscribed and associated with polycythaemia caused by ectopic secretion of erythropoietin.

LYMPHOMA

Primary cerebral lymphoma is very rare, and extra-cerebral involvement raises the possibility of secondary involvement of the brain (see chapters 16 and 20). It is associated with acquired immune-deficiency syndrome (AIDS) but also occurs sporadically. It has a very poor prognosis, even in non-AIDS patients, with a median survival untreated of 3–4 months rising to 15 months after cranial radiotherapy. There is a tendency for CSF spread, leading to involvement of the spinal cord and dura. In these circumstances, craniospinal irradiation may be of benefit. As with high-grade gliomas, long-term survivors are exceptional.

METASTASES

These usually originate from cancers of the lung, breast, kidney, colon, pancreas and melanoma. Lung cancer is the most common primary (50 per cent), particularly small-cell and large-cell variants, where one-quarter to one-half of patients will have cerebral metastases at autopsy. They are most frequent in the frontal and parietal lobes, usually rounded, well circumscribed and enhanced on CT and MRI with intravenous contrast. They are often associated with cerebral oedema (Fig. 12.10) and may occasionally be confused with a cerebral abscess.

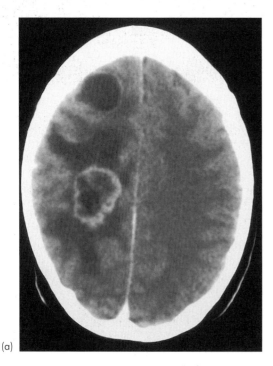

(a)

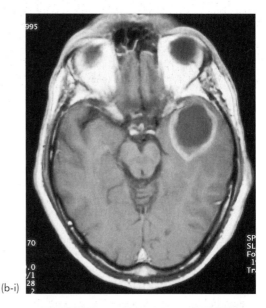

(b-i)

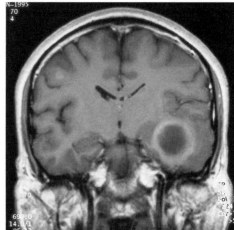

(b-ii)

Fig 12.10 Solitary brain metastasis. (a) Contrast enhanced computed tomography image of the brain showing a solitary metastasis arising in the right parietal region. This is typically well-circumscribed, hypodense with ring enhancement and associated with oedema of the surrounding brain. (b) Magnetic resonance image of the brain demonstrating a solitary brain metastasis: (i) transverse view; (ii) coronal view.

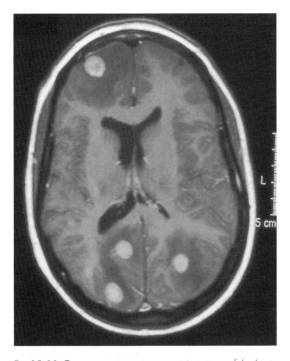

FIG 12.11 Transverse magnetic resonance image of the brain showing multiple cerebral metastases.

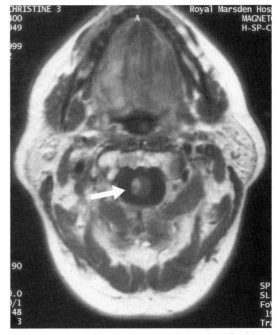

FIG 12.12 Intramedullary metastasis. Magnetic resonance image of base of skull. There is an eccentric area of contrast enhancement in the cervical spinal cord corresponding to a metastasis.

One-third to half of such individuals will die as a result of the cerebral component of their disease, and, therefore, attaining local control is a priority. The majority of patients will present with multiple cerebral/cerebellar metastases (Fig. 12.11). In these circumstances, radiotherapy is the most appropriate treatment. It is important to achieve neurological stability before proceeding with treatment. Judicious use of dexamethasone to treat raised intracranial pressure is essential as radiotherapy may exacerbate any pre-existing cerebral oedema. Radiotherapy fields are designed to treat the whole brain using a pair of opposed lateral fields with an inferior baseline running from the superior orbital ridge through the tragus of the ear. Evidence from well-conducted randomized trials indicates a response rate for most symptoms such as headache, epilepsy and neurological disability in the order of 80 per cent. The net result is an improvement in functional independence for the majority of treated patients. Cranial nerve palsies are often less responsive. In approximately two-thirds of responders, the improvement will be sustained for more than 12 months.

Potentially curable tumours such as germ cell tumours are managed aggressively, even if there are multiple sites of metastatic disease. Craniotomy and biopsy may be considered for the more common solid tumours if there is no known primary and no other malignant tissue to biopsy. Excision should be considered for a solitary brain metastasis in selected patients with solid tumours if they are of good performance status and there is no evidence of distant metastases elsewhere, or in a patient with previous cancer after a prolonged disease-free period. Excision of a solitary metastasis should be followed by radiotherapy to the whole brain and a boost to the site of excision.

Newer radiotherapy techniques such as stereotactic radiotherapy (SRT) using multiple non-coplanar arcs of radiation delivery, gamma-knife and IMRT allow dose escalation by virtue of their superior radiation dosimetry. Their role is this context is still being explored, but they hold much promise, particularly for treatment of one or several metastases. Evidence already suggests that in selected patients with solitary metastases, SRT yields 2-year actuarial control rates of 60–70 per cent.

Intramedullary metastases present with characteristic sensory dissociation and upper motor neurone signs. They are comparatively rare (Fig. 12.12).

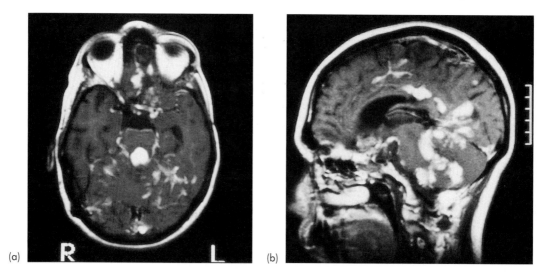

(a) R L   (b)

FIG 12.13 Magnetic resonance image of the brain showing meningeal carcinomatosis. (a) Transverse view; (b) sagittal view.

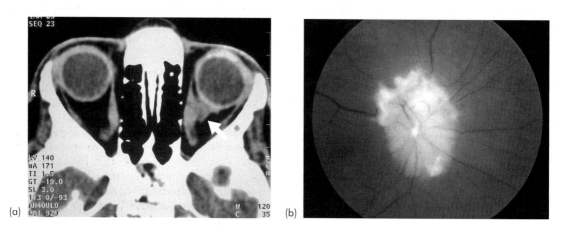

(a)   (b)

FIG 12.14 Optic nerve metastases. (a) Transverse computed tomography image showing irregular thickening of the optic nerve. (b) Fundoscopy showing irregular, pale plaque of tumour at optic disc.

CARCINOMATOUS MENINGITIS

Tumour spread to the CNS may manifest as diffuse involvement of the meninges around the brain (Fig. 12.13) and/or spinal cord. This is seen particularly in haematological malignancies (e.g. non-Hodgkin's lymphoma) and breast cancer. It may present with non-specific symptoms such as headache, vomiting, meningism lethargy, confusion or more focal neurological deficit, typically cranial nerve palsies. Such patients may have disease that extends along the optic nerves (Fig. 12.14). Its onset and presentation is insidious, and it is easy to mistake some of the symptoms for other conditions (e.g. opiate toxicity). Diagnosis may be made from typical appearances on a double-dose contrast-enhanced MRI, although lumbar puncture is often necessary to obtain CSF for cytology and confirm the diagnosis. Treatment options include intrathecal instillation of chemotherapy agents such as methotrexate at weekly intervals via lumbar puncture or an Ommaya intraventricular catheter, and/or cranial/craniospinal radiotherapy.

HEAD AND NECK CANCER

There are approximately 90 000 new cases of head and neck cancer and 35 000 deaths recorded in the European Union per annum. Nearly 90 per cent arise in the over-50s, the incidence increasing with age, and there is a strong male predominance, particularly for carcinoma of the larynx. Incidence rates vary greatly from region to region within each country, and the incidence and mortality rates are increasing. World-wide, the highest incidence is in India and Sri Lanka where in some areas they are the most common cancers, constituting up to 40 per cent of the total. Other pockets of high incidence include South America and the Bas-Rhine region of France (oral cancer), and Newfoundland (lip). The head and neck contain the origins of the respiratory and gastrointestinal tracts, both of which are exposed to environmental carcinogens through the air we breathe and the food and drink we ingest. Each site will be dealt with individually, although cancer of the oral cavity will be described in detail as many of the basic principles are applicable to head and neck cancer in general. As a general rule, the prognosis worsens as the tumour site moves further down the aerodigestive tract from the lips.

CARCINOMA OF THE ORAL CAVITY

The oral cavity extends from the skin–vermilion junction of the lips to the junction of the hard and soft palates above and to the line of circumvallate papillae on the tongue below. This includes carcinomas of the lip, anterior two-thirds of tongue, floor of mouth, buccal mucosa, hard palate, retromolar trigone and lower alveolus.

Aetiology

Inhalation of tobacco smoke from cigarettes, pipes and cigars is a major cause. As with lung cancer, the greater the amount smoked and the higher the tar content, the higher the risk. Chewing tobacco and 'snuff-dipping' carry a particularly high risk of carcinoma of the floor of the mouth where saliva pools. Heavy alcohol consumption is a major risk factor and high-alcohol mouthwashes have also been implicated. Alcohol acts synergistically with tobacco. Alcoholics also tend to have poor nutrition, and their low intake of vitamins A and C may add to their risk of developing cancer. Carcinoma of the lip is more common in those with outdoor occupations where ultraviolet exposure is greater, and this accounts for the predominance of this tumour on the lower lip. Physical trauma from poor dentition can lead to malignant transformation at the site of trauma, usually the lateral border of the tongue. Chronic heat trauma from claypipe smoking can lead to carcinoma of the lip. Asians frequently chew betel nut to relieve indigestion and as a social habit, but this substance also contains carcinogens. This habit is easily detected by the dark-brown staining between the teeth. During the nineteenth century, chronic syphilitic glossitis was a major cause of carcinoma of the tongue. This has declined with the advent of effective antibiotic treatment of syphilis at an early stage and it is no longer justified to check routinely the syphilis serology in all patients with oral cavity cancer.

Pathology

The tumours may be frankly ulcerated, with raised, everted, nodular edges. They may also be papilliform or appear as subtle areas of superficial denudation of the mucosa. Synchronous primaries sometimes occur either in the oral cavity or elsewhere in the aero-digestive tract. The tumour may be secondarily infected, and there may be surrounding white plaques – leucoplakia – which are premalignant (Fig. 13.1). Ninety per cent are squamous carcinomas, the remainder being adenocarcinomas, mucoepidermoid carcinomas, adenocystic carcinomas, lymphomas and melanomas. *In situ* carcinoma and/or dysplasia may be seen in the surrounding mucosa.

Natural history

The tumours spread to adjacent subsites of the oral cavity and invade the deeper layers of the mucosa, reaching muscle in the case of the tongue and cheek, and even the underlying bone of the maxilla or mandible. Tumours of the lower alveolus tend to spread along the alveolus by insidious submucosal spread, so that their microscopic extent can be much greater than appreciated macroscopically. A high proportion of patients have spread to the regional lymph nodes even when they are not palpable (e.g. 70 per cent in carcinoma of the tongue), the incidence being greater with increasing tumour size and increasingly undifferentiated tumours. Tumours

adjacent to the anatomical mid-line may spread to lymph nodes bilaterally. First station lymph nodes include those in the jugulo-digastric, submandibular and submental groups. Second station lymph nodes are those of the jugular, and the upper and lower posterior cervical groups. Haematogenous spread is uncommon at diagnosis and usually seen in the terminal phase of the disease, the lungs being the most common site, followed by bone.

Symptoms

Many patients are asymptomatic, the tumour having been noticed at a routine dental examination (Fig. 13.2), but some complain of soreness at the site of the tumour owing to chronic superficial ulceration and occasionally the presentation is a result of cervical lymph node enlargement. In locally advanced cases, pain may be more marked and may radiate to the ear, while a fungating tumour will lead to halitosis. Bulky tumours of the tongue (Fig. 13.3) will interfere with mastication and swallowing and lead to difficulty with speech.

Signs

Patients frequently have physical signs consistent with heavy smoking and alcohol intake. Oral hygiene is often poor with an increased incidence of dental decay and gum disease, and this should be noted as it is relevant to the planning of radiotherapy. A thorough ear, nose and throat (ENT) examination is mandatory, preferably by an ENT surgeon. The primary tumour should be described in detail with respect to its position (preferably supplemented by a

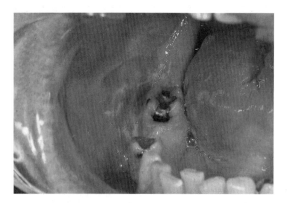

FIG 13.1 Leucoplakia. The retromolar region has a white, superficial, lace-like appearance. This may lead to the development of a squamous carcinoma.

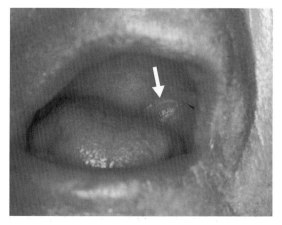

FIG 13.2 A T1 squamous carcinoma arising from the left side of the palate.

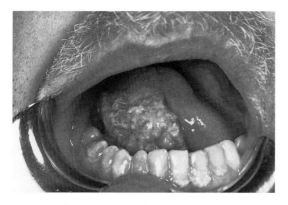

FIG 13.3 A large carcinoma of the tongue. Such tumours will interfere with speech and swallowing.

drawing), size and depth of invasion. Areas of leucoplakia should be sought and care taken to exclude another primary tumour. The tumour should be palpated with a gloved finger to complement inspection, feeling for induration and mucosal irregularity. All patients should have an indirect laryngoscopy. If available, direct fibre-optic endoscopy of the nasal fossa, nasopharynx, oropharynx, hypopharynx and larynx may give vital information regarding the site of origin and local tumour spread. The neck should be palpated very carefully to detect enlarged lymph nodes, recording their distribution (preferably with a diagram), size, number, consistency, degree of tenderness and fixation to surrounding structures. It is common for small, tender lymph nodes to be due to associated infection in the region of the tumour rather than lymph node metastases.

Differential diagnosis

Other causes of oral ulceration should be considered including:

- simple aphthous ulceration;
- lichen planus;
- herpes simplex;
- syphilis.

Investigations

Biopsy

A biopsy is essential to obtain tissue for histological analysis, and can be performed as an outpatient, by an ENT/oral surgeon.

Examination under general anaesthetic

This permits detailed palpation of the tumour to define its precise size, position and extent of local invasion.

Oral pantogram

An oral pantogram (OPG) is of value in excluding invasion of the mandible or maxilla, and provides a detailed survey of the teeth which will help plan any dental procedures that may be necessary prior to radiotherapy.

Fine-needle aspiration of any enlarged lymph nodes

This should be performed in the outpatient clinic and the specimen sent for immediate cytology. As the result may make a substantial difference to the proposed treatment, it is worth repeating the aspiration if a cytologically negative lymph node is still clinically suspicious.

Chest X-ray

This should be performed in all cases to exclude obvious lung metastases, although suspicious areas should be reassessed by a computed tomography (CT) scan of the chest.

Computed tomography/magnetic resonance imaging of the oral cavity and neck

These are useful for defining the local extent of the tumour, particularly when it arises from a site that is difficult to visualize or palpate (e.g. subglottic larynx). They also have an important role in lymph node metastases which may be impalpable or inaccessible (e.g. retropharyngeal lymph nodes). Identification of bone invasion is of particular importance with respect to staging and planning of treatment and this is an area where CT is superior to magnetic resonance imaging (MRI). Soft tissue and anatomical definition is greater with MRI. The head and neck CT protocol can be extended in selected cases to include the thorax to exclude pulmonary metastases.

Staging

The TNM staging (see Chapter 2) is used.

- Tis – carcinoma *in situ*.
- T0 – no evidence of primary.
- TX – primary cannot be assessed.
- T1 – 2 cm or less in greatest dimension.
- T2 – >2 cm but not >4 cm in greatest dimension.
- T3 – >4 cm in greatest dimension.
- T4 – invasion of deep (extrinsic) muscle of tongue, skin, cortical bone or maxillary sinus.
- N0 – no regional lymphadenopathy.
- N1 – single ipsilateral node 3 cm or less in greatest dimension.
- N2 – single ipsilateral node >3 cm but not >6 cm in greatest dimension or multiple ipsilateral nodes not >6 cm or bilateral/contralateral nodes not >6 cm in greatest dimension;
  - 2a – single ipsilateral node >3 cm but not >6 cm in greatest dimension;
  - 2b – multiple ipsilateral nodes none >6 cm in greatest dimension;
  - 2c – bilateral/contralateral node(s) >6 cm in greatest dimension.
- N3 – any node >6 cm in greatest dimension.
- M0 – no distant metastases.
- M1 – distant metastases.

Treatment

Patients should ideally be seen at a joint clinic attended by a clinical oncologist and a head and neck surgeon. Patients should be advised to stop smoking and drinking alcohol to lessen the risk of mucositis during radiotherapy or chest infections after an anaesthetic. Advice should be sought from a dietician, as patients are frequently malnourished at presentation owing to neglect, oral soreness or dysphagia and are therefore unlikely to tolerate either radical radiotherapy or surgery well. The patient may require a softer consistency of diet or liquid supplements. A liquidizer can be very useful. Patients having radiotherapy should be referred to a dentist to have mild degrees of dental decay immediately dealt with by conservative measures (e.g. filling), while any teeth with serious decay can be extracted prior to radiotherapy.

RADICAL TREATMENT

Surgery

The aim of surgery is to remove the primary tumour with a margin adequate to encompass all microscopic spread, and if necessary include an excision of the regional lymph nodes and reconstruct any major tissue deficits. Surgery may be used as the sole primary treatment, combined with radiotherapy or as salvage for local recurrence following radical radiotherapy. Surgery may be the treatment of choice for locally advanced tumours (i.e. T3 and T4 tumours), as these are bulky tumours which may invade adjacent bone when they are particularly difficult to eradicate by radiotherapy alone. There is also an increased risk of osteonecrosis after radiotherapy when the bone is invaded and this is a particularly difficult management problem. However, radical surgery may involve a major resection of tissue, leading to severe functional morbidity. For example, resection of part of the tongue will result in some degree of dysarthria and possibly difficulty in mastication of food and swallowing, and such symptoms may severely compromise the patient's quality of life. Therefore, T1, T2 and small bulk T3 tumours are usually best treated by radiotherapy with surgery reserved for local recurrence.

The surgeon may also elect to perform a radical dissection of the cervical lymph nodes when these are involved. This is a major procedure involving removal of the ipsilateral nodes *en bloc* together with the internal jugular vein (IJV) and some other tissues, such as the sternocleidomastoid and accessory nerve. The IJV cannot be sacrificed bilaterally although a modified radical dissection may be performed on the contralateral side if necessary (IJV preserved). It may be a curative procedure and provides valuable staging and prognostic information. Radiotherapy is advised after neck dissection if three or more nodes are involved or if there is any evidence of extracapsular spread outside a lymph node.

Improvements in surgical techniques have resulted in more patients being able to benefit from reconstructive procedures after radical cancer surgery. This has lessened considerably the functional morbidity experienced after major resections of the tongue and other structures of the oral cavity.

Speech therapy is of value after major resections in the oral cavity, particularly of the tongue, floor of mouth and lips, which may result in speech and swallowing difficulties.

Radiotherapy

As with surgery, radiotherapy may be used as the sole primary treatment, combined with surgery or for salvage of local relapse after surgery, and can be used to treat all stages of local disease. It has the advantage of preserving the voice, speech, swallowing and tissues that surgery would sacrifice, and is therefore the treatment of choice for T1 and T2 tumours.

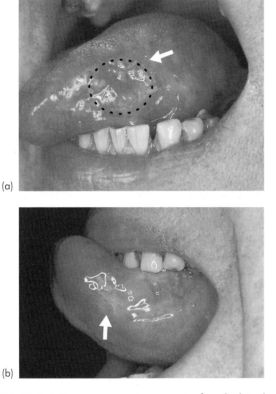

(a)

(b)

F$_{IG}$ 13.4 A T1 squamous carcinoma arising from the lateral edge of the tongue. (a) Before treatment; (b) 6 months after interstitial implant. Tongue function, speech and swallowing have been fully preserved.

Historically, brachytherapy using radioactive needles (e.g. caesium), wire (e.g. iridium) or grains (e.g. gold) was superior to external beam radiotherapy in terms of local control and cosmetic outcome for small primary tumours with no lymph node involvement (Fig. 13.4).

External beam radiotherapy is routinely used in current clinical practice. It has the advantage of including the first station lymph nodes adjacent to the primary tumour as a prophylactic measure to eradicate subclinical tumour deposits, and facilitates treatment of whole cervical lymph node chain at risk if there are palpable lymph node metastases. Radiotherapy gives poor local control when used alone for bulky T3 and T4 tumours, and therefore forms part of a combined modality approach with surgery. The most significant advance for radiotherapy in recent years has been the development of CHART (continuous, hyperfractionated, accelerated radiotherapy). This regime involves rapid completion of treatment combined with avoidance of breaks in radiotherapy at weekends. CHART involves treatment three times daily, 7 days a week for 2.5 weeks (54 Gy in 36 fractions). The rationale is that it does not allow the tumour to repopulate, as may occur when the tumour has a short potential doubling time and treatment is protracted and interrupted over the 6–7 weeks of a conventional course of radiotherapy. A large, well-conducted randomized trial comparing CHART with a conventional course of radiotherapy has the confirmed superiority of CHART for advanced laryngeal cancers. Unfortunately, the logistic difficulties inherent in CHART have precluded its widespread acceptance and implementation; further trials are in progress. Advances in the technology of radiation delivery such as intensity-modulated radiotherapy (IMRT) will undoubtedly play a role in these diseases. It allows the high-dose radiation envelope to be matched in three dimensions to the shape of the volume of tissue containing the tumour. It therefore spares the surrounding organs at risk, such as the spinal cord and parotid salivary glands. Apart from reduced morbidity from standard dose/fractionation schedules, IMRT may allow significant dose escalation for what is essentially a highly sensitive cancer to radiotherapy. Alternatively, it may allow retreatment following failure of a previous course of radiotherapy. These technical advances may also facilitate safe delivery of concurrent chemoradiotherapy (CRT), which is likely to be the preferred treatment over the next decade.

Chemotherapy

The most active agents are 5-fluorouracil (5-FU) and cisplatin, which in combination will give an objective response rate of 60–80 per cent. Chemotherapy alone cannot be used with expectation of cure, and adjuvant/neo-adjuvant chemotherapy has no proven survival benefit. For more locally advanced tumours, meta-analysis of over 60 trials suggests an 8 per cent absolute survival advantage for the subgroup receiving CRT. This is therefore a current standard of care in many countries.

PALLIATIVE TREATMENT
Surgery

Major resection is not justified for the palliation of symptoms in incurable cases because of the trauma sustained and the possibility of major postoperative morbidity with loss of function, but debulking may be necessary to avert respiratory obstruction or dysphagia. Tracheostomy may be indicated if there is upper airways obstruction as this is a particularly distressing symptom.

Radiotherapy

Radiotherapy may be used in cases of locally advanced disease, even when the prospect of cure is low, as it is of value in relieving obstructive symptoms.

Tumour-related complications

Locally advanced tumours are often necrotic and infected, which can lead to embarrassing halitosis, an unpleasant taste and local discomfort. A course of the appropriate antibiotic (usually metronidazole) and chlorhexidine mouthwash can help. Obstruction of the aerodigestive tracts is very distressing and warrants urgent consideration for a tracheostomy. Trismus, dysphonia, dysphagia and salivary fistulae are all recognized.

Treatment-related complications

Surgery

Difficulty in mastication, swallowing, dysarthria and dysphonia result from surgical resection of structures involved in these processes. Poor healing is a particular problem following extensive surgery when the vascularity of the tissue has been compromised, especially if the tissues have been previously irradiated. Osteomyelitis may complicate surgery when there has been a resection of bone (e.g. mandibulectomy) which has become secondarily infected. Treatment is with high doses of the appropriate antibiotic and further surgery may be required to remove the sequestrum.

Radiotherapy

The oral mucosa is very sensitive to radiation, the reaction beginning during the second week of radiotherapy as erythema and soreness, progressing to severe discomfort manifested as a fibrinous mucositis leading to dysphagia and difficulty in mastication. This can be lessened by advising patients to use a very soft toothbrush to avoid gingival trauma, regular mouthwashes to prevent secondary infection, avoiding smoking, alcohol, spicy foods and food or drink that is very hot or very cold. Soluble aspirin 600 mg gargled and swallowed q.d.s. can relieve oral and oropharyngeal discomfort, while a mucosal surface protectant (e.g. sucralfate) sipped slowly can also help the latter. Oral candidiasis should be treated promptly with a topical or systemic antifungal agent. Local anaesthetic lozenges are also useful. A dry mouth is very common during radiotherapy and may recover only partly or not at all. It results from radiation damage to the parotids and minor salivary gland(s) at the site of radiation beam entry and/or exit from the oral cavity, predisposing the patient to dental caries, making swallowing difficult and exacerbating any radiation mucositis. Artificial saliva sprays are the treatment of choice but oral hygiene is also important. Careful monitoring or nutrition is necessary and many patients will require nutritional support with some form of enteral nutrition.

Trismus is a late complication of both surgery and radiotherapy and is caused by fibrosis in and around the temporomandibular joint leading to restriction of jaw opening and closing. Osteonecrosis is a late complication of radiotherapy, usually affecting the mandible as the maxilla has a better blood supply. It may be precipitated by a dental infection or extraction many years after radiotherapy.

Prognosis

The prognosis varies greatly with site of origin, TNM stage and histological grade, and the reader should refer to a more specialized text for more detailed data. In general, there is a high expectation of cure for all T1 and T2 tumours with a 5-year survival of 60–90 per cent, falling to less than 30 per cent for T4 tumours.

Screening/prevention

Dentists play a vital part in screening because they have the opportunity to inspect the oral cavity in many people on a regular basis, but unfortunately the people most at risk of cancer tend to be those who are least likely to attend a dentist. Long-term survivors should be kept under close surveillance in the clinic as many will develop second primaries, usually in the head and neck but also in the lung and gastrointestinal tract. Many cases of oral cavity cancer could be prevented by better patient education, i.e. by reducing smoking, chewing tobacco and betel nut. There is some evidence that isotretinoin may prevent second primary cancers.

Rare tumours of the oral cavity

Other rare carcinomas

The palate and oral mucosa contain a number of minor salivary glands which may result in mucoepidermoid carcinomas, adenocarcinomas and adenoid cystic carcinomas, which are treated by surgery with radiotherapy after incomplete excision or for inoperable tumours.

Kaposi's sarcoma

The oral cavity, particularly the palate, is a common site for this disease and should prompt serological testing to exclude acquired immune-deficiency syndrome (AIDS; see Chapter 20).

Soft tissue and bone sarcomas

These are exceptionally rare but include leiomyosarcoma, rhabdomyosarcoma, fibrosarcoma, malignant fibrous histiocytoma, osteosarcoma and Ewing's sarcoma.

Metastases

Tumour cells may spread via the blood to the gingiva or lower alveolus, from which they may erode the overlying mucosa and mimic a primary carcinoma of the oral cavity. The lung is a common source of such metastases.

CARCINOMA OF THE OROPHARYNX

The oropharynx comprises the tonsils, posterior third of the tongue, soft palate and posterior wall of the oropharynx down to the level of the hyoid bone. Since the oropharynx is a direct extension of the oral cavity, tumours arising in this region are similar in their epidemiology, presentation and pathology. The structures do have a bilateral pattern of lymphatic drainage to the neck which should be considered when planning treatment. Radiotherapy is the preferred treatment for all but the earliest tumours, as radical resection of the tumour is likely to produce functional compromise greater than that from radiotherapy alone. It should be noted that the oropharynx is a site where lymphoid tissue is concentrated and where lymphoma may occasionally arise.

CARCINOMA OF THE LARYNX

There are 25 000 cases and 11 000 deaths recorded in the European Union per annum. These tumours are much more common in men with a male-to-female predominance of 10:1, predisposed to by smoking, and 95 per cent are squamous carcinomas. All

patients complaining of a hoarse voice which has persisted longer than a month should undergo indirect laryngoscopy to visualize the vocal cords directly. Glottic tumours arise on the vocal cords and present at an early stage, as distortion of the vocal cords rapidly manifests as dysphonia, which is noted by both patients and physicians alike. Tumours may arise above the cords (supraglottic) or below the cords (subglottic). These non-glottic tumours present later in their natural history as they grow insidiously and have to reach a large size before presenting with dysphagia, stridor or symptoms from direct invasion of the glottis. A tumour in the supraglottic larynx may lead to referred pain in the ipsilateral ear. The vocal cords have a poor lymphatic drainage and therefore lymph node metastases are less common at this site compared with a 70 per cent incidence from supraglottic tumours as the supraglottis has a rich lymphatic drainage. The TNM staging system is used for laryngeal tumours, the T-stage is outlined below (N-staging is the generic head and neck version cited above).

- TX – primary tumour cannot be assessed.
- T0 – no evidence of primary tumour.
- Tis – carcinoma *in situ*.

Supraglottis

- T1 – tumour limited to one subsite of supraglottis with normal vocal cord mobility.
- T2 – tumour invades mucosa of more than one adjacent subsite of supraglottis or glottis or region outside the supraglottis (e.g. mucosa of base of tongue, vallecula, medial wall of pyriform sinus) without fixation of the larynx.
- T3 – tumour limited to larynx with vocal cord fixation and/or invades any of the following: postcricoid area, pre-epiglottic tissues.
- T4 – tumour invades through the thyroid cartilage, and/or extends into soft tissues of the neck, thyroid, and/or oesophagus.

Glottis

- T1 – tumour limited to vocal cord(s) (may involve anterior or posterior commissure) with normal mobility:
  1a – tumour limited to one vocal cord;
  1b – tumour involves both vocal cords.
- T2 – tumour extends to supraglottis and/or subglottis, and/or with impaired vocal cord mobility.
- T3 – tumour limited to the larynx with vocal cord fixation.

- T4 – tumour invades through the thyroid cartilage and/or to other tissues beyond the larynx (e.g., trachea, soft tissues of neck, including thyroid, pharynx).

Subglottis

- T1 – tumour limited to the subglottis.
- T2 – tumour extends to vocal cord(s) with normal or impaired mobility.
- T3 – tumour limited to larynx with vocal cord fixation.
- T4 – tumour invades through cricoid or thyroid cartilage and/or extends to other tissues beyond the larynx (e.g. trachea, soft tissues of neck, including thyroid, oesophagus).

Laryngeal tumours may be treated by surgery or radiotherapy. A partial or total laryngectomy will have the disadvantage of changing the quality of the voice, and therefore radiotherapy is preferred for T1, T2 and small bulk T3 tumours. The prognosis from glottic tumours is excellent, reflecting their early presentation and low rate of lymphatic spread. Although there is a strong rationale for its use, neo-adjuvant chemotherapy has not been shown to confer a survival advantage in locally advanced laryngeal cancer, although it may facilitate laryngeal preservation in a higher proportion of patients.

CARCINOMA OF THE HYPOPHARYNX

The hypopharynx extends from the level of the tip of the epiglottis to the lower border of the cricoid and comprises the pyriform fossae, posterior pharyngeal wall and postcricoid region. The tumours are squamous carcinomas which tend to present late with dysphagia. There is an association with iron deficiency (Plummer–Vinson syndrome). The results of both radiotherapy and surgery alone are very poor, but the former is preferred unless the patient is physically fit for combined modality treatment.

CARCINOMA OF THE NASOPHARYNX

This disease has a marked geographical variation, being more common in the Far East, particularly southern China where it is endemic. There is very strong evidence that in areas of high incidence the disease is related to infection with the Epstein–Barr virus (EBV). In endemic areas it has a peak incidence at a younger age (15–25 years versus 40–60 years in developed countries and a predominance of anaplastic tumours (squamous in developed countries). There is a lesser association with excess alcohol and tobacco consumption compared with other head and neck sites. Routes of spread include:

- nose (produces epistaxis, nasal discharge and blockage);
- orbit (produces diplopia);
- Eustachian tube (blockage produces deafness);
- cavernous sinus (causes palsies of cranial nerves 3, 4, 5 and 6);
- cribriform plate (causes loss of smell);
- pterygoid muscles and parapharyngeal space (produces inability to open jaw fully [trismus]).

The TNM staging is employed (generic N-staging).

- TX – primary tumour cannot be assessed.
- T0 – no evidence of primary tumour.
- Tis – carcinoma *in situ*.
- T1 – tumour confined to the nasopharynx.
- T2 – tumour extends to soft tissues of oropharynx and/or nasal fossa:
  2a – without parapharyngeal extension;
  2b – with parapharyngeal extension.
- T3 – tumour invades bony structures and/or paranasal sinuses.
- T4 – tumour with intracranial extension and/or involvement of cranial nerves, infratemporal fossa, hypopharynx, or orbit.

Computed tomography or MRI are the investigations of choice for delineating the locoregional extent of the tumour (Fig. 13.5), CT being superior with respect to delineation of the skeletal anatomy which is frequently involved by the tumour. Seventy per cent will have overt or occult lymph node metastases with a tendency to bilateral involvement. The treatment of choice is radiotherapy. For the more advanced stages, chemotherapy (e.g. bleomycin, epirubicin, cisplatin) combined with radiotherapy may confer an advantage and make the tumour more easily encompassed

CARCINOMA OF THE PARANASAL SINUSES

These are rare, with sites of origin including the frontal, ethmoid, maxillary and sphenoid sinuses. The maxillary sinus is most frequently affected. They are usually squamous carcinomas, frequently presenting late as the symptoms are mistaken for those of chronic sinusitis. All too often, by the time of diagnosis they have spread beyond the bony walls of the sinus and have led to other symptoms owing to local invasion of adjacent structures such as diplopia from orbital involvement (Fig. 13.6), or epistaxis from nasal cavity involvement. They may also invade the cranial cavity. Radical surgery is hazardous due to adjacent vital organs and therefore radiotherapy is the treatment of choice. Approximately 40 per cent will survive 5 years after treatment. It should be noted that the sinuses are a potential site of extranodal lymphoma.

SALIVARY GLAND TUMOURS

The parotid gland forms the vast bulk of salivary gland tissue and therefore is the most common site for tumours, while the sublingual, submandibular and smaller glands distributed throughout the oral cavity are rarely involved. There are several variants:

- pleomorphic adenoma;
- adenolymphoma;
- carcinoma;
- lymphoma.

Pleomorphic adenoma

This is the most common salivary gland tumour constituting 75 per cent, with a peak incidence of 30–50 years. It usually arises in the superficial lobe of the gland. It is a benign tumour and therefore slow growing. There is never any associated facial nerve weakness – this feature should always suggest carcinoma or lymphoma. All cases are treated by superficial parotidectomy. Postoperative radiotherapy is indicated if there is capsular rupture at the time of surgery or incomplete microscopic clearance. There is a small risk of transformation of a recurrence into a carcinoma.

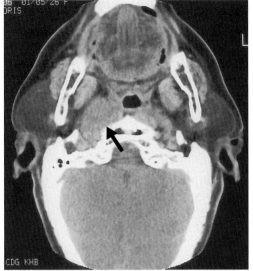

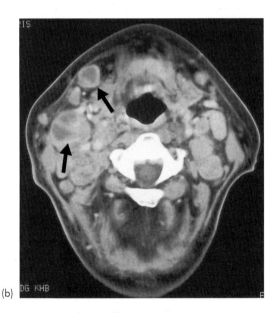

FIG 13.5 Nasopharyngeal carcinoma. (a) Transverse computed tomography (CT) image of the base of skull. There is soft tissue within the nasopharynx, particularly on the right side. (b) A CT image of the neck of the same patient, showing multiple enlarged, necrotic lymph nodes consistent with nodal metastases.

within acceptable radiotherapy fields. The prognosis for squamous carcinoma is poor, with a 5-year survival of less than 20 per cent versus up to 50 per cent for other histological types. The advent of IMRT will make retreatment of this particular site to high doses a real possibility.

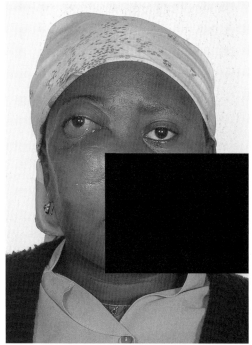

(a)

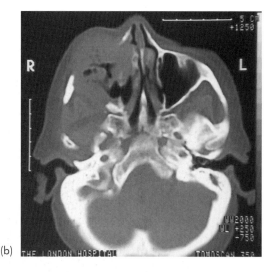

(b)

FIG 13.6 Carcinoma of the maxillary antrum. (a) Frontal view of face. Note the swelling of the right cheek due to anterior spread from the antrum. Superior spread into the orbit has lead to proptosis of the right eye. (b) Computed tomography image of the base of skull from the same patient showing destruction of the facial bones on the right side.

Adenolymphoma

This is a benign, slow-growing tumour most commonly arising in the lower pole of the superficial lobe of the parotid, and is bilateral in 5 per cent. The treatment of choice is surgery.

Carcinoma

This usually arises *de novo* but may develop in a pleomorphic adenoma. It may be distinguished clinically from benign tumours when a facial nerve palsy is present (Fig. 13.7). Variants include:

- adenoid cystic carcinoma (slow-growing and has a tendency for invasion along nerves and into the cranial cavity);
- acinic cell carcinoma arising from serous cells;
- mucoepidermoid carcinoma arising from mucin cells;
- adenocarcinoma;
- squamous carcinoma (must be distinguished from a metastasis);
- undifferentiated carcinoma.

The treatment of choice is resection of the lobe of origin followed by radiotherapy to the parotid. Five-year survival varies between 20 per cent and 80 per cent depending on tumour type and histological grade.

Lymphoma

The parotid is a common site of extranodal non-Hodgkin's lymphoma. Localized disease can be treated by radiotherapy, with chemotherapy used for more advanced disease.

ORBITAL TUMOURS

These are all very rare, presenting because of a mass effect leading to proptosis and diplopia. Benign tumours include haemangioma, leiomyoma, rhabdomyoma, lipoma, fibroma, meningioma, neurofibroma, Schwannoma, pseudotumour and 'malignant' granuloma (e.g. Wegener's granulomatosis). Malignant tumours include gliomas, rhabdomyosarcoma, leiomyosarcoma, malignant

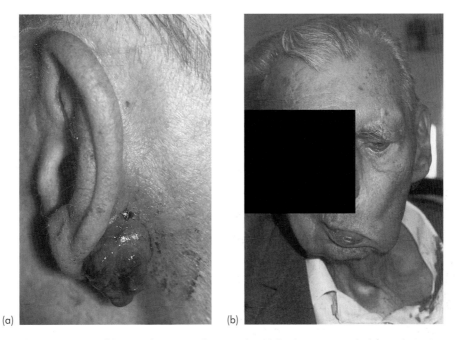

(a)   (b)

FIG 13.7 Adenoid cystic carcinoma of the parotid. (a) Tumour fungation through the skin posterior to the left ear. (b) Same patient. Dense left lower motor neurone facial nerve palsy characteristic of a malignant parotid tumour.

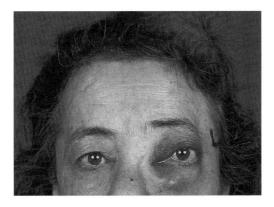

FIG 13.8 Orbital metastasis. This is most commonly seen in cancers of the breast, prostate and lung. The left eye demonstrates non-axial proptosis. The patient has severe diplopia.

fibrous histiocytoma, fibrosarcoma, osteosarcoma, chondrosarcoma, Ewing's sarcoma, lymphoma, Langerhans cell histiocytosis, melanoma, nephroblastoma, plasmacytoma and metastases, particularly from breast and lung cancers (Fig. 13.8).

Tumours within the eye itself are also very rare, presenting with visual loss and strabismus. Benign tumours include naevi, leiomyoma, haemangioma and hamartoma. Malignant tumours include retinoblastoma, medulloepithelioma, melanoma and metastases.

With both sites, optimum management will preserve vision in the affected eye as much as possible, and usually comprises radiotherapy alone, surgery alone or combined modality treatment.

THYROID CANCER

Epidemiology

There are 14 000 new cases of thyroid cancer and 3000 deaths recorded in the European Union per annum. The overall incidence increases with age, papillary, follicular and medullary types typically arising in young adults while anaplastic cancers are usually seen in the elderly. There is a female predominance of 4:1 and a particularly high incidence in Iceland, Israel and Hawaii.

Aetiology

Ionizing radiation is a recognized aetiological agent. Radiation-induced cancers have a latency of 5–40 years, with a peak 15 years after exposure. Radiation induces papillary cancer, which has been described following childhood irradiation for thymic hyperplasia, ringworm, cervical lymphadenitis and in atomic bomb survivors. A higher incidence of follicular cancer has been noted in endemic goitre areas where there is a dietary deficiency of iodine, while a higher incidence of papillary cancer is seen in areas where there is an excess of iodine in the diet. Multiple endocrine neoplasia (MEN) is a dominantly inherited condition, type I being occasionally associated with differentiated thyroid cancer, while type II is associated with medullary cancer which is more often multifocal and presents at a younger age than its sporadic counterpart.

Rare associations include:

- Pendred's syndrome (goitre and nerve deafness at birth);
- Gardener's syndrome (polyposis of the bowel, osteomas and sebaceous cysts);
- Cowden's disease (multiple hamartomas).

Pathology

The tumour usually appears as a firm, well-circumscribed lump, often with a pseudocapsule of compressed thyroid tissue at its periphery. The cut surface will have a characteristic glistening appearance of colloid if there is a significant follicular element. There may be haemorrhage and necrosis in anaplastic tumours, and it may be multifocal. Follicular, papillary and medullary cancers may grow very slowly over many years, while anaplastic cancers are usually fast-growing and locally invasive. Tumours may arise in ectopic thyroid tissue in the tongue, a thyroglossal cyst, sublingual, infrahyoid, pretracheal, mediastinal and pericardial regions. Microscopically, thyroid cancer is characterized by invasion of the capsule and/or thyroid vasculature. There are four main types:

- follicular carcinoma (50 per cent);
- papillary carcinoma (20 per cent);
- anaplastic carcinoma (25 per cent);
- medullary carcinoma (4 per cent).

The presence of papillary structures is diagnostic of papillary carcinoma, although these tumours also frequently contain a follicular component. Follicular carcinoma must be distinguished from an adenoma. It is usually well differentiated with colloid held within follicles and there are no papillary elements. Anaplastic carcinoma is very poorly differentiated, usually with no identifiable follicular elements. Medullary carcinoma arises from the parafollicular ('C') cells, with the inherited form often multifocal in origin. Amyloid may be identified within the stroma and immunocytochemistry will be positive for the hormone calcitonin. Squamous carcinoma, clear cell carcinoma and Hürthle cell carcinoma are also recognized.

Natural history

The tumour initially spreads within the lobe of origin, contained by the capsule, but may then invade the contralateral lobe via the isthmus. Capsular invasion will lead to infiltration of surrounding structures such as the trachea, larynx, recurrent laryngeal nerves and skin. Papillary and medullary carcinomas have a propensity to metastasize to lymph nodes, the affected groups comprising the deep cervical, supraclavicular and paratracheal chains. All may give rise to distant metastases, the lung being the most common site, followed by the skeleton, liver, skin, brain and kidney. Lung metastases are often very numerous and small, sometimes giving a 'snowstorm' appearance. Follicular and anaplastic variants are the types most often associated with distant metastases.

Symptoms

The most common presentation is with a painless solitary lump in the neck (Fig. 14.1). Some patients complain of a hoarse voice, which raises the suspicion of extracapsular extension leading to pressure on one or both of the recurrent laryngeal nerves innervating the vocal cords. Dysphagia may be noticed if the tumour is very large and causing extrinsic compression of the pharynx or upper oesophagus, and may suggest retrosternal extension if the neck mass is small. Patients with medullary carcinoma may complain of diarrhoea, which is thought to be caused by secretion of prostaglandins by the tumour.

Signs

The patient will be euthyroid. The thyroid lump is usually confined to one side of the neck, moving

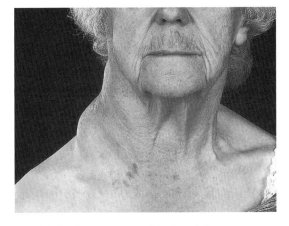

FIG 14.1 Papillary carcinoma of the thyroid. The tumour arises from the right lobe of the thyroid and has spread to lymph nodes on the same side of the neck.

with swallowing and protrusion of the tongue, non-tender, firm/hard in consistency and well circumscribed. Stridor may be heard because of either recurrent laryngeal nerve involvement or extrinsic tracheal compression. Vocal cord palsy may be confirmed by indirect laryngoscopy (IDL). Extracapsular invasion may lead to loss of the normal laryngeal mobility. Lymphadenopathy may be palpable in the deep cervical and supraclavicular regions, while anaplastic tumours may invade the overlying skin to produce induration, erythema and nodularity.

Differential diagnosis

This includes:

- benign tumours of thyroid (e.g. adenoma);
- other malignant tumours of thyroid (e.g. lymphoma and fibrosarcoma);
- metastases (e.g. carcinoma of the lung, hypernephroma and melanoma).

Investigations

Serum markers

Thyroglobulin is a useful marker of differentiated thyroid cancer after ablation of normal thyroid tissue. Calcitonin should be measured in any patient suspected of having medullary carcinoma (e.g. if there is a family history of thyroid carcinoma at a young age or associated diarrhoea). These patients should also be screened for other MEN type II tumours, i.e. parathyroid adenomas (serum calcium and phosphate) or phaeochromocytoma (urinary vanillylmandelic acid).

Chest X-ray

This should be performed in all patients to exclude obvious pulmonary metastases. Equivocal cases should undergo a full thoracic computed tomography (CT) scan.

Thyroid ultrasound and fine-needle aspiration

Carcinoma will give rise to a solid nodule rather than a cystic one and in either case fine-needle aspiration (FNA) should be performed to obtain a cytological diagnosis.

Fine-needle aspiration of enlarged lymph nodes

This is essential to distinguish reactive lymph node enlargement from metastatic infiltration.

Open thyroid biopsy

This is only required in inoperable tumours when an FNA has proven negative or given an equivocal histological diagnosis.

Isotope thyroid scan

In the case of thyroid cancer, administration of a tracer dose of technetium-99 or iodine-131 will give rise to a cold spot relative to the surrounding functioning thyroid tissue, providing useful information to the surgeon about location and extent. Functioning adenomas will produce a hot spot.

Computed tomography scan of the neck/upper chest

This may be of value in assisting the surgeon to make a decision regarding operability of a large mass, particularly when retrosternal extension is suspected (Fig. 14.2), or for radiotherapy planning.

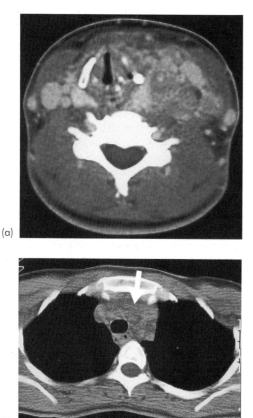

(a)

(c)

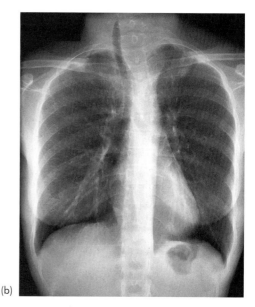

(b)

FIG 14.2 Medullary carcinoma of the thyroid. (a) Computed tomography (CT) scan of the neck showing a massive tumour arising from the left lobe of the thyroid, pushing the trachea to the right side of the neck. (b) Chest radiograph from the same patient. Note the soft tissue mass in the neck and tracheal deviation. (c) A CT scan of the thorax showing retrosternal extension of tumour that had not been appreciated from the chest radiograph.

Staging

The TNM staging (see Chapter 2) is used.

- TX – primary tumour cannot be assessed.
- T0 – no evidence of tumour.
- T1 – tumour 1 cm or less in greatest dimension, limited to thyroid.
- T2 – tumour >1 cm but not >4 cm in greatest dimension, limited to thyroid.
- T3 – tumour >4 cm in greatest dimension, limited to thyroid.
- T4 – tumour of any size extending beyond thyroid capsule.
  All categories may be subdivided into 'a' (solitary) and 'b' multiple.

Treatment

All patients should have some form of thyroid ablation followed by physiological hormone replacement therapy to prevent hypothyroidism and maintain thyroid-stimulating hormone (TSH) at very low ('suppressed') levels to minimize the likelihood of recurrence of a TSH-dependent tumour.

RADICAL TREATMENT

Surgery

This may be curative when used alone, all patients requiring a total thyroidectomy with the aim of removing all thyroid tissue and any extracapsular extension, taking care to preserve the parathyroid glands and recurrent laryngeal nerves if possible. A cervical lymph node dissection should be undertaken when there is overt lymph node invasion.

Unsealed source brachytherapy and external beam radiotherapy

Radioiodine is concentrated in the thyroid gland and can therefore be used for the diagnosis of locoregional and metastatic disease, for the ablation of a thyroid remnant and/or tumour persisting after surgery, and as a means of detecting early relapse. It is concentrated not only by normal thyroid tissue, but also by 70–80 per cent of well-differentiated thyroid carcinomas and their metastases (Fig. 14.3). Radioiodine is given as an oral preparation using strict radiation protection procedures, with the large doses used for ablation of thyroid and tumour being given as an inpatient treatment. It emits β-particles (electrons) with a tissue range of only 2 mm, and it is these that ablate the thyroid/tumour. It also emits low-energy γ-photons which are a radiation hazard to staff and visitors but allow external monitoring of

the distribution, concentration and excretion of the isotope. Radioiodine is given primarily to destroy any remaining normal thyroid tissue. If scans demonstrate any distant metastases, further doses are given to concentrate higher radiation doses at those sites. Most patients will require one to three such treatments, six being the maximum advisable because of the cumulative radiation burden. External beam irradiation to the neck is used when there is residual papillary or follicular carcinoma in the neck that is not concentrating iodine-131, and is necessary in all cases of anaplastic carcinoma and incompletely excised medullary carcinomas.

PALLIATIVE TREATMENT

Surgery

Tracheostomy is occasionally necessary, particularly with anaplastic tumours causing tracheal compression and when there are bilateral palsies of the recurrent laryngeal nerves leading to total vocal cord paralysis and upper respiratory obstruction.

Radiotherapy

Death from asphyxiation caused by a rapidly growing anaplastic carcinoma is particularly unpleasant and distressing, and under such circumstances, even if the patient has distant metastases, radiotherapy to the neck is justified.

Chemotherapy

This has no role in the curative treatment of thyroid cancer. Patients with anaplastic carcinoma and symptoms refractory to all other treatments may be considered for palliative chemotherapy. Adriamycin is the most active agent. Responses are short-lived and toxicity considerable.

Hormone therapy

Elderly patients unfit for surgery with small, well-differentiated tumours may be treated by thyroxine alone at a dose sufficient to suppress TSH, as the natural history of the disease is likely to exceed the patient's natural life expectancy.

Tumour-related complications

Respiratory obstruction is seen with anaplastic carcinomas as a result of extrinsic compression of the trachea or bilateral damage to the recurrent laryngeal nerves, while dysphagia may result from extrinsic compression of the cervical oesophagus and/or retrosternal extension. Superior vena cava obstruction is a rare complication associated with a large retrosternal tumour.

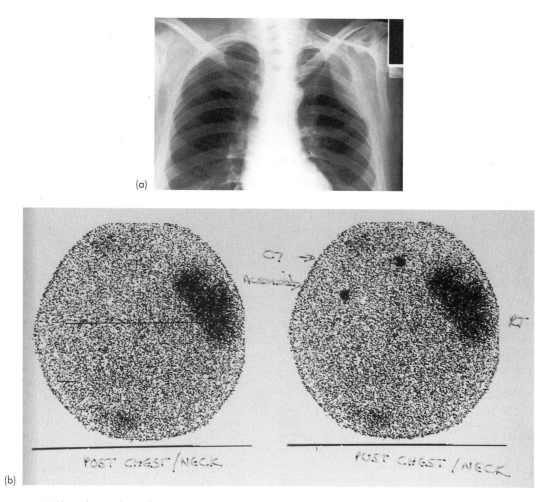

FIG 14.3 (a) Plain chest radiograph showing a left upper lobe pleural metastasis from a follicular carcinoma of the thyroid. (b) Iodine-131 uptake scan showing increased activity (dark) in the corresponding region.

Treatment-related complications

Surgery

Specific complications include risk of secondary haemorrhage during the postoperative period, laryngeal oedema, hypoparathyroidism (hypocalcaemia leading to perioral paraesthesiae, tetany, Trousseau's sign, Chvostek's sign) and vocal cord palsy due to damage to the recurrent laryngeal nerves leading to dysphonia and respiratory obstruction.

Radiotherapy

External beam irradiation to the neck will result in an acute radiation laryngitis characterized by sore throat, dysphagia and dysphonia. Late complications include chronic laryngeal oedema, intense subcutaneous fibrosis leading to restricted neck movements and radiation chondritis of the tracheal cartilage rings.

Radioiodine

Severe adverse reactions to radioiodine are rare. Possible complications include nausea, acute parotitis, sore throat due to radiation laryngitis, acute pneumonitis if there are miliary lung metastases, myelosuppression, leukaemogenesis and induction of cancer elsewhere (there is some uptake in the salivary glands, stomach, colon and bladder). Acute thyroiditis is also recognized – this may cause temporary upper airways obstruction in severe cases. It settles quickly with corticosteroid treatment.

Hormone replacement therapy

Inappropriate dosage or poor patient compliance may lead to either hypothyroidism or hyperthyroidism.

Prognosis

Differentiated thyroid cancer has a good prognosis. Papillary carcinoma has the best prognosis of all, with a 10-year survival of more than 90 per cent, followed by follicular carcinoma (80 per cent) and medullary carcinoma (60–70 per cent). Most patients with anaplastic carcinoma will die within 6 months after diagnosis. Children have an extremely good prognosis, young adults fare better than the elderly and women fare better than men, again reflecting the incidence of differentiated thyroid cancer in these groups. Extracapsular invasion, lymphatic invasion and distant metastases are poor prognostic signs.

Screening/prevention

Patients developing medullary carcinoma of the thyroid have a significant risk of having MEN type II, particularly if aged 20–40 years with a multifocal carcinoma. Regular screening of their first-degree relatives by measuring serum calcitonin may detect occult carcinomas which can be easily cured by surgery.

Rare tumours

LYMPHOMA

This constitutes less than 2 per cent of extranodal lymphomas, with a median age at presentation of 65 years and a female predominance. It is invariably a non-Hodgkin's lymphoma, usually diffuse high-grade and may be preceded by Hashimoto's thyroiditis. It is staged and treated using the same principles as for lymphoma elsewhere and has a 5-year survival of about 40 per cent.

TUMOURS OF THE PARATHYROID GLANDS

These are rare and may be part of MEN types I or II. Adenomas are usually impalpable, solitary and present with hyperparathyroidism (high serum calcium, low serum phosphate, hyperchloraemic metabolic acidosis, evidence of subperiosteal bone resorption

on plain radiographs, e.g. of phalanges). The glands can be imaged by radioisotope imaging using a technetium-99 scan (images the thyroid) followed by a thallium-201 scan (images both the thyroid and the parathyroids); subtraction of the two images gives an image of the parathyroids alone. Ultrasound or magnetic resonance imaging (MRI) of the neck are alternatives, and venous sampling for parathyroid hormone is useful for tumours that cannot be visualized. Parathyroidectomy is the sole treatment. Carcinoma is extremely rare.

TUMOURS OF THE ADRENAL GLANDS

Tumours of the adrenal gland are rare, accounting for approximately 100 deaths per year in the UK.

Phaeochromocytoma

This is a very rare tumour arising from the autonomic cells of the adrenal medulla, with a peak incidence at 35–55 years but may occur from infancy to old age. Recognized associations include:

- MEN type II;
- neurofibromatosis;
- von Hippel–Lindau syndrome;
- Sturge–Weber syndrome;
- tuberose sclerosis.

Ninety-nine per cent are found in the abdomen or pelvis: 90 per cent of these are in the adrenal medulla, the most common extra-adrenal site being adjacent to the aortic bifurcation. Other sites include the sympathetic chain, bladder, thorax (usually paravertebral) and carotid arch. The tumours may be very small or weigh several kilograms, are well circumscribed and slow-growing, with 10 per cent bilateral (70 per cent of those arising in familial cases); 90 per cent are benign and 10 per cent are malignant (more likely for extra-adrenal tumours). They are rich in lipid and therefore yellow in cut section. Phaeochromocytomas arise from chromaffin cells of neural crest origin. The cells therefore stain with chrome salts and enzymes such as dopa decarboxylase and contain neurosecretory granules. Since most tumours are benign, local invasion is unusual although malignant tumours may infiltrate the underlying kidney and retroperitoneum. Lymphatic spread is unusual but malignant tumours may spread to lung, bone and liver. The classic presentation is with paroxysms of headache, postural dizziness, feelings of apprehension and fear, pallor, sweating, tremor, chest pain and palpitations. Attacks last minutes to hours and are followed by a feeling of exhaustion and muscle pain, and may be precipitated by emotion, exertion, posture, bending, pressure on tumour, foods or handling of tumour at operation. Thyrotoxicosis should be excluded as it may present in a similar manner. Half the patients have sustained hypertension while 70 per cent have postural hypotension. Investigations include:

- urinary vanillylmandelic acid (VMA);
- meta-iodobenzyl guanidine (mIBG) imaging;
- CT/MRI scan;
- selective venous sampling;
- selective angiography.

Both VMA and catecholamine are measured using a 24-hour urine collection, and are useful screening tests during investigation of malignant hypertension. Urinary VMA is elevated in phaeochromocytoma, while high levels of adrenaline suggest an adrenal origin, high levels of noradrenaline suggest an extra-adrenal tumour, and high levels of dopamine suggest a malignant phaeochromocytoma. Computed tomography is the best investigation for delineating site and size of primary and excluding gross tumour in the contralateral adrenal, but is limited by its resolution of 0.5–1 cm which will miss some tumours.

Selective venous sampling is used to localize radiologically occult tumours, identifying their venous drainage using multiple venous samples which are tested for catecholamines. Selective arteriography is also of value when planning surgery as phaeochromocytomas have a rich vascular supply, but this may precipitate a hypertensive crisis.

Imaging with mIBG is not widely available. The compound is taken up by adrenergic tissue. It is of particular benefit in staging patients with malignant tumours, the iodine moiety being radioactive iodine-131 and therefore detectable by a gamma camera to give a whole-body image. Uptake of mIBG opens up an additional therapeutic option for malignant tumours.

Adrenalectomy is the treatment of choice. Expert anaesthetic advice and preoperative α- and β-blockade (e.g. phenoxybenzamine with propranolol or labetalol alone) is necessary as the tumour will be handled, leading to a release of catecholamines. At laparotomy it is important to inspect the contralateral adrenal for a second primary. In inoperable cases, phenoxybenzamine is a useful medical therapy, being an α-adrenergic receptor blocker. α-Methyltyrosine inhibits hydroxylation of tyrosine to dopa, an intermediate compound in the synthesis of catecholamines and is a more toxic alternative. External beam radiotherapy and chemotherapy have no role in the curative treatment of these tumours, although the former is of value in palliating local symptoms from metastases. Meta-iodobenzyl guanidine can be used to treat metastatic disease if the tumour concentrates enough of it. Only one-third of patients will concentrate mIBG to an adequate degree within their tumours and of these only one-third will show evidence of an objective response. With regard to prognosis, the vast majority will be cured by surgery alone. Even patients with malignant tumours may survive for many years, death often resulting from cardiovascular complications (e.g. myocardial infarction or cerebrovascular accident) rather than from metastatic disease.

Adrenal cortex tumours

Benign tumours are common at autopsy in the general population, but may be part of MEN type I disease. Most are non-functioning, the majority of functioning tumours arising in females. Of functioning tumours, those arising in prepubertal patients are virilizing, while those in postpubertal patients tend to produce Cushing's syndrome although Conn's syndrome (primary hyperaldosteronism) may also result. A CT scan will delineate the primary tumour if greater than 1 cm in diameter, although angiography is more sensitive, and treatment is by adrenalectomy.

Malignant tumours are rare arising at a younger age than most other carcinomas (median 35–55 years). Half are functioning and, as with benign tumours, are more frequent in females. Presentation is with vague abdominal symptoms, and up to one-third have signs of endocrine dysfunction, usually a combination of Cushing's syndrome and virilism. Half have metastatic disease at presentation, with haematogenous spread occurring to lung and liver. Investigation and treatment is as for benign tumours. In advanced disease, metyrapone (250–1000 mg q.d.s.) is useful for palliation of Cushing's syndrome by inhibiting 2β-hydroxylase, but it may exacerbate virilism and physiological glucocorticoid replacement is necessary. Aminoglutethimide may be added if control is insufficient. An alternative is mitotane (o,p'–DDD), which causes necrosis and atrophy of normal adrenal tissue and differentiated carcinoma cells, reducing steroid output in 70 per cent and giving objective tumour regression in one-third, although response is slow and glucocorticoid cover necessary.

CARCINOID TUMOURS

Carcinoid tumours form one of several types of gastroenteropancreatic (GEP) neuroendocrine tumours (see Chapter 9), although distinguished by their appearance, albeit rare, at sites outside the gastrointestinal tract.

Epidemiology

These are rare tumours arising at a younger age than carcinomas, with a peak incidence at about 50 years. There is no significant sex predominance or geographical pattern.

Aetiology

Carcinoid tumour may be a feature of multiple endocrine neoplasia type I.

Pathology

The primary tumour is often small compared with the bulk of liver metastases and symptoms of the carcinoid syndrome. They usually arise submucosally and appear as a nodule, often red/brown in colour, yellow in cut section, may be multifocal, and unlike carcinomas ulceration is uncommon. Carcinoid is most common in the small bowel – 90 per cent arise in the ileum, particularly the terminal segment, 7 per cent in the jejunum, 2 per cent in the duodenum and 2 per cent in a Meckel's diverticulum, but may arise elsewhere in the gastrointestinal tract, e.g. stomach, colon, rectum and other midline structures such as thyroid, lung, bladder, testes, ovaries, common bile duct and pancreas. An encasement reaction characterized by a massive fibrous stroma may occur when the tumour reaches the mesentery and this predisposes to bowel obstruction. Carcinoids arise from amine precursor uptake and decarboxylation (APUD) cells which are derived from the neural crest cells. Midgut-derived carcinoids characteristically stain with and reduce silver salts (argentaffin reaction), others stain with silver but cannot reduce it (argyrophilic reaction, e.g. gastric and bronchial carcinoids), while hindgut-derived carcinoids do not take up silver. Immunocytochemistry indicates staining for chromogranin which is useful when the diagnosis is in doubt.

Natural history

The tumours frequently behave in a benign manner and local infiltration of surrounding tissues is unusual. In contrast to a carcinoma, lymphatic spread is uncommon. Haematogenous spread is usually to the liver as most tumours will arise in the portal circulation. Ileal tumours frequently metastasize, especially if more than 2 cm in diameter, while appendiceal, rectal and bronchial carcinoids rarely metastasize. The metastases are characteristically multiple and bulky compared with the primary, and may undergo spontaneous necrosis. The skeleton is sometimes a site of distant metastases and these may be osteoblastic.

Symptoms

Symptoms depend on the site and size of the tumour. Carcinoids are often found incidentally at appendicectomy, when they are almost invariably benign and therefore very rarely metastasize to the liver. The patient may notice an abdominal mass if the tumour is large and superficial, or experience colicky abdominal pain if there is significant stenosis of the bowel lumen. Ultimately, there may be symptoms of subacute small bowel obstruction. Bronchial carcinoids present with haemoptysis or bronchial obstruction leading to recurrent chest infections. Carcinoid syndrome arises when there are liver metastases, so that the vasoactive tumour products, particularly 5-hydroxytryptamine (5-HT or serotonin), reach the systemic circulation, or in tumours arising outside the portal circulation. It comprises:

- flushing (distribution may vary with site of primary);
- weals (due to release of histamine);
- lacrimation;
- facial oedema;
- tachycardia;
- hypotension;
- wheezing;
- diarrhoea, borborygmi, abdominal colic and weight loss.

A given patient with liver metastases will not necessarily have all these symptoms and may complain of hepatic pain if a large subcapsular metastasis infarcts. Attacks may be precipitated by alcohol, stress, emotion, ingestion of food, infusion of calcium, noradrenaline or pentagastrin.

Signs

The patient with advanced disease often looks remarkably well bearing in mind the bulk of liver metastases. The patient may appear malnourished if diarrhoea has been a particular problem, an abdominal mass may be palpable or there may be signs in the chest of pulmonary collapse/consolidation depending on the site of the primary tumour. Hepatomegaly is expected in patients with carcinoid syndrome. Auscultation of the heart may reveal tricuspid or pulmonary valve disease, although left-sided cardiac lesions have been described with bronchial carcinoids, and there may be signs of heart failure.

Differential diagnosis

Other tumours arising at the site of the carcinoid should be considered, although none produce a syndrome akin to carcinoid when there are liver metastases. It should be noted that carcinomas at other sites may produce a carcinoid syndrome due to 5-HT production (e.g. medullary carcinoma of the thyroid or small cell lung cancer).

Investigations

Urinary 5-hydroxyindoleacetic acid

The 24-hour urinary 5-hydroxyindoleacetic acid (5-HIAA) is elevated in those with carcinoid syndrome, reflecting metabolism of 5-HT. A false-positive result may be obtained if the diet at the time of urine collection is rich in bananas, pineapples, avocados or walnuts. Malabsorption syndromes (e.g. coeliac disease) can also cause modest elevations in 5-HIAA. In addition to 5-HT, carcinoids may produce histamine, kallikrein, motilin, enteroglucagon, neurotensin, substance p, prostaglandins, insulin, ACTH, glucagon, parathyroid hormone and calcitonin, most of which can be assayed if clinically relevant.

Computed tomography/magnetic resonance imaging

A CT/MRI scan of the liver and site of primary defines the locoregional extent of the primary tumour and will exclude liver metastases.

Hepatic angiography

This is of value if resection of liver metastases or embolization is planned.

Staging

There is no formal staging system in routine clinical use.

Treatment

RADICAL TREATMENT

Surgery

The primary tumour should be completely excised as this offers the only chance of long-term cure. Radical lymph node resection is unnecessary, although obviously enlarged nodes should be cleared to ensure a complete resection of the tumour.

PALLIATIVE TREATMENT

Dietary advice

Referral to a dietician may help the patient to avoid ingestion of substances which may precipitate an attack of flushing and permit modification of the diet to lessen diarrhoea and protein-losing enteropathy.

Surgery

In patients with symptoms from one large liver metastasis or multiple metastases confined to one lobe of the liver, resection may be justified to reduce tumour bulk, thereby reducing secretion of vasoactive peptides and therefore palliating symptoms. Careful supervision is essential during the perioperative period to avert a hypotensive crisis when the tumour is handled. Bypass of an intestinal obstruction may also be necessary.

Radiotherapy

Carcinoids are not sensitive to radiation, although low doses of radiation are useful for the palliation of skeletal metastases.

Pharmacological measures

Codeine phosphate (30–60 mg t.d.s.) or loperamide (up to 16 mg daily) are both useful for the treatment of diarrhoea. Historically, drugs used for the palliation of symptoms refractory to more conventional measures include:

- parachlorophenylalanine (blocks conversion of tryptophan to 5-HT);
- cyproheptadine (blocks action of 5-HT on its receptors);
- ketanserin (a 5-HT2 receptor antagonist).

However, a somatostatin analogue such as octreotide is a potent inhibitor of the physiological effects of carcinoid tumours and should be considered the treatment of choice. The treatment may also have an antiproliferative effect on the tumour leading to disease stabilization.

Hepatic arterial embolization

This may be of benefit in up to 80 per cent with symptomatic hepatic metastases, with palliation lasting up to 3 years. This procedure may be repeated as necessary.

Chemotherapy

Streptozotocin is the most active chemotherapy agent with a partial response rate of 30 per cent.

Tumour-related complications

As with any other gastrointestinal tumour, perforation, obstruction or intussusception may all occur. Ectopic hormone production is recognized, the tumour producing growth hormone-releasing hormone leading to acromegaly, or ACTH leading to Cushing's syndrome. Pellagra is a rare syndrome characterized by glossitis, dermatitis in sun-exposed areas, diarrhoea and dementia, and is due to the tumour consuming tryptophan which is a precursor for nicotinic acid. Heart failure may ensue in advanced cases due to damage to the pulmonary and tricuspid valves.

Treatment-related complications

All cytoreductive treatments can release large amounts of vasoactive substances and therefore patients with bulky tumours should be pretreated with parachlorophenylalanine and cyproheptadine to avoid a serotonergic crisis.

Prognosis

Carcinoid tumours are usually very slow-growing so that even patients with heavy metastatic burdens may survive for many years. Appendiceal carcinoids have an excellent prognosis as they are small, easily removed and rarely metastasize.

MULTIPLE ENDOCRINE NEOPLASIA (MEN)

Type I

Described by Werner, MEN is dominantly inherited. Involved glands include:

- parathyroids (90 per cent; hyperplasia or adenoma);
- pancreatic islets (80 per cent; adenoma, carcinoma or more rarely diffuse hyperplasia);
- anterior pituitary (65 per cent; adenomas);
- adrenal cortex (40 per cent; hyperplasia or adenoma);

Carcinoid is also a rare association.

Type II

Originally described by Sipple, it has an autosomal dominant inheritance. Involved glands include:

- parafollicular cells of thyroid (medullary carcinoma);
- adrenal medulla (phaeochromocytoma);
- parathyroids (hyperplasia or adenoma).

Subtype A has no mucocutaneous features while subtype B is characterized by multiple small subcutaneous or submucosal neuromas of the oral cavity and lips, autonomic ganglioneuromatosis, and Marfanoid habitus.

Mixed multiple endocrine neoplasia

This demonstrates features of both types I and II.

SOFT TISSUE SARCOMAS

Epidemiology

Soft tissue sarcomas are rare tumours, with around 1000 cases reported in the UK each year divided equally between men and women. In children, the predominant tumour is a juvenile rhabdomyosarcoma, which will be considered in the section on paediatric tumours. It has very different characteristics to the soft tissue sarcomas of adults. In adults these tumours can occur at any age, the incidence being slightly more common in the 50- to 70-year age-group.

Aetiology

Usually, there is no identifiable cause but the following factors may be of importance:

- chronic mechanical irritation – sarcomas can be induced in animal models but this does not appear important in humans;
- radiation – a small number of sarcomas are undoubtedly related to previous therapeutic irradiation, with tumours developing several years after exposure;
- familial – these sarcomas form part of the Li Fraumeni syndrome where they are associated with tumours of breast, brain, adrenal cortex and leukaemias in close relatives under the age of 45 years; they are also seen in patients with von Recklinghausen's syndrome of familial neurofibromatosis with malignant change within pre-existing neurofibromata occurring;
- chemical – angiosarcoma is associated with vinyl chloride exposure.

Pathology

Sites for soft tissue sarcomas include:

- limbs (upper, 15%; lower, 40%);
- retroperitoneum (20%);
- viscera (bladder, bowel, uterus; 10%);
- trunk (10%);
- head and neck (4%).

Macroscopically, soft tissue sarcomas are often large, fleshy tumour masses with associated haemorrhage and necrosis. They are seen to invade local soft tissues, nerves and blood vessels.

Microscopic classification of soft tissue sarcomas is based on the finding of recognizable connective tissue elements within the tumour. The basis of the diagnosis is the finding of malignant spindle cells which may form characteristic patterns, as in a fibrosarcoma when a 'herringbone' pattern is described and malignant fibrous histiocytoma when a 'cartwheel' pattern may be seen. A classification of the soft tissue sarcomas is shown in Table 15.1.

Histological grade is an important prognostic feature of sarcomas and a three-point scale is used to describe the degree of differentiation. However, this must be interpreted in the light of the cell type. For example, angiosarcoma will usually appear well-differentiated but is usually a highly malignant tumour. Similarly, virtually all synovial sarcomas can be regarded as high-grade tumours irrespective of their grading.

Natural history

There is extensive local growth with infiltration of surrounding structures including blood vessels and nerves, and early blood-borne spread to lungs as the most common distant site.

TABLE 15.1 Classification of soft tissue sarcomas

Sarcoma subtype	Tissue type	Features
Fibrosarcoma	Fibrous tissue	Most common type, typically found in thigh
Liposarcoma	Fat	Lower extremity and retroperitoneum
Rhabdomyosarcoma	Skeletal muscle	Adult forms are alveolar or pleomorphic
Leiomyosarcoma	Smooth muscle	Uterus and gastrointestinal tract common, also limbs and retroperitoneum
Malignant fibrous histiocytoma	Histiocytes	Especially legs, buttocks and retroperitoneum
Neurogenic sarcoma	Neural tissue	Arise within large nerves, e.g. sciatic (neurofibrosarcoma), median, spinal roots
Synovial sarcoma	Uncertain	Arise around joints, especially thigh, foot, knee
Angiosarcoma	Blood vessels	Scalp, breast, liver
Lymphangiosarcoma	Lymph vessels	Sites of chronic lymphoedema, e.g. post-mastectomy arm

Lymph node spread is relatively uncommon except for synovial sarcomas and alveolar rhabdomyosarcoma.

Symptoms

Peripheral sarcomas present as a lump which may be present for some time before it becomes symptomatic. Retroperitoneal sarcomas may grow to a large size before causing symptoms, the most common of which is backache.

The rapid increase in size of a pre-existing neurofibroma should alert to the possibility of malignant change to a neurofibrosarcoma.

Signs

At presentation, peripheral sarcomas are often large masses within soft tissue. Figure 15.1 shows a large soft tissue sarcoma arising in the lower limb. Movement can become limited, particularly when close to joints. Retroperitoneal masses may be palpable per abdomen.

Differential diagnosis

Other benign soft tissue masses should be considered, such as a neurofibroma, lipoma or fibroma.

Investigations

Routine investigations such as full blood count and blood biochemistry are usually unremarkable.

Radiography

Chest X-ray may show pulmonary metastases (Fig. 15.2). If normal, a computed tomography (CT) scan of the chest should be performed to further exclude metastases.

Computed tomography scan or magnetic resonance imaging

Magnetic resonance imaging (MRI) of the primary site will give most precise definition of the soft tissue extent and involvement of local structures, as shown in Fig. 15.3. Spiral CT scan of the lungs is essential to exclude small volume lung metastases before considering radical treatment.

Biopsy

Biopsy of the primary lesion is essential to confirm the diagnosis and the type of sarcoma. Definition of a sarcoma may be difficult and if needle biopsy is not sufficient an open biopsy may be required. It is important that this is performed in consultation with the surgeon that will perform the definitive resection, as implantation at the biopsy site can occur and this should be included in the resection.

Staging

Staging (see Chapter 2) is based on the size of the primary tumour.

- Tl – tumour $\leqslant 5$ cm maximum diameter.
- T2 – tumour >5 cm maximum diameter.
- N0 – no nodes.
- N1 – regional nodes.
- G1 – low grade.
- G2 – intermediate grade.
- G3 – high grade.

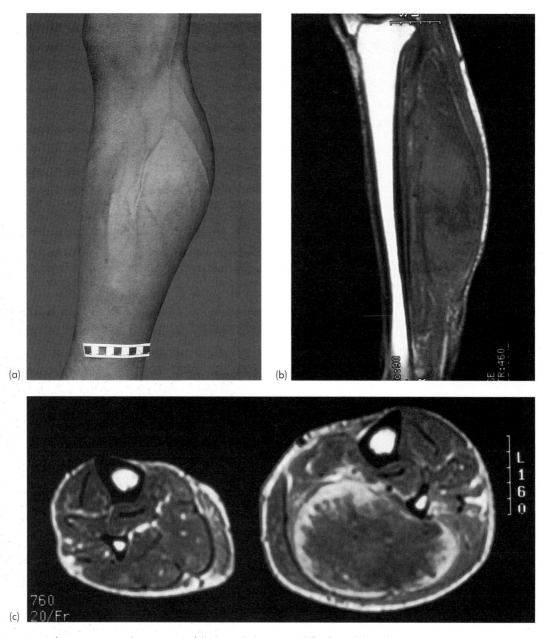

FIG 15.1 Soft tissue sarcoma (liposarcoma) of the lower limb seen (a) clinically and (b and c) on magnetic resonance imaging, demonstrating the extensive involvement of the muscle compartment.

Treatment

Sarcoma management is complex and these tumours are relatively rare. They should therefore be treated by specialized multidisciplinary teams incorporating surgical and oncological expertise in this field.

LOCAL TREATMENT

Wide surgical resection including excision of any previous biopsy scar, combined with radiotherapy which may be given pre- or post-operatively, enables conservation of the affected limb. Amputation is avoided if at all possible but may be necessary for

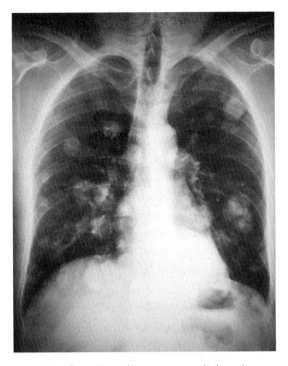

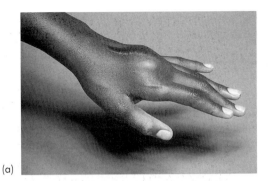

(a)

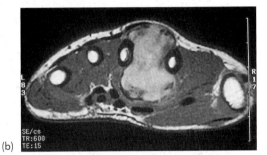

(b)

Fig 15.2 Chest X-ray demonstrating multiple pulmonary metastases from a soft tissue sarcoma.

locally advanced tumours or those that progress despite radiotherapy.

Retroperitoneal tumours present a more difficult surgical problem and resection may not be possible. High-dose irradiation is required, delivering doses of at least 60 Gy in 6 weeks.

Radiation alone may control a soft tissue sarcoma but is inferior to the combination of surgery with irradiation.

The role of adjuvant chemotherapy remains under investigation. Soft tissue sarcoma is not a particularly chemosensitive tumour but recent analyses suggest that there may be a small benefit for local and distant relapse-free survival, but not overall survival, from intensive adjuvant chemotherapy.

Isolated limb perfusion with drugs such as melphalan may be of benefit in locally advanced, unresectable limb tumours.

METASTATIC DISEASE

Chemotherapy has only limited activity. Responses are seen with cisplatin, Adriamycin and ifosfamide but long-term remissions are few and the toxicity of treatment is considerable.

Surgical resection (metastatectomy) is the most successful treatment of lung metastases if feasible.

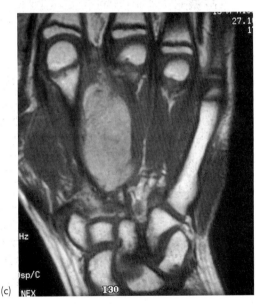

(c)

Fig 15.3 (a) Fibrosarcoma arising on dorsum of the hand. (b,c) Magnetic resonance imaging scans to show detail of precise anatomical location.

Tumour-related complications

Local effects due to tumour size are the main problem associated with soft tissue sarcomas. In general, paraneoplastic effects and systemic complications such as hypercalcaemia are not features of these tumours, although hypoglycaemia has been described as a rare association with massive retroperitoneal sarcomas.

Treatment-related complications

The emphasis of modern treatment is towards limb preservation. However, the effects of extensive resection and radiotherapy may lead to functional deficits in the limb, with joint stiffness, loss of muscle power and limb oedema.

Prognosis

The prognosis for peripheral limb tumours is better than that for sarcomas affecting the retroperitoneum, trunk or internal organs. With conservative limb-preserving treatment local control rates will be of the order of 80 per cent with 5-year survival around 60 per cent, depending on the tumour stage and grade. Patients with operable lung metastases have a 5-year survival of around 30 per cent following metastatectomy.

Future developments

The major change in the management of soft tissue sarcomas has been in the development of limb-preserving treatment instead of amputation. The main difficulty now lies in the management of systemic disease for which there is no satisfactory treatment. Adjuvant chemotherapy has been proposed as a possible way of reducing systemic relapse but trials to date demonstrate only small benefits.

Rare tumours

Extraosseous Ewing's and primitive neuroectodermal tumours

These are rare soft tissue tumours characterized by small round cells rich in glycogen morphologically identical to the classical Ewing's tumour of bone (see below). Extraosseous Ewing's is most common on the trunk and extremities, arising in soft tissue, distinct from bone, while primitive neuroectodermal tumour (PNET) is most common in the chest, when it may be termed Askin's tumour, and also the abdomen and pelvis. Management and prognosis follows that of classical Ewing's tumour of bone (see below).

Desmoid tumours

These classically arise in the abdominal wall of women postpartum but may occur at any site, presenting as a diffuse fibrous infiltrative tumour, which, while pathologically benign, may cause serious effects by virtue of its relentless local growth. Surgical resection is the treatment of choice but when inoperable, slow regression is achieved following a radical dose of radiotherapy.

Stewart–Treves tumour

This is the name given to the rare development of a lymphangiosarcoma in the upper limb of a woman having chronic lymphoedema secondary to the treatment of breast carcinoma. Treatment may be difficult owing to the pre-existing oedema and associated postoperative and post-radiotherapy changes. Amputation may be necessary.

Dermatofibroma

This is a benign tumour of the skin presenting as a fibrous nodule typically on the limbs, and distinct from simple fibromas because of the presence of histiocytes on microscopy. Its malignant counterpart is dermatofibrosarcoma protuberans, so called because of its microscopic appearance of an hourglass shape pushing the epidermis outwards. It is usually found on the trunk and histologically it is essentially a fibrosarcoma.

OSTEOSARCOMA

Epidemiology

Osteosarcoma is the most common malignant tumour of the bone, although it is rare in relation to other malignancies. It occurs mainly in adolescents, particularly during periods of active bone growth, with a second peak of incidence in those over 60 years when it is related to Paget's disease. It is almost twice as common in males as in females.

Aetiology

No recognizable aetiological agent is present for the majority of cases. Paget's disease may be a pre-existing feature in adult osteosarcoma, as shown in Fig. 15.4.

Osteosarcoma is a rare late effect following therapeutic irradiation. Historically, it is associated with radium dial painting and the use of thorium-based

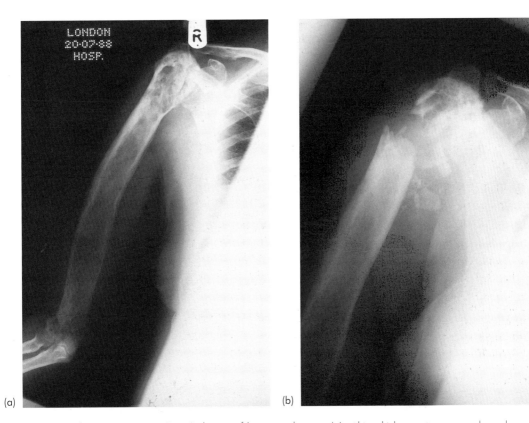

(a)   (b)

FIG 15.4 X-rays showing pre-existing Paget's disease of bone in a humerus (a) within which an osteosarcoma has subsequently developed (b).

contrast agents (e.g. Thorotrast) in diagnostic radiology.

It may occur as a component of the rare Li–Fraumeni syndrome, in which bone or soft tissue sarcomas are associated with a familial pattern of breast, brain and adrenal cortex tumours and leukaemia. In these cases, germ line mutations of the *p53* gene are found. An association with the retinoblastoma gene with deletions on the long arm of chromosome 13 and loss of heterozygosity on chromosome 17 has also been recognized. Survivors of hereditary retinoblastoma may have a relative risk of up to 500 for developing osteosarcoma with a latency of 10 years or more.

Pathology

The most common site for osteosarcoma is in a long bone, particularly around the knee, with 30 per cent arising from the lower femur and 15 per cent in the upper tibia. Ten per cent arise in the humerus and the remainder may affect any bone, including the axial skeleton. Two principal groups are described,

'central (medullary)' and 'surface (peripheral)' tumours. The classical osteosarcoma is a central tumour and accounts for 95 per cent of those seen.

Macroscopically, the tumour arises in the metaphysis and grows both eccentrically, expanding the cortex and raising the periosteum at its edges, and also along the medulla. Within the tumour will be areas of haemorrhage and necrosis, together with new bone formation in the subperiosteal regions to form the classic Codman's triangles and sunray spicules. Pathological fracture through the tumour-bearing bone may occur.

Microscopically, there are two main populations of cells: a background stroma of spindle-shaped sarcomatous cells containing a matrix which may be myxoid, cartilaginous or osteoid, together with multinucleate giant cells.

Natural history

There is local spread within the bone of origin, typically within the medullary cavity, and early blood-borne spread, particularly to the lungs. Other bones may also be affected through blood-borne spread. Lymph node disease is not a prominent feature.

Symptoms

There is usually pain in the bone and there may be a lump around the site of origin. There is sometimes a history of preceding trauma, although no causal relationship exists. Symptoms from metastases may include cough and haemoptysis but other features of malignant disease such as anorexia and weight loss are infrequent unless very advanced.

Signs

Swelling and deformity of the bone are seen. It is often hot and red and there may be an audible bruit. Thinning of the periosteum may result in a characteristic crackling on palpation and there may be crepitus if fracture has occurred. There is often an associated fever.

Differential diagnosis

Other causes of bone swelling should be considered, including benign tumours such as osteochondromas and other malignant tumours.

Investigations

Routine investigations are often unremarkable, although there may be a leucocytosis and the alkaline phosphatase will be inappropriately raised (note that in growing children and adolescents the normal range for alkaline phosphatase is increased during bone growth).

Radiography

Plain X-ray of the affected bone will show local destruction of bone with areas of new bone formation that may form the classic Codman's triangles and sunray spicules but more often are less well demarcated. There will be periosteal elevation and pathological fracture may be apparent. In adults, coexisting Paget's disease may be apparent, as illustrated in Fig. 15.4.

Computed tomography scan or magnetic resonance imaging

Further detail of the precise extent of bone destruction and spread within the medullary cavity will be found on CT or MRI scan, the latter being the investigation of choice. A CT scan of the lungs is important to identify pulmonary metastases.

Isotope bone scan

This will give further information on the extent of local bone involvement and also identify any bone metastases.

Staging

There is no widely used staging system for osteosarcoma.

Treatment

The mainstay of modern treatment for osteosarcoma is a course of intensive chemotherapy, together with local removal or irradiation of the site of origin.

CHEMOTHERAPY

Schedules based on the use of combination chemotherapy containing cisplatin, ifosfamide and Adriamycin have been shown to be as effective as the original chemotherapy regimes which used high-dose methotrexate in doses of between 8 g/m^2 and 12 g/m^2 of body surface area in combination with other drugs such as Adriamycin, bleomycin, vincristine, cyclophosphamide and dactinomycin.

LOCAL TREATMENT

Following induction chemotherapy with a satisfactory response, conservative limb-preserving resection of the bone is undertaken. This may entail the use of an appropriate prosthesis or excision of the entire bone if expendable, as in the case of a rib or the fibula. In children, a prosthesis which can be expanded to accommodate growth may be used, as shown in Fig. 15.5.

For surgically unresectable disease, local radiotherapy will be given with the aim of delivering a dose of up to 60 Gy in 6 weeks. In certain sites, particularly in the spine close to spinal cord, the dose may be limited by the tolerance of central nervous system (CNS) tissue. Following local treatment, chemotherapy will be continued for a total of around 20 weeks.

METASTASES

Patients presenting with lung metastases will be treated in a similar fashion if resectable, with metastatectomy being performed in addition to local surgery.

PALLIATION

Palliative treatment may be required for relapsed disease. Local irradiation may be valuable for local

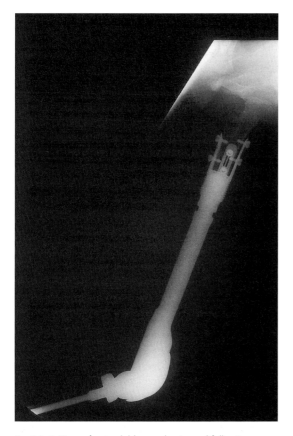

FIG 15.5 X-ray of extendable prosthesis used following resection of tumour from the lower femur.

pain and to arrest tumour growth through skin. Amputation may be considered for recurrent disease but only when there is thought to be a realistic chance of long-term salvage.

Metastatic disease may require further chemotherapy and limited pulmonary metastases may be resected.

Tumour-related complications

The principal complication is pathological fracture.

Treatment-related complications

The affected limb may have limitation of movement and muscle strength. Prostheses fitted to young patients that have not completed their growth may require revision from time to time. Following amputation, which may still be required in a small number of patients, specific problems may include

phantom limb pain and stump ulceration and chafing. Thoracotomy may result in limited respiratory reserve, depending on the extent of resection required, and postoperative pain in the thoracotomy scar is a well-recognized problem.

Chemotherapy will have considerable acute morbidity, including nausea, vomiting, alopecia and mucositis. Longer-term problems may arise from nephrotoxicity related to the use of methotrexate or cisplatin and neurotoxicity from cisplatin or vincristine. In children there may be growth retardation and effects on subsequent maturation and fertility.

Prognosis

Overall, using modern chemotherapy-based schedules for treatment, the 5-year survival for non-metastatic osteosarcoma is between 40 per cent and 50 per cent. In patients presenting with lung metastases, up to 20 per cent may become long-term survivors and as many as 40 per cent of those relapsing with pulmonary metastases may be salvaged. Elderly patients have a worse prognosis partly because of the limitations of delivering intensive chemotherapy to this group. Those with tumours secondary to Paget's disease have a 5-year survival of only 4 per cent.

Rare tumours

Parosteal sarcoma

This typically occurs in young adults, and is a peripheral tumour arising from the juxtacortical part of the bone metaphysis growing concentrically around the bone. The lower femur and upper tibia are the usual sites. Surgical excision is the treatment of choice. This is a low-grade malignancy with a low risk of metastases. Prognosis is better than that for an osteosarcoma, with 5-year survival figures of 50–70 per cent. Occasionally, transformation into a high-grade osteosarcoma is seen.

EWING'S SARCOMA

Epidemiology

Ewing's sarcoma is a tumour of bone affecting predominantly children and young adults, the maximum incidence being between the ages of 10 and 20 years. A rare extra-osseous form of this sarcoma also may be recognized. The incidence of Ewing's sarcoma in the UK is 0.6 in 100 000 and males are affected more than females. It is relatively rare in black populations.

Aetiology

There is no recognized aetiological agent but a specific chromosomal translocation in Ewing's sarcoma has been demonstrated between chromosomes 11 and 22, and other similar translocations between chromosome 22 and chromosomes 21, 7 and 17 have also been described.

Pathology

Ewing's may affect any bone and is found in long bones, vertebrae and limb girdles, especially the pelvic bones. Macroscopically, it arises in the diaphysis of the bone, growing subperiosteally. Periosteal reaction, as it traverses the length of the bone, may give rise to the characteristic onion-peel appearance of the bone on X-ray. To the naked eye the tumour contains areas of necrosis, and haemorrhage and cystic regions may also be seen.

Microscopically, Ewing's is composed of sheets of small round cells which are rich in glycogen. A surface marker, CD99 is characteristic for the Ewing's family of tumours.

Natural history

There is local growth, the primary often reaching a considerable size, and blood-borne dissemination, with metastases to lungs in particular. Lymph node metastases are not usually a major feature.

Symptoms

Ewing's is typically painful and, characteristically, pain is intermittent in the early development of the tumour mass. There may be a preceding history of trauma but no causal relationship is recognized. Pathological fracture may occur. Lung metastases may cause cough or haemoptysis.

Signs

The tumour mass will be apparent as a palpable mass, often tender to palpation. There may be associated fever, particularly in advanced cases.

Differential diagnosis

Ewing's must be differentiated from other primary tumours of bone. Other round cell tumours which can affect bone should also be excluded, in particular lymphoma, neuroblastoma and anaplastic carcinoma.

Investigations

Blood cell count

A full blood count may demonstrate a raised white cell count and occasionally a mild anaemia may also be present.

Biochemistry

Biochemical tests may be normal or show an inappropriately raised alkaline phosphatase level.

Radiography

An X-ray of the affected bone will show thinning of the diaphysis and in later stages extensive bone destruction (Fig. 15.6). The characteristic onion-peel appearance of successive layers of periosteal reaction may also be seen.

Chest X-ray and, if normal, CT scan of the lungs should be performed to evaluate the possibility of lung metastases.

Computed tomography scan or magnetic resonance imaging

Greater detail of the tumour mass, in particular soft tissue invasion and spread along the marrow cavity of the bone will be seen with MRI. Spiral CT of the lungs is essential to exclude small-volume lung metastases.

Biopsy

Biopsy of the primary lesion is essential to confirm the diagnosis.

Staging

There is no recognized staging system for Ewing's sarcoma.

Treatment

CHEMOTHERAPY

The common chemotherapy schedule used is based on the use of VAC (vincristine, Adriamycin and cyclophosphamide). Recently, more intensive schedules alternating VAC with ifosfamide and etoposide have been developed. The role of

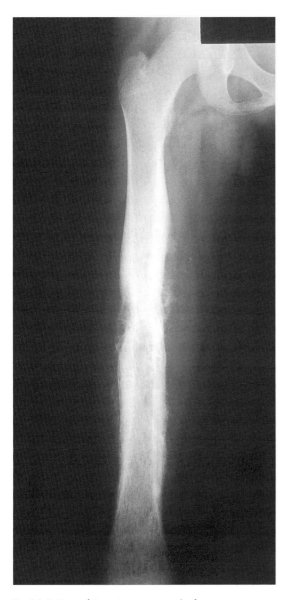

FIG 15.6 X-ray of Ewing's sarcoma in the femur.

intensive high-dose schedules remains under evaluation.

LOCAL TREATMENT

After 2–3 months of chemotherapy, radiotherapy will be the treatment of choice for most patients to deliver a total dose of between 50 Gy and 60 Gy in 5–6 weeks.

Surgery may be used instead, particularly for bones such as rib and fibula which can be removed *in toto*. Chemotherapy is then continued for several months following local treatment.

PALLIATIVE TREATMENT

Standard chemotherapy, as described above, is appropriate for widespread symptomatic metastases. Local symptoms of pain or bleeding may be better dealt with by local radiotherapy. In selected patients, high-dose chemotherapy with autologous marrow transplant may be an option.

Tumour-related complications

These include pathological fracture and spinal cord compression from rapid growth of spinal tumours.

Treatment-related complications

Chemotherapy may result in acute nausea, vomiting and alopecia. In the longer term, vincristine can be associated with a peripheral neuropathy and in high doses Adriamycin is cardiotoxic. For this reason, actinomycin D is substituted once a tolerance dose has been reached.

High-dose radiotherapy to a limb may result in joint stiffness, skin changes and lymphoedema.

Prognosis

The overall 5-year survival for patients without metastases treated with modern chemotherapy-based regimes is around 50 per cent. This is determined particularly by tumour size ranging from 70 per cent in tumours less than 500 cm^3 to 35 per cent in tumours greater than 500 cm^3.

Local control rates may approach 90 per cent and are greater in long bones than in the pelvis.

OTHER BONE TUMOURS

Chondrosarcoma

This is a tumour typically affecting the pelvic bones, although it may also occur in the femur, humerus and scapula. It is a tumour of adults and is usually slow growing. Rarely, tumours may arise within a pre-existing chondroma. Initial treatment is radical surgical resection or, if inoperable, radiotherapy. Well and moderately differentiated forms have a good prognosis and only metastasize late, if at all. There is, however, a high-grade variant which has an aggressive course and these patients may be selected for treatment with early chemotherapy using drugs similar to the osteosarcoma schedules. The overall 5-year survival is around 35 per cent.

Osteoclastoma (giant cell tumour)

This is a tumour arising in adults, usually between the ages of 30 years and 50 years, the most common sites being the long bones around the knee, radius and humerus. There is a characteristic 'soap bubble' appearance on X-ray with eccentric thinning of the cortex. Clinically, this may be demonstrated, albeit rarely, by 'eggshell crackling' on palpation.

It is composed of two populations of cells, a background stroma of spindle cells, the differentiation of which defines the activity of the tumour, and scattered multinucleate giant cells. The majority are of low-grade malignancy and present a problem of local control rather than disseminated disease.

Wide surgical excision is the treatment of choice. Around one-third will recur locally and a further one-third will be high-grade tumours that ultimately metastasize. Local irradiation may be of value for local recurrence; chemotherapy is not usually successful in metastatic disease. The overall 5-year survival is around 65–70 per cent.

Spindle cell sarcoma

Tumours histologically identical to fibrosarcoma or malignant fibrous histiocytoma of soft tissue may be found as primary bone tumours. They are usually tumours of adults in the 30- to 60-year age-group. Treatment is radical surgical excision. There has been some interest in giving adjuvant chemotherapy in this group of patients but, to date, there is no evidence that this improves survival. Overall 5-year survivals are in the range 25–40 per cent.

Angiosarcomas may also arise in bone and will be treated in the same way as the other spindle cell sarcomas of bone.

Malignancies of the lymphoproliferative system can be broadly classified into Hodgkin's disease and all other lymphomas, which are termed the non-Hodgkin's lymphomas. The classification of these is complex and many different systems have been described. A simplified clinical view is shown in Fig. 16.1.

HODGKIN'S DISEASE

Epidemiology

There are around 1400 cases per annum in the UK with an incidence of 25 per million population. There is a bimodal age distribution, the two peaks of incidence occurring in young people aged 20–30 years and in later life between 60 years and 70 years.

Overall, it is almost twice as common in men as it is in women. In children, the sex difference is even more extreme, occurring almost exclusively in boys under the age of 10 years. It is rare in the Japanese and in the USA black population, and particularly high in the Jewish populations of the USA and the UK.

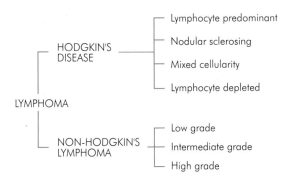

FIG 16.1 Clinical types of lymphoma.

Aetiology

There is no proven aetiological agent responsible for the development of Hodgkin's disease.

Pathology

Macroscopically, Hodgkin's disease is usually found in lymph nodes, the spleen and liver. More rarely, infiltration of the lungs, bone marrow, skin or central nervous system may occur. Typically, the nodes are relatively soft and uniformly enlarged. The spleen and liver appearances are of multiple nodules within their substance, the cut surface of which has been likened to that of a German sausage.

Microscopically, the diagnostic feature is the presence of binucleate cells called Reed–Sternberg cells. In addition a wide variation of other cells including lymphocytes, neutrophils, plasma cells, eosinophils, histiocytes and fibroblasts are also found infiltrating the node or affected organ. There are four major histological subclassifications, as shown in Table 16.1.

Natural history

Typically, stepwise involvement of adjacent node groups occurs. The most common nodes involved are those in the neck. In this situation, spread is to adjacent nodes in the supraclavicular fossa, the axillae and the mediastinum before involving para-aortic nodes below the diaphragm. Extranodal involvement as a sole manifestation is rare and usually occurs in the context of extensive or bulky node disease.

Symptoms

Typically, the patient is aware of a painless enlarged node in the neck. This may be present for many weeks or months but may develop more rapidly.

TABLE 16.1 Histological subtypes of Hodgkin's disease

Subclass	Features	Prognosis
Lymphocyte predominant	Infiltrate of many small lymphocytes	Good
Nodular sclerosis	Node divided by fibrous bands. Cells may be rich in lymphocytes (type 1) or be of mixed type (type 2)	Type 1 – good Type 2 – moderate
Mixed cellularity	Mixed population of cells	Moderate
Lymphocyte depleted	Fibrous node with Reed–Sternberg cells but few other cells seen	Poor

'B' symptoms are characteristic of lymphomas and are:

- fever greater than 38°C often with typical remittent pattern (Pel-Ebstein fever);
- weight loss of more than 10 per cent body weight;
- night sweats.

Other uncommon but characteristic symptoms include generalized and often intractable itching and alcohol-induced pain in the enlarged nodes. Although the lymph nodes themselves are usually painless, there may be backache from para-aortic nodes and left-sided abdominal pain from splenic enlargement.

Signs

Enlarged lymph nodes may be present in any site. They are most common in the neck. Typically, the nodes of Hodgkin's disease are described as firm and rubbery as opposed to the hard craggy nodes of carcinoma. There may be palpable hepato-splenomegaly or an abdominal mass due to para-aortic or mesenteric nodes. Inguinal and pelvic lymphadenopathy may be associated with oedema of the lower limbs, although arm oedema is an unusual complication of axillary lymphadenopathy due to lymphoma. Mediastinal lymphadenopathy may present with the signs of superior vena cava obstruction (SVCO).

Differential diagnosis

The main differential diagnosis is between Hodgkin's disease and non-Hodgkin's lymphoma. Other causes of lymphadenopathy will also be considered, including infection which can be either pyogenic, tuberculous or viral e.g. Epstein–Barr (EB) virus or cytomegalovirus (CMV), toxoplasmosis and other neoplastic conditions such as leukaemia or carcinoma.

Investigations

Blood count

A full blood count may show mild anaemia and leucocytosis with a raised lymphocyte count but is frequently normal.

Erythrocyte sedimentation rate

The erythrocyte sedimentation rate (ESR) may be raised, particularly in more aggressive forms of the disease.

Biochemistry

Routine biochemical blood tests may show evidence of hepatic infiltration with raised alkaline phosphatase and gammaglutamyltransferase. More profound hepatic disturbance is rare. Obstruction of the renal tracts by enlarged nodes may cause renal failure. Hypercalcaemia is a recognized but rare finding in Hodgkin's disease. Serum lactate dehydrogenase is a sensitive index of disease activity and of prognostic importance.

Bone marrow examination

Unlike non-Hodgkin's lymphoma, bone marrow involvement is unusual in the absence of other soft tissue involvement (i.e. stage 4 disease). Bone marrow examination is no longer routine for those patients presenting with stage 1–3 nodal disease in the absence of B symptoms.

Radiography

Chest X-ray may show widened mediastinal shadow due to enlarged nodes or, more rarely, lung parenchymal infiltration. Pleural effusion is also a recognized finding.

Computed tomography and magnetic resonance imaging

Computed tomography (CT) scan of the chest, abdomen and pelvis will give the most accurate assessment of internal lymphadenopathy and has now superseded the use of bipedal lymphangiography as the imaging of choice for staging in lymphoma. There is less experience of magnetic resonance imaging (MRI) scanning in Hodgkin's disease but wider availability and the use of new contrast agents may broaden its role in the future.

Biopsy

A tissue diagnosis is mandatory to confirm the diagnosis and define the histological subtype of Hodgkin's disease. This will usually take the form of an open lymph node biopsy from an accessible node in the neck, supraclavicular fossa or groin.

Splenectomy

Splenectomy was previously a standard procedure to complete the staging of Hodgkin's disease. It is now performed only rarely because current indications for systemic treatment mean that information about splenic status will rarely influence management, and imaging with ultrasound, CT and MRI will give an accurate picture of subdiaphragmatic disease for which laparotomy was once required.

Staging

The staging of Hodgkin's disease follows the Ann Arbor classification.

- Stage 1 – involved lymph nodes limited to one node area only.
- Stage 2 – involved lymph nodes encompassing two or more adjacent areas but remaining on one side of the diaphragm only.
- Stage 3 – involved lymph nodes on both sides of the diaphragm.
- Stage 4 – involvement of extranodal organs denoted by the following suffixes: M, bone marrow; D, skin; H, liver; S, spleen.

   Each stage is further subclassified 'A' or 'B' according to the absence or presence, respectively, of B symptoms (see above).

Treatment

Hodgkin's disease is both radiosensitive and chemosensitive and most patients can expect to be cured of their disease. Because this is a disease frequently affecting young people who will live for many years after successful treatment, there is now considerable emphasis not only on the efficacy of treatment but also on achieving cure with minimal long-term morbidity.

LOCALIZED DISEASE (STAGES 1A AND 2A)

Radical radiotherapy alone will cure many patients. This may take the form of 'involved field' irradiation where a volume including only those areas known to be affected is treated, or wide-field irradiation. The former approach is associated with less morbidity but a greater chance of regional relapse. This may be overcome by a short course of chemotherapy equivalent to two to four cycles rather than six to eight as in advanced disease followed by involved field radiotherapy.

The usual wide-field radiotherapy treatments are a 'mantle' field above the diaphragm and an 'inverted Y' below the diaphragm (Fig. 16.2). Involved field treatments are much smaller and cover only areas of known disease.

Hodgkin's disease is much more sensitive to radiation than the common epithelial cancers and requires only 35–40 Gy given over 4–4.5 weeks (compared with 60–70 Gy for a squamous carcinoma).

Relapse in these patients can in most cases be salvaged using chemotherapy.

ADVANCED DISEASE (STAGES 1B, 2B, 3 AND 4)

Although there may be only limited nodal disease apparent, the presence of B symptoms is a poor prognostic feature and implies more widespread disease. For this reason, stages 1B and 2B disease are included in this category, together with those patients that have widespread node disease or involvement of systemic organs. Chemotherapy is given to these patients.

Prior to starting chemotherapy male patients should have the opportunity to consider sperm banking as subsequent fertility, although frequently preserved, cannot be guaranteed after chemotherapy.

All patients having chemotherapy should be well-hydrated and started on allopurinol to prevent tumour lysis syndrome (see Chapter 22). Response may be dramatic and rapid; an example of a chemotherapy response on treating bulky mediastinal nodes from Hodgkin's disease is shown in Fig. 16.3.

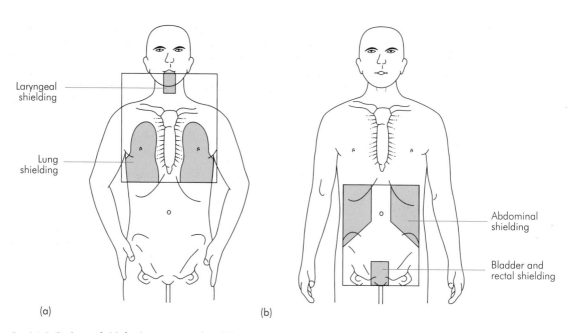

FIG 16.2 Radiation fields for the treatment of Hodgkin's disease: (a) mantle fields for nodes above the diaphragm; (b) inverted Y field for nodes below the diaphragm.

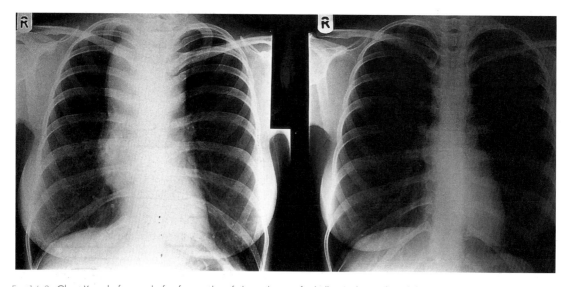

FIG 16.3 Chest X-ray before and after four cycles of chemotherapy for bulky mediastinal Hodgkin's disease.

SPECIFIC CHEMOTHERAPY

Early schedules used were based upon MOPP (mustine, vincristine, procarbazine and prednisolone). While effective in giving complete remission rates of up to 80 per cent, there is significant toxicity and modifications have been developed to minimize this morbidity.

LOPP or ChIVPP replaces the mustine by chlorambucil and in the case of ChIVPP, vincristine is replaced by vinblastine.

Anthracycline-based (i.e. Adriamycin or its analogues) schedules such as ABVD (Adriamycin, bleomycin, vincristine and dacarbazine) are also highly active and are now recognized as the chemotherapy of choice for Hodgkin's disease. These schedules are associated with less long-term toxicity and randomized trials have shown cure rates to be at least equivalent to earlier schedules. Most patients will receive six to eight courses of standard chemotherapy. Radiotherapy is then often given following (or sometimes in the middle of) chemotherapy to initial sites of bulky lymph node disease, except for those patients with stage 4 disease affecting major organs or bone marrow.

A new generation of chemotherapy regimens have emerged over recent years using a more intensive weekly schedule of drugs alternating, seven agents and followed by involved field radiotherapy. Examples of these are 'Stanford V' and BEACOPP. Over the next few years these will be compared in trials with ABVD representing the current gold standard.

TREATMENT FOR RELAPSE

Relapse after radiotherapy will generally be treated with chemotherapy and response rates similar to other patients receiving primary chemotherapy are to be expected, with around 80 per cent going back into remission. Relapse after chemotherapy is not so easy to treat. Of those patients given initial chemotherapy for advanced disease around 40 per cent will either relapse or fail to achieve a sustained complete remission. Retreatment with the same or alternative chemotherapy regimens may result in further regression of disease for around 50 per cent but, of these, only 15–20 per cent will achieve long-term remission. It is therefore in this group of patients that more intensive treatment using high-dose chemotherapy and bone marrow autograft or peripheral blood progenitor cells (PBPC) (see below) may be indicated. With such techniques, long-term survival may be achieved in over 30 per cent of patients relapsing after conventional chemotherapy for Hodgkin's disease.

Tumour-related complications

Massive lymphadenopathy may have consequences as a result of local pressure, although in general lymphoma tends to grow around structures rather than directly invade them. In the mediastinum dysphagia and SVC obstruction may occur. In the abdomen, renal failure owing to ureteric obstruction and lower limb oedema owing to pelvic node enlargement are seen.

Treatment-related complications

RADIOTHERAPY

Wide-field irradiation may have various long-term effects, although it should be emphasized that for most patients there are few if any sequelae. The potential problems are shown in Table 16.2. Mediastinal fibrosis following mantle radiotherapy is shown in Fig. 16.4.

TABLE 16.2 Late effects of radiotherapy for Hodgkin's disease

Site	Late radiation effects
Neck	Hypothyroidism, laryngeal oedema or fibrosis Treatment in puberty may induce thyroid cancer, loss of muscle and soft tissue bulk causing asymmetry
Mediastinum	Pneumonitis and lung fibrosis Pericarditis
Spinal cord	Myelitis
Abdomen	Increased incidence of peptic ulceration
Pelvis	Amenorrhoea in women and sterility if gonads included in radiation field

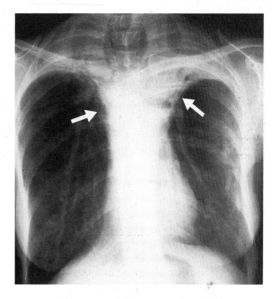

Fig 16.4 Chest X-ray following mantle radiotherapy (as demonstrated in Fig. 16.2) showing post-radiation fibrosis in the mediastinum and lung apices.

CHEMOTHERAPY

Acute toxicity includes nausea and vomiting, alopecia and bone marrow depression. Neutropenic sepsis is a potential hazard of any such treatment. Peripheral neuropathy may develop from the use of vincristine or less commonly vinblastine.

Adriamycin has specific dose-related cardiotoxic effects and bleomycin may cause lung damage at high doses. Neither of these effects will be expected in standard treatment schedules but may become a potential hazard in patients requiring retreatment.

Bleomycin also results in characteristic changes to the nails and skin.

The anthracycline-containing schedules such as ABVD have the advantage of preserving fertility whereas after MOPP-type regimes most patients are sterile, men being more sensitive than women.

There is increasing concern regarding the incidence of second malignancies in patients that are cured of their Hodgkin's disease. There is an ongoing risk with time from treatment which appears to be rising to over 15 per cent in patients that have survived for 20 years or more. In the early years,

Case history: Hodgkin's disease

A 23-year-old man presented to his general practitioner (GP) with a 1-month history of an enlarging lump in the left side of his neck. On examination he was found to have a 3 cm enlarged gland in the left deep cervical region with a further 2 cm node in the left supraclavicular fossa. These were non-tender and there were no associated foci of infection to find. On further questioning, however, he admitted to episodes of fever and several nights when he awoke drenched with sweat. A biopsy of the lymph node was undertaken and this showed nodular sclerosing Hodgkin's disease. Further investigations showed a normal full blood count but an erythrocyte sedimentation rate (ESR) of 53 mm/hour and normal biochemistry; a computed tomography (CT) scan showed other areas of enlarged lymph nodes in the anterior mediastinum and para-aortic region with marked splenomegaly. A bone marrow examination was clear. A diagnosis of stage IIIB Hodgkin's disease was made. He was recommended to receive combination chemotherapy. Prior to starting chemotherapy he was counselled with regard to future fertility and an initial sperm count being normal, semen was taken for cryopreservation.

He underwent combination chemotherapy using Adriamycin, bleomycin, vinblastine and dacarbazine (ABVD) for which he attended the hospital outpatient chemotherapy unit on a fortnightly basis. After each visit he had 24 h of nausea which was controlled by taking ondansetron 4 mg twice daily for the first 2 days after chemotherapy. By the fourth week of chemotherapy his hair was thinning and he needed to shave only once every other day.

One week after the third chemotherapy injection he developed a high fever and felt generally unwell. As instructed by the chemotherapy unit he attended there for a blood count which showed that he had a haemoglobin of 10.3, a total white count of 0.9 with a neutrophil count of 0.2 and a platelet count of 73. Admission to the oncology ward was arranged that day and he was treated with intravenous cefotaxime. Within 24 h his temperature had settled. He was treated with 5 days of high-dose intravenous antibiotics, by which time his neutrophil count had risen to 1.3 and he could be safely discharged from hospital. He proceeded with his next course of chemotherapy uneventfully.

After his eighth injection given at fortnightly intervals, representing four monthly courses of ABVD chemotherapy, a further CT scan was undertaken. This showed that he was in complete remission, that is no abnormal lymphadenopathy could be detected. He was therefore recommended to receive two further months of treatment to complete his programme. His further chemotherapy was completed uneventfully. On completion of chemotherapy he noted that his nails had developed marked changes with loosening of the nail bed and a brownish discoloration. He was reassured that these were normal reactions to the bleomycin drug in the chemotherapy and over the next few months these changes grew out as new nail advanced. His hair regrew normally and he returned to a normal lifestyle.

A repeat CT scan 3 months after completion of his chemotherapy showed that he was still in remission. He continued to attend the oncology clinic initially at 3-monthly intervals but later at less frequent intervals. Five years later he remains fit and well with no signs of active disease. He is seen at the clinic on an annual basis. He has recently married and his wife is pregnant with their first child, his fertility having been preserved despite his chemotherapy.

occasional leukaemias or non-Hodgkin's lymphomas are diagnosed but the major problem appears to be an increasing risk of solid tumours as the years pass. The exact cause for this remains unclear. The greatest incidence is in those patients receiving both radiotherapy and chemotherapy drugs such as mustine, chlorambucil and procarbazine and in those patients that have splenectomy compared with those that retain their spleen. It is thought that the newer anthracycline-containing schedules may be safer in this respect but this may be balanced by an increased risk of cardiac disease, especially in those that also receive mediastinal radiotherapy.

Prognosis

Overall, the prognosis for patients diagnosed with Hodgkin's disease is good. Virtually all patients presenting with stage 1A disease will be cured and with intensive chemotherapy over 80 per cent of those with advanced disease (stages 3B or 4) can also expect cure.

Future prospects

Increasingly, the emphasis in Hodgkin's disease now is to maintain the very high cure rates obtained while reducing morbidity. This is achieved by developing new, less toxic chemotherapy schedules, reducing the routine use of radiotherapy and, where needed, using smaller fields and lower doses of radiation.

For those patients with advanced disease more intensive weekly drug schedules combined with involved field radiotherapy may achieve even higher cure rates and for those that relapse or fail to achieve remission, high-dose salvage treatment with PBPC support is well established.

NON-HODGKIN'S LYMPHOMA

Epidemiology

There are around 7000 cases of non-Hodgkin's lymphoma (NHL) in the UK each year, with an incidence of 12 per 100 000 population and accounting for 2 per cent of all maligancies. It occurs equally in men and women and the incidence increases with age, being relatively unusual under the age of 50. As with Hodgkin's disease there is a marked low incidence in the Japanese and the USA black population. The overall incidence is increasing

and this is amplified by the effects of an ageing population.

Aetiology

No single aetiological agent has been identified to account for the common forms of lymphoma found in the UK.

Infective agents

Epstein–Barr virus is associated with Burkitt's lymphoma found predominantly in Africa. Human T-cell lymphotropic virus type 1 (HTLV-1) virus is associated with T-cell lymphoma found in the Caribbean and Japan. Human immunodeficiency virus (HIV) infection is also associated with an excess of lymphomas, which is probably a feature of the immunosuppressed status rather than a direct causation by virus.

Helicobacter is closely associated with gastric mucosa-associated lymphoma (MALT)-type lymphomas and eradication of *Helicobacter* has been accompanied by regression of gastric lymphoma in a high proportion of cases.

Altered immune status

In addition to HIV, NHL is also increased in other disease states associated with a depressed immune system, including rheumatoid arthritis, coeliac disease, hypogammaglobulinaemia and following iatrogenic immune suppression after renal transplantation. There are also associations with autoimmune disease such as Hashimoto's thyroiditis and thyroid lymphoma, and Sjögren's disease and salivary gland lymphoma.

Irradiation

This may also be a factor in the development of NHL and increased incidences are seen following exposure in Hiroshima and Nagasaki, and after low-dose therapeutic irradiation to the spine for ankylosing spondylitis.

Pathology

Non-Hodgkin's lymphoma, describes a spectrum of neoplastic conditions, as a result of which many complex and confusing classifications have arisen. The majority of NHL arise from the B lymphocyte but there is a well-recognized group which are T-cell derived neoplasms. Rare forms of histiocytic neoplasm also occur.

Macroscopically, NHL, will occur as a mass of neoplastic lymphoid tissue which may reach a considerable size. Ulceration, necrosis and haemorrhage are unusual. It may arise in recognized lymph node chains but, unlike Hodgkin's disease, extranodal lymphoma is relatively common with up to 50 per cent involving sites such as Waldeyer's ring, the gastrointestinal tract, skin and bone.

Microscopically, the appearances are complex and interpretation can be difficult. In broad terms, lymphomas may be low-grade or high-grade. Features of low-grade lymphoma are the preservation of follicular architecture and cellular composition of well-differentiated small lymphocytes. In contrast, high-grade lymphomas are characterized by diffuse infiltration of the gland or extranodal site with large undifferentiated lymphoid cells. The current international classification for NHL is the WHO World Health Organization–Revised European American Lymphoma (WHO–REAL) classification shown in outline in Table 16.3; this classification attempts to define disease entities rather than a pure morphological categorization. It also introduces some new definitions, such as mantle zone lymphoma and the mucosa-associated lymphomas (MALT).

The histological diagnosis of lymphoma is now supported by a range of specific monoclonal antibody stains. Distinction from a poorly differentiated small cell carcinoma is made using the leucocyte common antigen (LCA). Distinction of one subtype of lymphocyte from another has become a complex science. Monoclonal antibody stains to identify surface markers can differentiate B cells from T cells from histiocytes, and a large library of stains has now been built up to enable subtyping of a suspected lymphoma.

Despite this relatively complex classification, in practice most lymphomas can be divided into low grade or intermediate/high grade, which will define their natural history, management and prognosis as shown in Table 16.4.

Natural history

Low-grade lymphoma may be very indolent, remaining asymptomatic for many years and, in the elderly, having little impact upon their life expectancy.

A high-grade immunoblastic or lymphoblastic lymphoma is an aggressive often rapidly fatal condition.

Extranodal lymphoma may have a relatively benign course, as in a low-grade skin lymphoma, existing as purplish nodules requiring little other than gentle local treatment from time to time, or an

TABLE 16.3 Simplified WHO–REAL classification of non-Hodgkin's lymphoma

B-cell neoplasms

I   Precursor B-cell neoplasm
    Precursor B-lymphoblastic leukaemia/lymphoma

II Peripheral B-cell neoplasms
    1. Small lymphocytic lymphoma/chronic lymphocytic lymphoma
    2. Lymphoplasmacytic lymphoma
    3. Mantle cell lymphoma
    4. Follicular lymphoma
    5. Marginal zone lymphoma including MALT (mucosa associated lymphoid tissue) lymphomas
    6. Splenic marginal zone lymphoma
    7. Hairy cell leukaemia
    8. Plasma cell myeloma
    9. Diffuse large B-cell lymphoma
    10. Burkitt's lymphoma

T-cell neoplasms

I   Precursor T-cell neoplasm
    Precursor T-lymphoblastic lymphoma/ leukaemia

II Peripheral T-cell and natural killer (NK)-cell neoplasms
    1. T-cell chronic lymphocytic leukaemia (CLL)/prolymphocytic leukaemia
    2. Large granular lymphocytic leukaemia
    3. Mycosis fungoides/Sézary syndrome
    4. Peripheral T-cell lymphomas, unspecified
    5. Angioimmunoblastic T-cell lymphoma
    6. Angiocentric lymphoma
    7. Intestinal T-cell lymphoma
    8. Adult T-cell lymphoma/leukaemia
    9. Anaplastic large cell lymphoma

aggressive course as in a high-grade lymphoma of the bowel or central nervous system.

In general, NHL, unlike Hodgkin's disease, does not have a clear pattern of contiguous spread from one area to the next. Dissemination is often wide and unpredictable following a pattern closer to that of a carcinoma, with frequent hepatic and lung involvement.

Symptoms

Non-Hodgkin's lymphoma usually presents with a painless lump in a lymph node area, most commonly the neck but also the axilla or groin. There may

TABLE 16.4 Simplified clinical classification of common forms of non-Hodgkin's lymphoma

Low-grade (40%) having long natural history but rarely if ever cured:
Follicular lymphoma with any of the following cell types:
   small cleaved cells
   mixed small and large cleaved cells
Well-differentiated diffuse small cell lymphocytic lymphoma

Intermediate grade/high grade (50%) being relatively aggressive, requiring combination chemotherapy but with a proportion of long-term cures:
Follicular lymphoma containing predominantly large cells
Diffuse lymphoma containing any of the following cell types:
   small cleaved cells
   mixed small and large cells
   predominantly large cells
Immunoblastic
Peripheral T-cell lymphoma

Rarer types requiring different management:
Lymphoblastic; aggressive requiring leukaemia-type treatment
Small non-cleaved cell as in Burkitt's lymphoma: poorly responsive to standard chemotherapy requiring more intensive schedules
Mycosis fungoides: skin lymphoma having long natural history
MALTomas, arising in mucosal surfaces, usually low grade. In stomach respond to anti-*Helicobacter* therapy

be backache due to enlarged para-aortic nodes or upper abdominal pain from hepatosplenomegaly.

'B' symptoms, as described for Hodgkin's disease, are also an important feature – namely weight loss, fever and night sweats.

Other symptoms relate to the site of origin of an extranodal lymphoma. Non-Hodgkin's lymphoma arising in Waldeyer's ring therefore will cause local symptoms similar to those of a carcinoma in these regions, with local pain or discomfort and epistaxis or nasal discharge where the nasopharynx is involved. Gastrointestinal lymphoma usually presents with an acute abdominal event owing to haemorrhage, perforation or obstruction. Central nervous system (CNS) lymphoma may cause symptoms of raised intracranial pressure with headache, vomiting and fits. Focal neurological features may cause bulbar palsy, diplopia, limb weakness and altered sensation. Skin lymphoma usually presents as asymptomatic lumps but mycosis fungoides has a characteristic pre-tumour phase often lasting many years with chronic skin change, which may be itchy and resemble dermatitis in its clinical picture.

Signs

Enlarged lymph nodes will be palpable, typically painless, firm, 'rubbery' nodes clinically indistinguishable from those of Hodgkin's disease but different from the hard craggy nodes of carcinoma. At extranodal sites lymphoma often has a characteristic purplish appearance, stretching overlying surfaces and ulcerating only rarely. Hepatosplenomegaly is a common finding in both nodal and extranodal lymphoma.

Investigations

Blood count

A full blood count may show signs of mild anaemia or pancytopenia if there is bone marrow involvement. A high white cell count composed predominantly of lymphocytes may also be found and is a relatively poor prognostic sign.

Erythrocyte sedimentation rate

The ESR will be raised; an ESR greater than 40 mm/hour is a further poor prognostic feature.

Biochemistry

Routine biochemistry may show signs of hepatic infiltration. Renal failure is an infrequent complication of massive para-aortic node enlargement causing ureteric obstruction. Serum lactate dehydrogenase (LDH) level is a marker of disease activity.

Radiography

The chest X-ray may show mediastinal or hilar lymphadenopathy; more rarely infiltration of the lung parenchyma, pleural nodules or a pleural effusion may be found.

Computed tomography

Imaging of the abdominal and pelvic lymph nodes is best performed using a CT scan, which has now superseded the use of bipedal lymphangiography. Figure 16.5 demonstrates extensive lymphadenopathy in the neck and para-aortic region on CT scan.

Bone marrow examination

Bone marrow examination will be required to assess the possibility of marrow infiltration.

Other imaging

Other imaging may be indicated depending on the site of origin. For bowel lymphoma, a full barium series is performed since multiple foci of disease are well-recognized. A CT scan of the brain will be performed for CNS lymphoma which may be further supplemented by an MRI scan to image potential spinal disease. Where there is equivocal evidence for lymphoma for example a slightly enlarged spleen or marginally enlarged lymph nodes, then positron emission tomography (PET) using fluorodeoxyglucose may be of value.

CEREBROSPINAL FLUID EXAMINATION

Cerebrospinal fluid examination for lymphoma cells will be required for CNS lymphoma and may also be considered for other types considered to have a high risk of CNS involvement, in particular diffuse large cell and lymphoblastic lymphomas and those affecting the testis, tonsil or nasal sinuses.

Differential diagnosis

The main differential diagnosis rests between NHL and Hodgkin's disease. Epithelial tumours may be considered where NHL arises in extranodal sites. It may be difficult to distinguish clinically a low-grade lymphoma with extensive bone marrow involvement from chronic lymphocytic leukaemia and lymphoblastic lymphoma from acute lymphoblastic leukaemia.

Staging

The Ann Arbor staging system is used for NHL, as for Hodgkin's disease, with the further addition

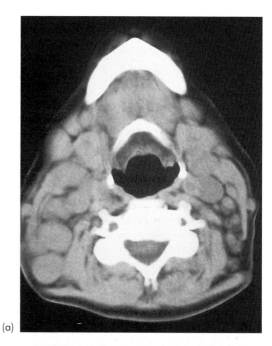

(a)

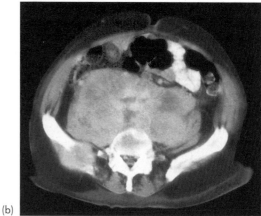

(b)

FIG 16.5 Computed tomography scans showing (a) extensive cervical lymphadenopathy and (b) para-aortic lymphadenopathy in non-Hodgkin's lymphoma.

of a suffix 'E' where the lymphoma has arisen in an extranodal site. For example, an NHL arising in the tonsil with involved nodes in the neck would be stage 2 by virtue of the presence of two or more sites all on the same side of the diaphragm and be designated stage 2E, having arisen in an extranodal site.

Treatment

Treatment is based on histological grade and stage.

Case history: Non-Hodgkin's lymphoma

A 53-year-old man presents to his general practitioner (GP) having for the past few weeks had a sore throat with discomfort on swallowing. On examination he is found to have enlargement of the left tonsil and a 2 cm lymph node palpable in the left side of the neck. He is referred urgently to an ear, nose and throat surgeon who performs an excision biopsy of the tonsil. Histology of the tonsil shows diffuse large cell non-Hodgkin's lymphoma. He is referred to the oncologist who undertakes various staging investigations. A computed tomography (CT) scan shows no evidence of further lymphadenopathy other than that detectable clinically in the neck. His bone marrow is normal and other blood tests including a full blood count, erythrocyte sedimentation rate (ESR), biochemical profile, immunoglobulins and serum lactate dehydrogenase are all normal. He is recommended to receive a short course of chemotherapy to be followed by radiotherapy.

Chemotherapy is started with a cycle of combination treatment using cyclophosphamide, Adriamycin, vincristine and prednisolone (CHOP). He is warned about the possibility of infertility but has decided he does not wish to store sperm having completed his family many years ago. An echocardiogram is also performed to check cardiac function before receiving anthracyclines and this is also normal. Following his first cycle of CHOP chemotherapy he has some transient nausea but otherwise no significant side-effects. Three weeks later he receives a second cycle of CHOP chemotherapy. By this time he has noted marked thinning of his hair but otherwise remains well and reports that the lump previously palpable in his neck has already disappeared. A third course of CHOP chemotherapy is repeated after three more weeks.

Two weeks later he attends the radiotherapy planning clinic where a cast for a head shell is made. His head is placed in the correct position for the treatment and a cast made of his features. This is later used to create a positive impression of his head and neck from which a close-fitting plastic shell is cast. A week later he attends for the shell to be fitted and minor adjustments made to the setting of the shell on the treatment couch of the radiotherapy machine. X-ray pictures are then taken of him wearing the shell and the beams to treat Waldeyer's ring and neck defined and marked on the shell for his subsequent treatment. A week later he attends for his first of 15 daily radiotherapy treatments. During each treatment he is placed in position wearing the shell and the X-ray beams from the linear accelerator are set up by the light beam against the marks on the shell. He is treated by a total of three beams, two lateral beams covering the Waldeyer's ring area and a beam from the front covering the lower neck below this. Each beam exposure takes about 1 min and the whole process around 10 min. He feels perfectly well during the procedure other than some minor discomfort on being kept still in the shell. By the end of the first week he notices some slight discomfort on swallowing again and as he continues treatment in the second week he becomes increasingly uncomfortable with pain on swallowing particularly hot foods. He also notices that the skin where the X-ray beams enters his face and neck has become red and starts to feel tight and uncomfortable as if he had been exposed to excess sun. He is given dietary advice and later soluble aspirin to take before food. He continues treatment on a daily basis through the third week. At completion of treatment he has marked skin reddening and some early peeling of the skin over the neck. Swallowing is very uncomfortable and he is warned to expect this to continue for a few days before a slow improvement develops. Two weeks later the skin is feeling itchy and peeling but he is otherwise comfortable. His throat has improved considerably and he is starting to return to a normal diet without the need for regular medication any longer.

Three months after treatment his symptoms have resolved completely and the follow-up CT scan shows no evidence of detectable lymph node enlargement or other abnormalities. Examination of his oropharynx shows no abnormalities either. He is told that he is in complete remission.

He is seen regularly in the outpatients clinic. Five years later he remains well with no signs of recurrence of his lymphoma.

LOW-GRADE NHL

This is a condition which is rarely curable but usually has a long indolent course. (Common types are follicular and diffuse small cell lymphoma in WHO-REAL classification.) Localized low-grade NHL (stage 1A) is treated using local radiotherapy. The involved area only is treated, using low doses of 20–30 Gy in 2–3 weeks.

Other stages are treated only when symptomatic using single-agent oral chemotherapy, of which the most popular is chlorambucil. There is no advantage to adding other drugs to chlorambucil in this setting. Alternatively, single-agent cyclophosphamide may be used and 70–80 per cent of patients will enter remission with either agent. A newer alternative to chlorambucil is fludarabine given orally or intravenously for five consecutive days every 4 weeks but randomized trials have yet to show any additional advantage for fludarabine as a single agent over simpler alkylating agent schedules such as oral chlorambucil. Trials are underway to determine whether fludarabine in combination with Adriamycin or mitozantrone and dexamethasone (FAD or FMD), which appear more active than the single drugs alone has any advantages over other established drug schedules.

A major new development in recent years has been the use of monoclonal antibody directed against the B-cell surface marker CD20 in the treatment of low grade follicular lymphoma. This drug, rituximab, has been shown to be effective against drug-resistant disease in around 50% of cases and its role in the primary management of low grade NHL alongside conventional chemotherapy is now being evaluated in clinical trials.

Relapse

Low-grade lymphoma which is not localized is never cured, although survival for many years is to be expected. At some point, however, relapse is inevitable. Retreatment with chlorambucil is often successful and local sites causing symptoms can be irradiated. Patients that fail to respond to successive courses of chlorambucil may be treated with fludarabine or alternatively combination chemotherapy such as CHOP (see Table 6.4 and below) in the same way that a high-grade lymphoma will be treated (see below). Rituximab (see above) will also achieve responses in chemotherapy-resistant disease.

Transformation

Richter's syndrome refers to the transformation from a low-grade to a high-grade lymphoma, which may occur in up to 15 per cent of patients presenting initially with low-grade lymphoma. For this reason re-biopsy of recurrent disease, particularly where there has been a period free from detectable disease or a change in growth rate is observed, should be considered before treatment.

Palliation

Steroids alone in moderate doses (40–60 mg of prednisolone) may have a valuable anti-tumour effect as well as their general effects in improving appetite and general well-being.

Single-agent etoposide or vincristine may be used for subsequent relapses. Hemi-body irradiation is a valuable palliative treatment for widespread NHL no longer responsive to chemotherapy.

HIGH-GRADE LYMPHOMA

This is a much more aggressive condition than low-grade lymphoma and in general requires more intensive therapy. The common type is diffuse large cell lymphoma in WHO–REAL classification.

Nodal lymphoma

Localized high-grade NHL (stage 1A and 2A) is best treated with a short course of chemotherapy (typically three courses of CHOP – see below) followed by local irradiation to the involved sites, delivering a dose of 30–40 Gy in 3–4 weeks.

Advanced disease (stage 1B, 2, 3 or 4) is treated with chemotherapy. As for Hodgkin's disease, consideration should be given to sperm banking for young males and all patients should be maintained well-hydrated and started on allopurinol to prevent tumour lysis syndrome (see Chapter 22).

Specific chemotherapy

Usually, combination chemotherapy is given of which the most widely used is CHOP (cyclophosphamide), Adriamycin (hydroxydaunorubicin), vincristine (Oncovin) and prednisolone. This is given as injections of the first three drugs on day 1 of a 21-day cycle with oral steroids on the first 5 days. A total of six to eight courses is usually given, the standard dictum being to deliver two courses of chemotherapy beyond complete clinical remission. Rapid responses may be seen after only one cycle of treatment, as illustrated in Fig. 16.6.

Alternative schedules give weekly drugs over a 12-week course. These cycles are, in general, associated with greater toxicity, in particular neutropenia with the risk of sepsis and mucositis, and, to date, no advantage over standard chemotherapy in terms of patient survival has been shown.

There is some evidence emerging from current trials that rituximab given at completion of a course of CHOP chemotherapy to those in complete remission may result in improved remission periods and survival.

Combined modality treatment

Sites of original bulky disease are often irradiated on the basis that these are frequently the sites of

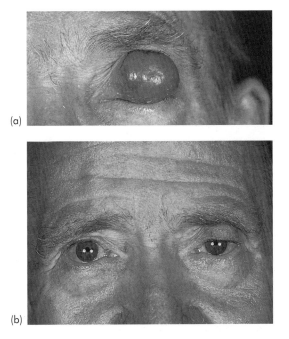

(a)

(b)

FIG 16.6 Conjunctival lymphoma (a) before and (b) after one cycle of CHOP chemotherapy.

initial relapse. There is no good evidence that this practice significantly improves survival, particularly in those patients that achieve a complete response to chemotherapy but where a reduced rate of local relapse in the irradiated area is seen.

High-dose chemotherapy

Intensive chemotherapy using drug schedules such as BEAM (BCNU, etoposide, cytosine arabinoside and melphalan) which result in ablation of the bone marrow are playing an increasing role in the management of NHL. This has been made easier in recent years by the development of PBPC collection from the blood, which can then be used to reseed the marrow after treatment. This technique has replaced autologous bone marrow transplantation in many centres, being simpler and associated with quicker recovery of bone marrow function after treatment and therefore a shorter high-risk period of pancytopenia.

Peripheral blood progenitor cells are obtained by using bone marrow stimulation with cyclophosphamide and colony-stimulating factors such as GCSF. This increases the number of PBPCs in the peripheral circulation which are then 'harvested' during plasmaphoresis. These cells are stored in liquid nitrogen until needed for reinfusion after an ablative dose of chemotherapy (or radiotherapy).

The role of high-dose chemotherapy in the initial treatment of poor-risk advanced high-grade NHL is under evaluation.

In recurrent disease, challenge with conventional dose chemotherapy is essential to select those with chemosensitive disease. In this group, further treatment with high-dose chemotherapy will result in prolonged remission in over 60 per cent. There is, however, no value in proceeding to such treatment in those patients having relapsed disease unresponsive to initial chemotherapy.

While expertise in this type of treatment is increasing, there is considerable associated morbidity and it is rarely considered for patients over the age of 65 years.

Lymphoblastic lymphoma

This form of high-grade lymphoma has a particularly aggressive course and resembles acute lymphoblastic leukaemia (ALL) in many of its features (e.g. a propensity to spread to the CNS). Results from standard lymphoma chemotherapy as described above are poor and most of these patients will be treated in protocols similar to those for ALL, including CNS prophylaxis.

Burkitt's lymphoma

This is a distinct high-grade lymphoma defined histologically as a diffuse small non-cleaved cell lymphoma. It is common in certain parts of Africa, where an association with Epstein–Barr virus infection is apparent, but is a rare lymphoma in Europe and the USA. Results from standard lymphoma treatment are poor and current schedules use more intensive chemotherapy.

Extranodal lymphoma

In general, these lymphomas are intermediate grade and will be treated in the same way as lymphomas arising in nodes as described above. There are, however, certain features of management particular to specific sites.

Waldeyer's ring lymphomas

These usually arise in the tonsils or nasopharynx. If early and non-bulky, radiotherapy alone may be used, including the whole of Waldeyer's ring in the treatment volume. More advanced disease will receive four to six courses of chemotherapy (e.g. CHOP followed by irradiation).

Gastrointestinal tract lymphomas

These often present as a surgical emergency and proceed to laparotomy at which bowel resection is performed. The diagnosis of NHL having been made, these patients will be treated with chemotherapy. A well-recognized hazard of initial chemotherapy in these patients is that of intestinal perforation as the lymphoma in the bowel wall regresses and careful observation as an inpatient is usually recommended for the first course of treatment. Irradiation is difficult in these patients as it is difficult to demarcate clearly the affected area using standard localization techniques and the bowel tolerates irradiation poorly.

A distinct pathological entity now recognized is the MALToma (mucosa-associated lymphoid tissue) found particularly in the stomach and small bowel. Initial management of MALTomas in the stomach should be a course of anti-*Helicobacter* therapy using antibiotics such as ampicillin or tetracycline with metronidazole and omeprazole. Responses are seen in over 90 per cent of patients but close gastroscopic surveillance is required to detect those patients that relapse and then require standard lymphoma chemotherapy.

Skin lymphomas

These are often low-grade (lymphoma cutis) and require only gentle local treatment from time to time, but more extensive high-grade lymphoma may develop, as shown in Fig. 16.7. Mycosis fungoides is a characteristic T-cell skin lymphoma which has a long pretumour phase before developing into the characteristic skin infiltration, which may be widespread. It responds poorly to chemotherapy. Less severe forms may respond to PUVA (psoralens and ultraviolet A exposure) and for others local irradiation is required. In widespread disease the entire body may be affected, when irradiation of the whole body with electrons will be required.

Primary cerebral lymphoma

This has a poor prognosis and has a propensity to seed throughout the CNS via the cerebrospinal fluid circulation. Conventional treatment includes irradiation of the entire CNS axis from the cerebral hemispheres to the sacral region but this has only limited success. Chemotherapy may improve results but most patients will still relapse after only a relatively short time. Two distinct populations have now emerged, those with sporadic primary CNS lymphoma and those where it is associated with HIV infection. The prognosis for the latter is particularly poor.

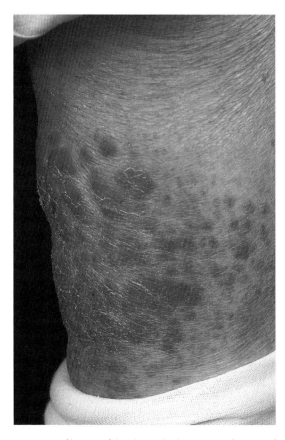

FIG 16.7 Infiltration of the skin with characteristic features of primary skin lymphoma.

Primary lymphoma of bone

This may, if still localized to the bone of origin, be cured by local radiotherapy alone but will usually be treated with a combined schedule of CHOP chemotherapy followed by radiotherapy. Conventionally, the entire bone is included in the radiation field.

Tumour-related complications

Given the great heterogeneity of NHL, a vast range of clinical complications may arise, most of which have been covered in the above text.

Mass effects may be caused by malignant nodes or lymphomatous tissue compromising normal function so that, for example, mediastinal disease may cause (SVC) obstruction or dysphagia, abdominal disease may cause renal failure as a result of a ureteric obstruction and pelvic disease may cause oedema of the lower limbs.

Gastrointestinal lymphoma may cause bowel haemorrhage, obstruction or perforation.

Central nervous system lymphoma may cause focal neurological damage or obstructive hydrocephalus.

Treatment-related complications

Radiotherapy

This may cause late toxicity related to site (e.g. irradiating Waldeyer's ring may cause dry mouth, taste loss and dental problems). Abdominal and pelvic irradiation may result in post-radiation bowel and bladder changes.

Chemotherapy

During treatment, bone marrow depression, with the risks of neutropenic sepsis, occurs together with nausea, vomiting, alopecia and mucositis.

Rapid tumour regression may result in complications, in particular perforation at the site of gastrointestinal lymphoma, which is estimated to occur in around 5 per cent of patients with lymphoma in this site, and tumour lysis syndrome (see Chapter 22).

In the longer term, Adriamycin may cause dose-related cardiotoxicity, and bleomycin is associated with dose-related pneumonitis and lung fibrosis together with peripheral skin changes.

Infertility may result, particularly in males, after combination chemotherapy, although pregnancy is seen in women even after high-dose chemotherapy.

Second malignancy in patients with NHL is becoming more apparent as the results of treatment improve and more patients survive to develop a new malignancy. It is estimated that the risk of developing acute myeloblastic leukaemia in the first 5 years following treatment is between 6 per cent and 8 per cent and, as with Hodgkin's disease, appears most marked in patients treated with both chemotherapy and radiotherapy. There is a less clear association with the development of solid tumours (i.e. cancers or sarcomas), but since it is known that this risk increases with time over 20 or 30 years, an association is likely to emerge as cohorts of cured patients are followed for this length of time.

Prognosis

There are four major independent prognostic features in NHL:

- age;
- performance status;
- stage (3 or 4 worse than 1 or 2);
- serum lactate dehydrogenase.

These have been validated and are referred to as the International Prognostic Index (IPI), outcome being related to the number of IPI features present.

The prognosis for low-grade lymphoma is better than that for intermediate or high-grade lymphomas, with median survival of 8–10 years reported from most centres.

Intermediate-grade localized lymphoma will be cured by local radiotherapy in around 60 per cent of patients.

Extranodal lymphoma, even when localized, tends to have a worse prognosis than nodal lymphoma; Waldeyer's ring and skin has a better prognosis than gastrointestinal tract, which has a better prognosis than CNS.

More advanced intermediate and high-grade NHL will respond to chemotherapy in most patients with complete regression of disease in 70–80 per cent; however, long-term survival figures tend to fall below 50 per cent at 5 years from treatment.

Future prospects

The main areas of development in the management of NHL are concerned with defining the place of high-dose chemotherapy with bone marrow or peripheral stem cell autograft for those patients requiring intensive therapy. The further development of monoclonal antibody-based agents such as rituximab and radiolabelled monoclonal antibodies will undoubtedly evolve into an important additional treatment modality for NHL. Another approach under evaluation is the development of 'anti-sense' compounds specifically targeted to the *BCL2* gene found in follicular lymphoma as a means of targeting these cells with cytotoxic agents.

Rare tumours

Malignant histiocytosis

This is a rare form of lymphoma characterized by systemic symptoms of fever, weight loss, generalized lymphadenopathy, hepatosplenomegaly and pancytopenia. Histiocytic lymphoma is typically associated with coeliac disease when it presents as a multi-centric bowel lymphoma. It may respond to lymphoma-type chemotherapy but the prognosis is generally much worse than other forms of lymphoma.

Castleman's disease

This is probably not a neoplasm but a hamartomatous condition of lymphoid tissue. It may present in a similar fashion to lymphoma and histological differentiation can be difficult. It is uncertain whether active treatment other than simple excision of affected nodes is of value, although there are reports of successful regression after irradiation.

Waldenstrom's macroglobulinaemia

This is lymphoplasmacytic lymphoma typically producing an IgM paraprotein and as such needs to be distinguished from myeloma. This is usually clear from the clinical findings, which are those of a lymphoma with lymph node and splenic involvement. Bone marrow examination shows infiltration with lymphoma rather than plasma cells. Haemolytic anaemia due to cold agglutins is a further rare feature. Management and prognosis is similar to that of other low-grade non-Hodgkin's lymphomas.

LEUKAEMIA

Neoplastic conditions of the haemopoietic and lymphoid systems are closely related. Subclassifications of leukaemias and lymphomas tend to be complex, but clinical management is usually based on a more simple and pragmatic division of leukaemias into acute or chronic, lymphoid or myeloid. There are around 4800 cases of leukaemia registered per year in the UK and these account for around 4000 deaths each year.

Acute leukaemia may be subclassified by its cell of origin into two broad groups: lymphoblastic and myeloblastic. Chronic leukaemias are malignancies of cells that have differentiated beyond the blast stage. They are subdivided into chronic granulocytic leukaemia and chronic lymphocytic leukaemia. Despite their name, they do not necessarily have a more protracted natural history and the prognosis for chronic leukaemia is, overall, no better than for acute leukaemia.

ACUTE LYMPHOBLASTIC LEUKAEMIA

Epidemiology

Acute lymphoblastic leukaemia (ALL) is less common than acute myeloid leukaemia, affecting males and females in equal proportions. It is predominantly a malignancy affecting children with 40 per cent occurring in the 3- to 5-year-old age group when it predominates in boys.

Aetiology

Down's syndrome is associated with a higher incidence.

Environmental agents (e.g. viruses) may be implicated. Clustering of cases in certain areas of the UK has been described but it is uncertain whether this is related to any specific environmental agent.

Chromosomal translocations have been identified which are thought to activate the oncogene *c-myc* following translocation of its sequence from chromosome 8 where it normally resides.

Radiation exposure may be implicated, although post-radiation leukaemia is usually myeloblastic.

Pathology

Lymphoblastic leukaemia is characterized by the presence of large immature lymphoblasts throughout the reticuloendothelial system. These cells are distinguished from other cells such as myeloblasts by their staining, as shown in Table 17.1.

Acute lymphoblastic leukaemia is also subclassified according to the type of lymphoid cell which has become neoplastic and by the cell morphology, as shown in Table 17.2.

In addition to *de novo* ALL, up to 15 per cent of cases represent transformation into an acute phase from chronic granulocytic leukaemia (CGL). These are characterized by possessing the Philadelphia chromosome (see below). Other chromosomal changes which may be identified and relate to a worse outcome are translocations affecting

TABLE 17.1 Staining characteristics of acute lymphoblastic leukaemia (ALL) compared with acute myeloid leukaemia (AML)[1]

	PAS	TdT	Sudan black
ALL	+	+	–
AML	–	–	+

[1] PAS, periodic acid–Schiff reagent;
TdT, terminal deoxyribonucleotidyl transferase.

TABLE 17.2 Subclassification of acute lymphoblastic leukaemia (ALL)

Morphological	
L1	Small uniform blast cells with high nuclear/ cytoplasmic ratio
L2	Larger blast cells, lower nuclear/cytoplasmic ratio
L3	Vacuolated blasts, basophilic cytoplasm

	Surface Ig	Rosette formation	Proportion (%)
B cell	+	–	2
T cell	–	+	15
Common	+	+	75
Null	–	–	8

chromosome 4, t(4;11), and chromosome 9, t(9;22), deletions of chromosome 7 and trisomy 8.

Natural history

Progressive infiltration of the bone marrow and subsequent bone marrow failure ensues. It may also affect other sites, in particular the central nervous system (CNS), where diffuse meningeal infiltration may be seen, and in males, the testes.

Symptoms

Patients present with bone marrow failure which results in:

- malaise, lethargy, effort dyspnoea or angina due to progressive anaemia;
- infection due to leucopenia;
- bleeding in the form of epistaxis, haematuria or haemoptysis due to thrombocytopenia.

Bone pains may also be present. There are also general symptoms of malignancy including fever, sweats and weight loss.

Signs

Peripheral lymphadenopathy is common and splenomegaly may be present. Other signs include:

- the liver may be palpable;
- purpura may be apparent, particularly on the lower limbs, as may other signs of recent haemorrhage from the nose or oral cavity;
- signs of infection may be present, with fever and oropharyngeal or chest signs.

Differential diagnosis

Other types of acute leukaemia or high-grade non-Hodgkin's lymphoma should be considered. Other causes of pancytopenia must also be considered, including aplastic anaemia. Infection with Epstein–Barr virus may give a similar picture, with abnormal blast cells seen in the peripheral blood.

Investigations

Blood count

A full blood count will show pancytopenia. The blood film will reveal the presence of lymphoblasts.

Erythrocyte sedimentation rate

The erythrocyte sedimentation rate (ESR) will be raised.

Liver function

Liver function tests may be abnormal.

Radiography

Chest X-ray may show evidence of leukaemic infiltration or more commonly infection. A mediastinal mass of lymph nodes may be demonstrated.

Bone marrow examination

A bone marrow aspirate and trephine is required to confirm the diagnosis with an excess (>5 per cent) of abnormal lymphoblasts. Specific stains will then be applied to subtype the cells into common, T, B or null ALL.

Staging

There is no formal staging system for the leukaemias. However, the important features which determine prognosis are:

- subtype, common ALL having a good prognosis;
- total white blood cell count, a total count of more than 20 000 being associated with a poor prognosis.

Other favourable features are female sex, young age and the absence of a mediastinal mass.

Treatment

The treatment of acute leukaemias can be considered in three phases: induction, consolidation and maintenance. Alongside this, intensive supportive treatment may be necessary using blood products and antibiotics. In the UK, most centres will treat patients within the national UKALL protocols through which modifications to treatment schedules have been tested in prospective randomized studies.

INDUCTION

Using vincristine and prednisolone with the addition of other agents such as Adriamycin, daunorubicin or L-asparaginase this can improve response rates from 50 per cent with vincristine and prednisolone alone to around 70 per cent. Induction therapy will usually continue over a period of 8 weeks.

CONSOLIDATION

This may be necessary once remission is achieved, i.e. when abnormal leukaemic cells are no longer detectable in the peripheral blood and bone marrow. This will take the form of prophylactic treatment to the CNS using intrathecal injections of methotrexate.

MAINTENANCE

Chemotherapy will then be given with methotrexate and mercaptopurine which may be continued for a total of 2–3 years.

BONE MARROW TRANSPLANTATION

Increasingly, high-dose chemotherapy with bone marrow transplantation is being considered for poor-risk patients who achieve initial remission. This is particularly the case for adults, who have a much worse prognosis from ALL than children, especially those with Philadelphia chromosome present on the leukaemic cells. Bone marrow transplantation is also indicated for children that relapse with bone marrow disease after initial chemotherapy.

Bone marrow transplantation is an intensive treatment which involves exposure of the patient to very high doses of chemotherapy, usually cyclophosphamide or melphalan and whole-body irradiation. This has the effect of completely ablating the bone marrow, which then has to be replaced. This may be from a matched donor (allograft) or from the patient's marrow previously collected and stored while in remission (autograft). The patient's marrow may be treated with monoclonal antibody techniques in an attempt to purge it further of residual leukaemic cells.

Intensive support is required for the period from marrow ablation to the re-establishment of the grafted marrow, which may be 3–4 weeks. During this time, blood and platelet transfusions are required. Antibiotic prophylaxis is given with aggressive treatment of any febrile episode using high-dose broad-spectrum antibiotics for bacterial, viral and fungal infections. Despite this, even in experienced units, a mortality rate of around 5 per cent may be expected from the procedure, usually due to neutropenic infection or pneumonitis. Mortality is in general related to age, and bone marrow transplantation is a hazardous undertaking in patients over the age of 40 years.

A further complication of allograft bone marrow transplantation is that of graft-versus-host disease in which the graft marrow reacts against the host tissues. This may manifest in a number of ways, most commonly through hepatic dysfunction, gastrointestinal disturbance and skin rashes. Various attempts have been made to reduce this event by treating the donor marrow to remove T lymphocytes which are the principal cell type involved and by the use of immunosuppressive agents such as methotrexate or azathioprine.

RELAPSE TREATMENT

When ALL has failed to respond to first-line chemotherapy or has relapsed following initial treatment, the usual pattern of relapse is with bone marrow disease. Central nervous system relapse occurs in up to 10 per cent of cases despite CNS prophylaxis and will require treatment with local irradiation and intrathecal therapy. Testicular relapse will be treated with local irradiation.

Salvage chemotherapy may take the form of using standard induction chemotherapy as above with alternative drugs added such as cytosine arabinoside. For those with a matched donor available then bone marrow transplant is indicated.

Tumour-related complications

Pancytopenia with consequent anaemia, leucopenia predisposing to infection and thrombocytopenia-related haemorrhage may occur.

Treatment-related complications

Complications include:

- tumour lysis syndrome (this is a rare complication arising as a result of the breakdown of large numbers of lymphoid cells when chemotherapy is initiated; it is discussed fully in Chapter 22);
- bone marrow suppression with the particular risk of neutropenic sepsis; bone marrow transplantation carries the added risks of graft-versus-host disease and prolonged immunosuppression;
- total-body irradiation during marrow transplantation may cause pneumonitis;
- CNS prophylaxis in young children may have effects on later intellectual development (attempts are constantly being made to minimize this effect by reducing the use of CNS irradiation);
- testicular irradiation will result in sterility but not impotence.

Prognosis

The prognosis for childhood ALL is for around 70 per cent of children to be long-term survivors cured of their disease. In adults, only about half this number will survive free from relapse 3 years after diagnosis. Bone marrow transplantation in this group may improve on these figures. Philadelphia-positive ALL has a worse outcome than other types of ALL.

ACUTE MYELOID LEUKAEMIA

Epidemiology

Acute myeloid leukaemia (AML) has an incidence of around 4 in 100 000 in the UK affecting males and females in approximately equal proportions. It is most common in young children under the age of 4 years and in adults over 40 years.

Aetiology

The vast majority of cases of AML (over 90 per cent) have no clear association with environmental agents and appear to arise *de novo*.

Increased incidence of AML appeared in populations exposed to radiation after the nuclear explosions in Hiroshima and Nagasaki. It is a rare but recognized event after therapeutic or diagnostic use of radiation.

Chemotherapy agents, in particular alkylating agents such as chlorambucil and procarbazine, have been associated with an increased incidence of AML. More recently, it has been recognized that etoposide is also associated with an increased incidence of secondary AML.

Pathology

Acute myeloid leukaemia encompasses a much broader pathological spectrum of disease than ALL. The characteristics of the myeloblast are positive staining with Sudan black and peroxidase stains. Eight subtypes based on morphological and cytochemical differences are now recognized; their features are outlined in Table 17.3. The common forms are M1 and M2.

Clinically, all these forms of AML behave in a similar fashion. Around half of all patients with AML will have chromosomal abnormalities. Recognized changes include trisomy of chromosome 8, deletions affecting chromosomes 5 or 7 and abnormalities of chromosome 11, all of which are poor prognostic features.

Natural history

There is progressive infiltration of the bone marrow with subsequent bone marrow failure. Testicular and

TABLE 17.3 Subtypes of acute myeloid leukaemia (AML)

AML subtype	Cell type
M0	Undifferentiated myeloblastic
M1	Undifferentiated myeloblastic without maturation
M2	Differentiated myeloblastic
M3	Promyelocytic
M4	Myelomonocytic
M5	Monoblastic
M6	Erythroleukaemia
M7	Megakaryoblastic

CNS involvement is relatively rare. Involvement of the latter is most common in monoblastic AML. Extramedullary involvement is more common than with ALL, with infiltration of liver and spleen in over 50 per cent and characteristic skin and gum infiltration in myelomonocytic and monoblastic leukaemias.

Symptoms

Symptoms include bone marrow failure causing fatigue, recurrent infections and haemorrhage. There is also associated fever, sweats and weight loss. Scattered bone pains may also occur.

Signs

These may include:

- signs of anaemia, bruising, purpura and recurrent infection;
- hepatosplenomegaly;
- lymphadenopathy (less common than with ALL);
- gum hypertrophy with associated gum bleeding, particularly in myelomonocytic and monoblastic forms of AML.

Differential diagnosis

Other forms of acute leukaemia and non-Hodgkin's lymphoma together with aplastic anaemia and myelofibrosis should be considered.

Investigations

Blood count

A full blood count will show pancytopenia with the presence of primitive blast cells on examining the blood film.

Biochemistry

Routine biochemistry may show abnormalities in liver function owing to infiltration.

Radiography

Chest X-ray may show signs of infection or more rarely leukaemic infiltration.

Coagulation studies

There may be coagulation abnormalities, particularly with promyelocytic leukaemia which is associated with disseminated intravascular coagulation (DIC).

Bone marrow examination

The diagnosis will be confirmed on examination of the bone marrow and the subtype of AML determined by specific stains.

Treatment

INDUCTION

This consists of chemotherapy in the form of daunorubicin, cytosine arabinoside and thioguanine (DAT) or etoposide. This will produce complete regression in up to 85 per cent of patients on first exposure to these agents.

CONSOLIDATION

Consolidation therapy in AML is less standardized than for ALL and may either consist of further courses of DAT or alternative chemotherapy such as high-dose cytosine arabinoside. Patients with CNS disease will also require cranial irradiation and intrathecal methotrexate but prophylactic CNS treatment is not generally recommended in contrast to ALL.

MAINTENANCE

Maintenance therapy has not been shown to have great value in AML and chemotherapy is not usually continued beyond 6 months after achieving initial remission.

BONE MARROW TRANSPLANTATION

This has a role in the management of AML and is considered in some centres as the consolidation treatment of choice for young adults, using either an allograft or autograft. It may also be considered in selected patients that relapse after primary treatment, particularly those that achieve a second remission with standard chemotherapy.

Tumour-related complications

These include, in particular, the effects of pancytopenia, including anaemia, susceptibility to infection and haemorrhage.

Treatment-related complications

Chemotherapy may be associated with further bone marrow depression and in particular the risk of neutropenic sepsis. Bone marrow transplant has its own specific risks of infection, graft-versus-host disease and radiation-induced pneumonitis.

Prognosis

The prognosis for AML is not as good as for ALL but has improved considerably in recent years with the use of bone marrow transplantation. Overall, around 40 per cent of all patients are cured of AML. Cure rates of around 50 per cent are to be expected in those undergoing transplantation in first remission and 25 per cent for those that are transplanted in second remission. Poor prognostic features at presentation include a high white count greater than $100 \times 10^9/l$ and disseminated intravascular coagulation associated with M3 (see Table 17.3). The outlook is worse for older patients (over 40 years) who have a lower rate of initial remission and are less able to tolerate intensive chemotherapy regimes or bone marrow transplantation. Other features associated with a poor prognosis are AML secondary to previous treatment, previous myelodysplasia and tumours expressing CD34 or bcl-2.

Rare tumours

Chloroma or isolated granulocytic sarcoma is a localized tumour of myeloblasts. Around two-thirds will progress to widespread AML; localized treatment with surgery or radiotherapy is not appropriate and these tumours should be treated as AML.

Screening and future prospects

Patients at risk of treatment-related AML, typically survivors from intensive chemotherapy treatment for germ cell tumours or lymphoma are screened with regular examination of the peripheral blood.

For promyelocytic leukaemia (M3) there is currently considerable interest in the use of all-*trans* retinoic acid (ATRA), which can alone induce remissions similar to chemotherapy and which may have a role as an adjuvant alongside chemotherapy.

CHRONIC GRANULOCYTIC LEUKAEMIA

Chronic granulocytic leukaemia typically affects adults between the ages of 30 years and 60 years. Its annual incidence in the UK is around 0.8 in 100 000 and it affects men and women equally.

Aetiology

There are no recognized environmental agents. Philadelphia chromosome is present in around 80 per cent of patients; it is formed by a translocation from chromosome 22 to chromosome 9 or less frequently another chromosome. Additional chromosomal abnormalities frequently develop in the acute phase of CGL (the blast crisis).

Pathology

Chronic granulocytic leukaemia represents neoplastic proliferation of granulocyte precursors and is characterized by an excess of metamyelocytes and myelocytes in the peripheral blood. Promyelocytes and myeloblasts may also be present and often there is an excess of basophils and eosinophils.

Natural history

An initial indolent period gives way to a fulminating blast crisis indistinguishable from an acute leukaemia but, in general, it is less responsive to treatment.

Blast crisis is usually myeloblastic in type, although lymphoblastic crises may occur. Occasionally, the blast crisis may be the first clinical manifestation of the disease, when it can be distinguished from a *de novo* acute leukaemia by the presence of Philadelphia chromosome.

Symptoms

Symptoms may include the following:

- chronic-phase CGL may present with symptoms of anaemia or thrombocytopenia due to bone marrow failure;
- abdominal distension and discomfort may occur owing to splenic enlargement, which may be massive;
- bone pain may also be present;
- general features of an active leukaemic process such as fevers and weight loss may occur and patients may also complain of itching;
- the very high white count may result in hyperviscosity of the blood, causing confusion and headaches;
- priapism is a further rare complication.

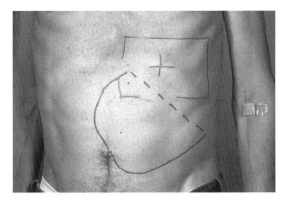

Fig 17.1 Massive hepatomegaly outlined in a patient with chronic granulocytic leukaemia.

Signs

These may include:

- clinical signs of anaemia and purpura;
- massive splenomegaly (Fig. 17.1);
- hepatomegaly;
- lymphadenopathy (not usually prominent).

Differential diagnosis

Myelofibrosis may also present with a large spleen and pancytopenia. In the acute phase differentiation between *de novo* acute leukaemia and blast crisis of CGL may be difficult unless the preceding history is known, but can be resolved by the finding of Philadelphia chromosome.

Investigations

Blood count

The peripheral blood usually has a characteristic picture with a very high white blood cell count of between 100 and $1000 \times 10^9/l$ of which the majority will be metamyelocytes with other granulocyte precursors. This is usually associated with a mild thrombocytopenia and anaemia.

Bone marrow examination

This will show a hypercellular picture with an excess of granulocyte precursors. Areas of myelosclerosis may also be seen. Philadelphia chromosome may be demonstrated in myeloid, erythroid and megakaryocytic cell lines.

Ultrasound

Abdominal ultrasound may be performed to confirm the extent of hepatomegaly and splenomegaly.

Other investigations

Other characteristic abnormalities are a low leucocyte alkaline phosphatase and raised serum B_{12} and B_{12} binding proteins. Blast crisis is characterized by the appearance of more primitive blast cells and on bone marrow these will comprise over 50 per cent of the myeloid population.

Treatment

CHRONIC PHASE

Initial treatment is aimed at reducing the peripheral blood white cell count to under $15 \times 10^9/l$ and to alleviate symptoms of splenomegaly. Chemotherapy using busulphan taken as a daily oral dose of 4 mg may be used until the white cell count reaches satisfactory levels. This is usually paralleled by a reduction in spleen size and a return to normal of other markers of CGL such as leucocyte alkaline phosphatase and B_{12} binding proteins.

Following initial induction chemotherapy, α-interferon maintenance therapy giving 3–12 MU subcutaneously three times weekly adjusting the dose to platelet and white cell count has been shown to result in better survival than low-dose maintenance oral chemotherapy.

Ultimately, patients relapse with disease resistant to further challenge with busulphan at which time alternative agents may be introduced such as hydroxyurea, 6-mercaptopurine, chlorambucil or cyclophosphamide.

Splenic irradiation may be useful in the palliation of local symptoms from a large spleen and the effects of hypersplenism in disease refractory to chemotherapy.

Leucophoresis will achieve rapid reduction of very high white cell counts. The patient's blood is passed through a cell separator, being returned through a continuous flow into a second intravenous cannula. This results, on average, in a 35 per cent reduction in white cell count with each procedure, and also has the advantage of providing large numbers of redundant granulocytes which can be used for therapeutic transfusion in other patients. However, no effect on the natural history of the CGL process is achieved by regular leucophoresis and it is therefore generally used only when hyperviscosity is a predominant feature.

The role of more intensive chemotherapy in the chronic phase of CGL, is still under evaluation but allogeneic bone marrow transplantation is the only treatment known to result in cures from the chronic phase. However, it is not clear which patients should be selected for this and at which stage in their disease.

ACUTE PHASE

The treatment of the blast crisis is essentially that of the acute leukaemia into which the CGL transforms. In around 70 per cent this will be an acute myeloid leukaemia, around 5 per cent may have a mixed picture and the remaining 25 per cent will manifest ALL. As with *de novo* acute leukaemia an ALL blast crisis has a better prognosis, with around 40 per cent of patients reverting to a chronic phase with simple induction therapy such as vincristine and prednisolone. Bone marrow transplantation may be of value in those patients achieving remission from their acute phase.

Tumour-related complications

There may be bone marrow failure resulting in anaemia, reduced resistance to infection and a bleeding tendency due to thrombocytopenia. This may be exacerbated by the effects of gross spleno-megaly, causing the phenomenon of hypersplenism, with pooling of blood within the large spleen. Massive splenomegaly may also cause local pain and may impair gastric emptying. Local areas of infarction may occur within the spleen, causing acute pain.

Large numbers of white cells in the circulation may cause hyperviscosity with headache, confusion, visual disturbance and priapism.

Treatment-related complications

Busulphan is associated with a rare Addisonian-like syndrome in which there is pigmentation, hypo-natraemia and weakness. Other features that are occasionally seen include pulmonary fibrosis, amen-orrhoea, gynaecomastia and testicular atrophy.

Bone marrow depression may occur after chemo-therapy, resulting in further anaemia, infection and bleeding.

Splenic irradiation or surgical splenectomy may be hazardous because of thrombocytopenia and a sub-sequent predisposition to infection, particularly pneumococcal pneumonia.

Rapid lysis of large populations of leukaemic cells may result in hyperuricaemia although florid gout is rare, as is tumour lysis syndrome. This is prevented by the use of allopurinol with chemotherapy and ensuring adequate fluid input.

Prognosis

The median survival of patients with CGL is around 4 years, with death usually occurring in the acute blast crisis. However, this masks the fact that some patients may live for many years in the chronic phase and an increasing number of patients are entering durable remissions in the acute phase with high-dose treatment and bone marrow transplantation.

Future prospects

A new drug acting as a competitive inhibitor of the abl-kinase system, imatinib mesylate (STI571), appears to have remarkably high levels of activity against resistant CML and is under investigation in randomized trials; it is likely to have a major role in its management in years ahead.

CHRONIC LYMPHOCYTIC LEUKAEMIA

Chronic lymphocytic leukaemia (CLL) represents the end of the leukaemic spectrum where the classi-fication merges with that of non-Hodgkin's lymph-oma. It is a neoplastic proliferation of the same cell type as lymphocytic lymphoma, the differentiating feature being the extent of bone marrow infiltration.

Epidemiology

Chronic lymphocytic leukaemia affects a somewhat older age group than CGL, with patients predom-inantly over 60 years. Males and females are affected in approximately equal proportions.

Aetiology

No specific aetiological factors for the common form of CLL seen in Europe and North and South America have been recognized.

The rarer T-cell variant may be associated with human T-cell lymphotropic virus type 1 (HTLV-1) infection, as found in Japan and the Caribbean.

Around half of all patients with CLL have demonstrable chromosomal abnormalities. The most common of these is trisomy of chromosome 12, with chromosome 14 being abnormal in other patients.

Pathology

The cell of origin for CLL is in most cases a B lymphocyte, although in 5 per cent there may be markers of T-cell origin. The B-cell type will demonstrate surface immunoglobulin which may be either κ or λ. The characteristic finding in the peripheral blood is of large numbers of mature lymphocytes with a total lymphocyte count of over $5000 \times 10^9/1$ being required to confirm the diagnosis. This is associated with bone marrow infiltration by immature lymphocytes which should account for more than 30 per cent of the total marrow. Three patterns of marrow involvement have been described: interstitial, nodular or diffuse. As with non-Hodgkin's lymphomas diffuse appearance is associated with a worse prognosis than the more focal forms.

Natural history

The natural history spans many years. Ultimately, death may occur owing to bone marrow failure or to transformation into a high-grade lymphoma.

Symptoms

Chronic lymphocytic leukaemia may be asymptomatic for some time. When symptoms do appear they include:

- painless lymphadenopathy;
- anaemia;
- recurrent infections;
- fever;
- sweats;
- weight loss.

Signs

These include:

- peripheral lymphadenopathy;
- splenomegaly;
- hepatomegaly (usually only mild).

Investigations

Blood count

A full blood count will reveal anaemia, thrombocytopenia and a high total white cell count, which, on examination of the blood film, is predominantly small, round, lymphocytes.

Bone marrow examination

This will confirm the diagnosis with the finding of excess lymphoid cells, at least 30 per cent of which will be immature forms.

Biopsy

Lymph node biopsy may be performed which will show infiltration of involved nodes with well-differentiated lymphocytes, usually in a diffuse pattern.

Other tests

Hypogammaglobulinaemia is a common association. Haemolytic anaemia may be associated with CLL with elevated conjugated bilirubin and a positive Coombs test. In HTLV-associated CLL, hypercalcaemia and hyponatraemia are characteristic features.

Differential diagnosis

Non-Hodgkin's lymphoma should be considered, particularly the diffuse small cell types.

Treatment

Because CLL has a long indolent course, in most patients treatment is only considered when symptomatic or when there are signs of bone marrow failure in the presence of very high peripheral white cell counts. There is usually a good response to gentle oral chemotherapy using chlorambucil or cyclophosphamide or to intravenous fludarabine, with no advantages in long-term outcome apparent for any particular approach to date. Steroids may also be used and are of value when the disease becomes refractory to alkylating agents. However, there is no evidence that adding them to chemotherapy in the early management of the disease is of value. Other combinations have also included vincristine or vinblastine, but again no significant advantage over single agent therapy has emerged. Chronic lymphocytic leukaemia is also responsive to rituximab, the anti-CD20 antibody.

Low-dose irradiation will result in rapid shrinkage of enlarged node masses or splenomegaly. Doses as low as 20 Gy or 30 Gy over 2–3 weeks are usually sufficient and associated with little or no morbidity.

There is no evidence that high-dose intensive treatment produces better results than more gentle therapy and bone marrow transplantation has no established role in CLL at present.

Tumour-related complications

The associated hypogammaglobulinaemia results in a high incidence of infections. There may be chronic anaemia, which can have a haemolytic component requiring regular transfusions. Thrombocytopenia may also persist.

The rare HTLV-related CLL may be associated with hypercalcaemia.

Treatment-related complications

Oral alkylating agents are usually relatively trouble free, provided that careful attention is paid to the blood count and treatment stopped when there are signs of significant bone marrow depression.

With a large tumour burden there is always the possibility of provoking hyperuricaemia due to cell lysis on initiation of chemotherapy. This should be prevented by administration of allopurinol and ensuring adequate fluid intake.

Prognosis

While remissions are usually readily achieved in CLL, cures are rare. Many patients will live with their disease for several years, the median survival being around 8 years.

The HTLV-associated T-cell form of CLL is a far more aggressive disease, however, and some patients may succumb within a few months, although a more chronic form similar to sporadic CLL is also seen.

RARE FORMS OF LEUKAEMIA

Prolymphocytic leukaemia

This is related to CLL, presenting in elderly men with splenomegaly and very high white cell counts. The cells are larger than the mature lymphocytes seen in CLL and the disease has a more aggressive course.

Hairy cell leukaemia

This is a chronic leukaemia occurring in the middle aged and is more frequent in men than women. It is rare, accounting for around 2 per cent of all cases of adult leukaemia. Typically, it presents with massive splenomegaly and pancytopenia. The characteristic finding is of 'hairy cells' in the peripheral blood and bone marrow. These are B lymphocytes with cytoplasmic projections giving them a 'hairy' appearance under the microscope.

Hairy cell leukaemia usually has a long indolent course. It responds to treatment with interferon with which it may remain in remission for many years before it becomes resistant and bone marrow failure develops. The new purine analogue drugs pentostatin and cladribine are also highly active in this disease and may be used instead of interferon.

MULTIPLE MYELOMA

Epidemiology

The incidence of multiple myeloma in the UK in men is around 55 per million with approximately 3000 cases diagnosed each year. Men and women are affected in equal proportions. There has been an apparent increase in incidence over the past 30 years from only 5 per million in 1960 which probably reflects improved diagnostic abilities rather than a true increase in the prevalence of the disease.

Aetiology

There are no recognized aetiological agents for multiple myeloma. It has been suggested that the origin of the paraprotein production may be as a host antibody response to a foreign protein but no consistent antigen has been identified.

Pathology

Multiple myeloma is one of a spectrum of plasma cell neoplasms which range from benign monoclonal gammopathy to solitary plasmacytoma to multiple myeloma. All these conditions are characterized by a neoplastic proliferation of B cells producing a characteristic paraprotein. Transformation within this group of conditions is well-recognized, with around 20 per cent of benign monoclonal gammopathies and 70 per cent of apparent solitary plasmacytomas eventually developing multiple myeloma.

Natural history

Three phases in the evolution of multiple myeloma have been described, not all of which may be seen in an individual patient:

- monoclonal gammopathy;
- smouldering myeloma, which is usually asymptomatic, with low levels of paraprotein and 10–20 per cent plasma cells in bone marrow;
- typical myeloma, with symptoms, rising paraprotein levels and >20 per cent plasma cells in bone marrow.

Once established, myeloma affects the bone marrow, bones and kidneys. Bone invasion is facilitated by release of chemicals which act as osteoclast-activating factors, including interleukins (in particular IL-1 and IL-6), tumour necrosis factor (TNF) and macrophage colony-stimulating factor (MCSF). Renal damage occurs as a result of deposition of paraprotein and amyloid formation, hypercalcaemia and hyperuricaemia.

Symptoms

Symptoms of multiple myeloma typically arise in three ways:

- bone marrow infiltration;
- bone destruction;
- metabolic and biochemical disturbance.

Bone marrow infiltration causes anaemia; thrombocytopenia is usually not prominent but more commonly there may be a bleeding disorder due to the effects of macroglobulinaemia.

Bone destruction results in local pain, pathological fracture or neurological complications such as nerve root or spinal cord compression; bone pain is present in two-thirds of patients presenting with myeloma.

Metabolic and biochemical disturbance occurs, including: high levels of paraprotein causing hyperviscosity, resulting in confusion and headache; renal failure, which is present in around one-third of patients and defined by a raised blood urea and creatinine, causing nausea, vomiting, malaise, fluid retention or itching; and hypercalcaemia, which is present in around one-third of patients that present with myeloma, resulting in thirst, polyuria, dyspepsia, nausea, vomiting, constipation or confusion.

Signs

Clinical signs of myeloma may be few. Patients may be clinically anaemic and bone lesions may present as locally tender or even swollen areas. There may be rib or spinal tenderness.

Patients presenting with pathological fracture will have obvious signs of swelling, tenderness and deformity.

Cord compression may present with weakness of the lower limbs, sphincter disturbance and neurological signs of an upper motor neurone lesion. In contrast cauda equina compression from disease in the lumbosacral spine will result in lower motor neurone weakness.

Hyperviscosity causes confusion. Papilloedema and retinal haemorrhage are also described.

Differential diagnosis

There are few conditions outside the spectrum of plasma cell neoplasms which will mimic myeloma, however there are rare forms of non-Hodgkin's lymphoma which may produce high levels of paraprotein and cause initial confusion.

Waldenstrom's macroglobulinaemia will also present with a paraprotein but none of the other features of myeloma and must be distinguished from benign monoclonal gammopathy (see Chapter 16).

Other causes of bone metastases including primary tumours of the breast, lung, thyroid and prostate should be considered.

Patients that present with a solitary plasma cell lesion may have a true solitary plasmacytoma as shown in Fig. 17.2, but 70 per cent will eventually manifest the characteristic features of widespread multiple myeloma.

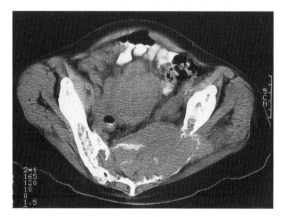

Fig 17.2 Solitary plasmacytoma arising in the ileum showing large soft tissue mass and bone destruction. This patient has an associated plasma paraprotein but no evidence of other sites of bone involvement and a normal bone marrow.

Investigations

Blood count

A full blood count may show anaemia and the ESR will be raised. The blood film may have rouleaux formation.

Biochemistry

Biochemical tests will show a raised total protein and there may be hypercalcaemia, renal failure with raised urea and creatinine and hyperuricaemia.

Protein electrophoresis

This will demonstrate the characteristic M band containing the paraprotein, which may also be quantitatively measured. This will be IgG in around 50 per cent of patients, IgA in 20 per cent, IgM in 10 per cent and light chain only in 10 per cent. Other rare types of paraprotein include IgD (2 per cent) and heavy chain fragments (1 per cent). In 1 per cent of patients there may be two different M proteins and in 1 per cent the paraprotein may be absent.

Serum β_2-microglobulin

The serum β_2-microglobulin is also raised in many patients and is an important marker of disease both for prognosis and for monitoring treatment.

Urine tests

There may be proteinuria and Bence–Jones protein may be detected on electrophoresis of the urine.

Bone marrow examination

This will show infiltration with plasma cells; infiltration with more than 20 per cent plasma cells is diagnostic.

Radiography and scans

An X-ray skeletal survey may show lytic bone lesions, many of which are asymptomatic. Typical appearances are shown on the skull X-ray in Fig. 17.3. Because the bone metastases of myeloma are usually predominantly lytic with little osteoblastic reaction, they often do not show on isotope bone scan or may be seen as cold areas rather than hot spots.

Other tests

Other investigations may be considered where indicated, including plasma viscosity, plasma volume, and rectal biopsy for amyloid.

Staging

A number of criteria for the diagnosis of myeloma have been defined as follows.

1. Presence of a monoclonal 'M' protein in serum or urine.
2. Bone lesions due to a plasma cell infiltrate.
3. Marrow plasma cells accounting for >10 per cent of marrow infiltrate.
4. Associated features: anaemia, hypercalcaemia or renal failure.

Diagnosis is confirmed on demonstration of any two of 1–3.

Staging of myeloma is based on recognized prognostic factors which include haemoglobin, blood urea, serum calcium, extent of bone lesions and level of paraprotein. The usual classification applied in the UK is the Durie–Salmon staging system.

- Stage 1 – haemoglobin (Hb) >10 g/dl; calcium normal; normal bone skeletal survey (or solitary plasmacytoma); low serum and urine paraprotein (serum IgG <6 g/dl; IgA < 3 g/dl; urine <4 g/24 h).
- Stage 2 – neither stage 1 nor stage 3.
- Stage 3 – Hb <8.5 g/dl; calcium >12 mg/dl; multiple lytic bone lesions; high paraprotein levels (serum IgG >7 g/dl; IgA >5 g/dl; urine >12 g/24 h).

There is a further subclassification into 'A'(normal renal function) or 'B' (raised serum creatinine).

It is proposed that the staging correlates with plasma cell mass, increasing from $<0.6 \times 10^{12}/m^2$ for stage 1 to $>1.2 \times 10^{12}/m^2$ for stage 3.

Serum β_2-microglobulin is a further important prognostic indicator.

Treatment

There is a small group of patients with indolent myeloma indicated by a few asymptomatic bone lesions or mild anaemia who require no specific treatment. They are managed by transfusion when appropriate and occasional monitoring of the serum paraprotein and β_2-microglobulin.

Solitary lesions (true plasmacytomas) are usually treated with local radiotherapy alone.

The remainder of patients will require treatment with chemotherapy and, where indicated, radiotherapy to sites of painful bone lesions.

CHEMOTHERAPY FOR MYELOMA

There are four main approaches to the drug treatment of myeloma.

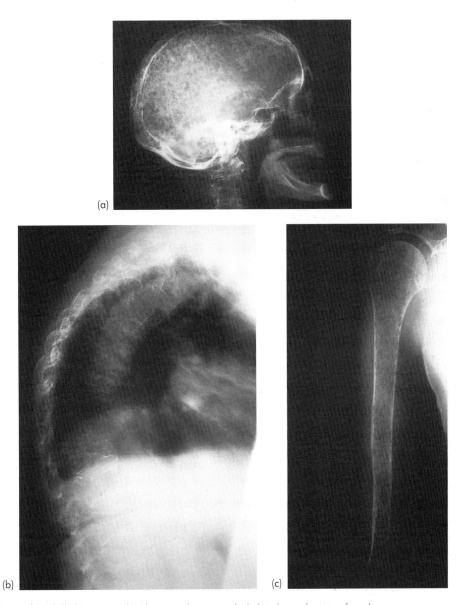

(a)

(b)

(c)

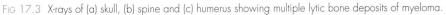

Fig 17.3 X-rays of (a) skull, (b) spine and (c) humerus showing multiple lytic bone deposits of myeloma.

Melphalan

This is given as an intermittent oral regime for 5–7 days. Steroids or vincristine may be added to oral melphalan but there is no evidence that this is of any value. Weekly cyclophosphamide is sometimes used as an alternative, with equivalent results.

Combination chemotherapy

There remains some controversy as to the role of combination chemotherapy over single-agent alkylating agents such as melphalan. One randomized trial in the UK has shown that a four-drug combination therapy is superior to melphalan alone in some patients and this may be chosen for young patients with advanced stage disease. One such combination is ABCM which comprises Adriamycin, BCNU, cyclophosphamide and melphalan.

Steroid-based regimes

It has been shown that continuous infusions of steroids such as dexamethasone are active in myeloma. The addition of other drugs may improve the results of this slightly as in the VAD schedule (vincristine, Adriamycin and dexamethasone) or CVAMP (cyclophosphamide, vincristine, Adriamycin, methyl prednisolone).

High-dose chemotherapy

This is perhaps the single most effective modality for initial treatment, although long-term overall survival may be little better. High-dose melphalan has been used in this context with bone marrow autograft or peripheral blood progenitor cell support following the high-dose chemotherapy. Some patients have also been treated by allogeneic bone marrow transplantation with a small number of long-term survivors reported.

The choice of treatment for an individual patient will depend on both the nature of the disease in that patient and their age and general health. For stage 1 myeloma, melphalan alone or in a younger patient ABCM, VAD or CVAMP may be chosen. For stage 3 myeloma, high-dose therapy should be considered for young patients (<50 years). For older patients high-dose therapy has considerable morbidity and mortality from the procedure and combination therapy with ABCM, VAD or CVAMP will be more appropriate.

Interferon maintenance therapy is sometimes recommended once initial treatment has achieved a response, usually defined by the paraprotein level reaching a plateau for at least 3 months.

Adjuvant bisphosphonate therapy (clodronate or pamidronate) has been shown to reduce the likelihood of complications such as pathological fracture due to bone deposits and should now be regarded as standard therapy in addition to chemotherapy.

SUPPORTIVE TREATMENT

Alongside chemotherapy, management of the complications of myeloma will have a considerable impact on both the quality of life and the survival of the patient.

- anaemia will require blood transfusion;
- infections will require prompt treatment with appropriate antibiotics;
- hypercalcaemia will require active hydration, diuresis and the use of bisphosphonates.
- renal failure will require management of fluid balance and in severe cases dialysis pending definitive chemotherapy may be justified;
- pathological fracture will require internal fixation followed by local radiotherapy;
- spinal canal compression will require steroids and urgent radiotherapy or surgical spinal stabilization;
- active rehabilitation is also important as immobility is a further adverse prognostic factor.

Tumour-related complications

These have been covered in the above discussion on supportive treatment in myeloma.

Treatment-related complications

Chemotherapy will cause bone marrow depression and the blood count must be carefully monitored with aggressive treatment of neutropenic infections. This is particularly the case when high-dose therapy is given where there will be a period of 2–3 weeks when the patient is pancytopenic.

Steroid infusions may cause 'Cushingoid' symptoms and, particularly in the elderly, fluid retention, causing cardiac failure.

Prognosis

The median survival for patients with stage 1 disease is around 4 years falling to only 2 years for stage 3. Those with solitary plasmacytoma in a site other than bone, usually in the head and neck region, have the best prognosis. Poor renal failure and a high β_2-microglobulin are associated with a poor prognosis with survival of less than 1 year.

Case history: myeloma

A 68-year-old man presents to his general practitioner (GP) with a 3-month history of increasing back pain. His GP elicits local tenderness in the thoraco-lumbar spine and sends him for an X-ray. This shows scattered lytic abnormalities in the vertebral bodies and it is commented that similar lesions are seen in adjacent ribs taken on the thoracic spine views. His GP proceeds to take blood for a full blood count, erythrocyte sedimentation rate (ESR), biochemical profile and paraproteins. A urine sample is tested at the local surgery and found to be positive for protein. A further sample is therefore sent to the pathology laboratory for detection of Bence–Jones proteins. In addition to this being positive he is found to have a paraprotein consisting of an immunoglobulin G with a level of 48 g/l. His other tests show that he is mildly anaemic with a haemoglobin of 10.3 but his other blood count parameters are normal. His ESR is 97 mm/hour. His urea is marginally elevated at 7.5 with a serum creatinine of 160. Serum calcium and other biochemical parameters are normal. He is referred to the haemato-oncology clinic. Further investigations performed there include an X-ray skeletal survey which shows scattered bone lesions and his bone marrow is reported as consisting of 35% plasma cells. A formal diagnosis of multiple myeloma is confirmed.

He is started on treatment with oral chemotherapy using melphalan 10 mg daily for 7 days given every 28 days. He finds this treatment is surprisingly easy to take with no significant side-effects. He is advised to take plenty of fluids each day and also started on clodronate tablets daily. He finds these are more troublesome than the chemotherapy, causing him nausea and occasional abdominal colic. He also finds it difficult to space the tablets between meals and other snacks, having been instructed that he must not take them within 1 hour of calcium-containing food or drink.

His paraprotein level falls satisfactorily and after his third month of treatment has reached 12 g/l. Over the next 2 months he continues with his treatment but no further change in the paraprotein level is seen and his paraproteins having reached a plateau, treatment is discontinued. He does however remain on the oral clodronate tablets which he is tolerating better. He remains well for the next 8 months, being seen occasionally in the clinic.

A paraprotein level measured after 6 months starts to show a slight rise and when seen at 8 months after completing his first course of chemotherapy he is complaining of some new back pain. X-rays show that he still has quite extensive lytic abnormalities in the bone. He is started back on melphalan 10 mg daily for 7 days every month. When seen at the end of the first month of restarting treatment his back pain is becoming more and more troublesome and he is referred for local radiotherapy. He attends the radiotherapy department and receives a single treatment to the thoraco-lumbar spine treating the painful area. That night he has quite troublesome nausea despite the dose of steroids and ondansetron given to him at the time of radiotherapy treatment. This however settles over the next 24 h taking regular metoclopramide tablets. He notices little change in the pain over the first few days but after 10 days there has been some gradual improvement and two weeks later he is left with a mild ache but otherwise untroubled by the previous pain.

However, when seen in the clinic 2 weeks later it is noted that his paraprotein is continuing to rise despite two further cycles of melphalan and he is advised that a change in treatment is indicated. He starts intravenous chemotherapy with vincristine, Adriamycin and high-dose dexamethasone (VAD). He finds this treatment much more troublesome, with quite marked constipation developing and troublesome nausea during the 4 days of intravenous drugs. He also finds the high-dose steroids give him a very large appetite and make him very restless. Sleeping is increasingly difficult during the week of treatment. After three cycles of VAD chemotherapy however his paraprotein has fallen once again to its plateau level and he perseveres with a further two cycles of treatment before this is discontinued. Within a few weeks of the treatment discontinuing he feels much improved, having recovered from the steroid side-effects. He is left with some numbness in his finger ends and occasional tingling but is reassured this is an expected side-effect of the vincristine in VAD and that a slow improvement can be expected.

He remains well again for a period of 8 months. He returns to the clinic complaining of general malaise and lack of energy. It is found that his haemoglobin has fallen to 8.6 and his white count is only 2.9 with a neutrophil count of 1.2. His platelet count is 112. His paraprotein level has risen once more to 42 g/l. He is given a 3-unit blood transfusion. The role of further chemotherapy is discussed with him and he is told that it is unlikely he will get a long response to further treatment but he is anxious to try further alternatives and is started on weekly injections of cyclophosphamide. He finds these are much better tolerated than his previous VAD chemotherapy but after the first month his paraprotein level has risen to 56 g/l and his haemoglobin is once again falling. He is started on erythropoietin injections given subcutaneously three times a week which improve his haemoglobin and maintain it at a level between 10.5 and 11 g/dl which he finds tolerable and free from symptoms. His paraprotein however continues to rise inexorably and the weekly cyclophosphamide injections are discontinued. It is noted that his creatinine level has risen to 230. He starts

Case history: myeloma *(cont.)*

complaining of increasing pain in the ribs with localized tenderness in several sites. He is started on diclofenac tablets, with some improvement in his pain. The next week he stumbles while coming down stairs at home and has severe pain in the right hip following which he can no longer bear weight. An ambulance is called and he is admitted through casualty. X-rays show that he has a pathological fracture of the right femur through a large lytic lesion. He is taken to the operating theatre and the bone is fixed internally. The following day he is found to have a postoperative temperature and to be rather chesty. His blood count shows that while the erythropoietin has maintained his haemoglobin, his white count has fallen with a neutrophil count of 0.9. He is started on intravenous antibiotics. However, his chest infection progresses with signs of widespread pneumonia. Three days later he has become semiconscious and confused with widespread signs of bronchopneumonia on his chest X-ray. His serum creatinine has risen to 380. The role of further antibiotics is discussed with his family who agree that in this circumstance it is unlikely to improve the situation and they are discontinued. He lapses into unconsciousness and dies peacefully over the next 24 h.

18 PAEDIATRIC CANCER

Malignant tumours are rare in children, with an incidence of around 100 per million children per year in the UK. Despite this, they are the most common cause of death in the age groups up to 14 years. The greatest incidence is under the age of 5 years, when around half of all paediatric cancers are diagnosed.

Tumours in children differ from those in adults with relatively more leukaemias and lymphomas and fewer solid epithelial cancers. The general distribution is shown in Table 18.1.

Overall, the outlook for paediatric malignancy is far better than for adults, with a cure rate of over 50 per cent. Because of the high cure rate there is now increasing emphasis on the long-term effects of treatment, in particular the influence of chemotherapy and radiotherapy on growth and both physical and intellectual development.

LEUKAEMIA

Leukaemias in childhood are predominantly acute lymphoblastic or less frequently acute myeloblastic leukaemias. Chronic leukaemia, while recognized, is extremely rare. Details of these conditions have been covered in Chapter 17.

CENTRAL NERVOUS SYSTEM TUMOURS

Around 70 per cent of childhood central nervous system (CNS) tumours are astrocytomas, predominantly low grade, the management of which has been covered in Chapter 12. Of the remainder, the most common is medulloblastoma which accounts for 15–20 per cent of the total.

MEDULLOBLASTOMA

Epidemiology
Medulloblastomas are more common in children under 5 years than over 5 years and occur in twice as many boys as girls.

Aetiology
There are no recognized aetiological factors in the development of this tumour other than the small proportion which develop within the context of Gorlin's syndrome.

Pathology
Typically, medulloblastoma is a tumour of the posterior fossa arising within the cerebellum.

TABLE 18.1 Frequency and type of common paediatric cancers

Cancer	Incidence (%)
Leukaemia	30
Central nervous system tumours	20
Bone and soft tissue	15
Lymphoma	10
Neuroblastoma	7
Nephroblastoma (Wilms')	7
Others	11

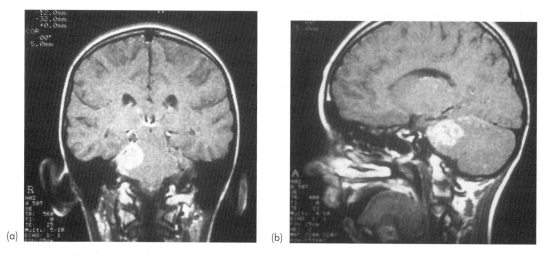

(a)   (b)

Fig 18.1 Magnetic resonance imaging scan showing medulloblastoma arising in posterior cranial fossa.

Obstruction of the fourth ventricle or aqueduct may result in secondary hydrocephalus. A characteristic feature of this tumour is its propensity to seed throughout the neuroaxis so that meningeal deposits may be found at any site both within the skull and down the spinal cord. Blood-borne metastases have been described, particularly in bone, but these are rare.

Microscopically, the cells are derived from precursors of neuronal tissue and have a characteristic appearance likened to short carrots, forming circles or rosettes.

Symptoms

In children, CNS tumours may have an insidious onset with irritability and failure to achieve appropriate milestones. Children or their parents may complain of specific difficulties with walking or headache. Spinal disease may cause nerve root pains and arm or leg weakness.

Signs

Posterior fossa tumours may cause specific signs of cerebellar dysfunction with incoordination, ataxic gait and scanning dysarthria. There may also be lower cranial nerve signs.

Spinal involvement will cause weakness of limbs and sensory changes, particularly the development of nerve root pains.

Hydrocephalus, causing raised intracranial pressure, may, in the young child, result in bulging of the fontanelle and increased head circumference.

Differential diagnosis

Other tumours of the posterior fossa should be considered, of which the most common is a low-grade astrocytoma. Other rarer tumours include ependymoma and germ cell tumours. Unlike adults, metastases in the posterior fossa are rare in children.

Investigations

Routine tests such as a full blood count and biochemical screen are usually unremarkable as is routine radiology, including a skull X-ray.

Computed tomography scan

The tumour will be seen on computed tomography (CT) scan which should be enhanced with intravenous contrast. A CT will also demonstrate any degree of hydrocephalus.

Magnetic resonance imaging

A magnetic resonance imaging (MRI) scan is often superior to CT in imaging the posterior fossa and should be used where available. (Fig. 18.1). Some form of spinal imaging is essential to complete the staging process. Previously this has required a myelogram but this can now be replaced by MRI scan, as demonstrated in Fig. 18.2.

Staging

There is no TNM staging (see Chapter 2) for medulloblastoma, although various other staging systems

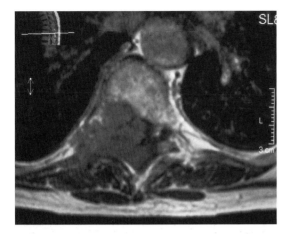

FIG 18.2 Magnetic resonance imaging scan demonstrating spinal metastases from medulloblastoma.

have been proposed. Essentially, patients can be divided by certain prognostic factors into two groups.

- Good risk – age <3 years; posterior fossa tumour with no dissemination; total excision or < 1.5 cm³ residual tumour postoperatively.
- Poor risk – age <3 years; primary site outside posterior fossa; metastatic disease; subtotal resection (i.e. >1.5 cm³ residual tumour).

Treatment

Initial treatment following the diagnosis of a posterior fossa tumour will be surgery. Surgery has three roles in the management of this tumour:

- to confirm the histological diagnosis from resected tissue;
- to remove all visible tumour if technically possible; and
- to relieve hydrocephalus if present by the insertion of a ventriculoperitoneal shunt.

Following surgery, postoperative radiotherapy will be given. This involves treatment of the whole craniospinal axis (i.e. the whole brain and spinal column down to the level of S2, where the thecal sac terminates).

There may also be some benefit from chemotherapy for high-risk patients (i.e. those with brainstem involvement, incomplete surgical removal, supratentorial tumour or spinal tumour).

Tumour-related complications

Obstructive hydrocephalus may occur. There may be permanent neurological deficits, in particular incoordination and ataxia. Spinal disease may result in permanent limb weakness.

Treatment-related complications

Ventriculoperitoneal shunts may become infected or block, requiring surgical revision. Craniospinal irradiation may cause significant bone marrow depression, particularly in those patients receiving chemotherapy. Late effects of this treatment include impaired growth, particularly of the spine, resulting in a disproportionate reduction in sitting height compared with standing height. The ovaries are usually included in the sacral radiation field, resulting in sterility in young girls.

Pituitary irradiation within the whole-brain volume may result in varying degrees of hypopituitarism, requiring appropriate replacement therapy.

Late results of whole-brain irradiation may result in some blunting of intellectual development and failure to reach the full potential, which may have been predicted pretreatment. Despite this, many patients achieve good results and function normally within society.

Prognosis

The overall long-term cure rate is 40–50 per cent.

Rare tumours

Ependymomas

These account for around 8 per cent of childhood brain tumours. When occurring in the posterior fossa they behave in a very similar fashion to medulloblastomas and the principles of treatment are the same. Cure rates are also similar.

BONE AND SOFT TISSUE TUMOURS

The common bone tumours in children are osteosarcoma and Ewing's sarcoma, both of which are discussed in Chapter 15.

The common soft tissue tumour to occur in children is the embryonal rhabdomyosarcoma. This differs significantly from the alveolar and pleomorphic forms of rhabdomyosarcoma found in adults.

RHABDOMYOSARCOMA (EMBRYONAL TYPE)

Epidemiology

These tumours are usually seen in the first five years of life and have an overall incidence of 3 per million children under 15 years of age in the UK. They may arise in any site, the most common being the head and neck region and the genitourinary tract.

Aetiology

There are no known aetiological factors.

Pathology

Approximately one-third arise in the head and neck region, one-third in the genitourinary tract and a quarter in the soft tissues of the trunk or extremities. The orbit is also a relatively frequent site, accounting for 10 per cent of the total.

Macroscopically, they appear as pink fleshy masses and proliferative forms may be likened to bunches of grapes ('sarcoma botryoides').

Microscopically, they are embryonal cells which are rich in glycogen and within which myofibrils can be demonstrated. They are distinct from the alveolar rhabdomyosarcoma of adult, although this type can be seen in older children and adolescents.

A specific chromosome deletion has been identified at chromosome 11p15 associated with embryonal type distinct from the other subtypes of rhabdomyosarcoma.

Natural history

The natural history of this form of rhabdomyosarcoma is for rapid local growth with infiltration along tissue planes and early blood-borne metastases. Around one in five will have bone marrow infiltration at presentation. Lymph node spread may also occur, particularly in those tumours arising in the genitourinary tract and limbs.

Symptoms

Presenting symptoms depend on site of origin. Many arise as rapidly enlarging but painless masses. Other local symptoms may be present including nasal obstruction and epistaxis from the nasopharynx, haematuria from the urinary tract, vaginal bleeding from the vagina or uterus and visual disturbances from the orbit.

Signs

Clinical signs will go along with the presenting symptoms. There may be an obvious mass visible. Vaginal tumours may present with a fleshy mass of 'botryoid' tumour at the introitus.

Differential diagnosis

In childhood there are few other tumours which are likely to arise in similar sites to rhabdomyosarcoma. Other causes of presenting symptoms such as epistaxis or haematuria in the absence of an obvious mass will be sought.

Investigations

Routine tests such as full blood count and biochemistry may well be normal.

Radiography

Chest X-ray may demonstrate lung metastases.

Computed tomography scan and magnetic resonance imaging

A CT scan or MRI of the affected site will be valuable in delineating the extent of local tumour most accurately.

Bone marrow examination

Bone marrow examination should be performed in view of the high incidence of marrow involvement and skeletal X-ray survey or isotope bone scan should also be performed.

Biopsy

A full examination of the affected site under anaesthetic with biopsy of the tumour is essential to confirm the diagnosis.

Staging

A TNM staging (see Chapter 2) is used and is based on post-surgical status.

- T1 – tumour limited to site of origin with microscopic margins of excision clear.
- T2 – tumour extending beyond site of origin but complete microscopic clearance of tumour.
- T3 – tumour extending beyond site of origin with incomplete excision.
- N0 – regional nodes negative.
- N1 – regional nodes involved.
- M0 – no metastases.
- M1 – distant metastases.

In practice, group staging as used by the Intergroup Rhabdomyosarcoma Studies (IRS) may be of more value.

- Stage I – localized disease completely resected.
- Stage II – either localized disease with residual microscopic disease, or
  node involvement completely resected (IIB), or
  node involvement with microscopic residual disease (IIC).
- Stage III – incomplete resection or biopsy only.
- Stage IV – distant metastases at diagnosis.

Around half of patients will be stage III at diagnosis and 20% will present with metastases.

Treatment

RADICAL TREATMENT

Chemotherapy

Chemotherapy is given to all cases using VAC (vincristine, actinomycin D and cyclophosphamide). One or two courses are given followed by definitive surgery or radiotherapy and then chemotherapy is continued for a period of up to 1 year.

Surgery

This is the treatment of choice in the absence of advanced distant metastases. For urogenital, truncal and limb rhabdomyosarcoma, wide resection is usually performed.

Radiotherapy

This is used for inoperable tumours such as orbit and nasopharynx, delivering doses of around 50 Gy in 5 weeks.

PALLIATIVE TREATMENT

For recurrent disseminated disease a course of palliative chemotherapy or radiotherapy may be valuable in minimizing symptoms. Second-line chemotherapy using drugs such as ifosfamide and etoposide may achieve good responses, although further relapse is usual. Local recurrence particularly in patients with the botyroid type of tumour should be treated actively as there is a high salvage rate in this group.

Tumour-related complications

These will depend on the site. Urogenital tumours may permanently affect renal, urinary and reproductive function and orbital tumours may affect sight.

Treatment-related complications

Chemotherapy using VAC may cause nausea, vomiting and alopecia during the period of administration. In the longer term, peripheral neuropathy from vincristine can persist.

Radical surgery may have late sequelae depending on the type of procedure. There are obvious effects of cystectomy or hysterectomy for urogenital tumours.

Radical radiotherapy may have late sequelae also, in particular growth impairment in the treated area. In a young child this can result in quite marked disfigurement if significant asymmetry develops, as may be the case following, for example, orbit irradiation.

Prognosis

The overall prognosis for embryonal rhabdomyosarcoma which is confined to the site of origin is good, with cure rates of around 80 per cent. Once metastatic, the outlook is poor with less than 20 per cent surviving.

Age and site is an important predictor of cure. The best prognoses are associated with tumours of the orbit, paratesticular region and vagina. Poor prognosis sites are parameningeal, prostate and perineum. Patients with metastatic disease aged <10 years have a significantly better outcome than older patients.

LYMPHOMA

Both Hodgkin's disease and non-Hodgkin's lymphoma (NHL) may occur in children. While they obey the general rules discussed in Chapter 16 there are certain features of paediatric lymphomas which should be considered.

Non-Hodgkin's lymphoma

In children this is usually high-grade nodal disease with a particular propensity for diffuse lymphoblastic or undifferentiated tumours and also T-cell lymphomas associated with a mediastinal mass. Low-grade NHL is rare in children.

Treatment usually involves combination chemotherapy; for extensive high-grade disease bone marrow transplant may be considered. Local radiotherapy may also be given in doses of 25–30 Gy.

Hodgkin's disease

Hodgkin's disease is relatively more common in boys than in girls which contrasts with a more even sex distribution in adults. Lymphocyte predominant histology is relatively more common and the less favourable lymphocyte-depleted form is uncommon.

Treatment is based on the same principles as in adult Hodgkin's disease but with even greater emphasis on minimizing late effects. For this reason, chemotherapy is often preferred for relatively early disease, avoiding the local growth problems after radiotherapy. Where irradiation is used, lower doses of around 20–30 Gy are given compared with 35–40 Gy in adults.

NEUROBLASTOMA

Epidemiology

Neuroblastoma is a tumour of young children, 50 per cent occurring before the age of 2 years. It has an annual incidence of 8 per million in the UK and is slightly more common in boys than in girls. There is some geographical variation; it is rare in Africa compared with Europe and the USA.

Aetiology

There is an association with von Recklinghausen's disease (multiple neurofibromatosis) and colonic aganglionosis, but most cases have no recognizable causal factor. There is some evidence that it may arise as a congenital anomaly and cases *in utero* have been reported.

Specific chromosome abnormalities have been identified in neuroblastoma, including amplification of the *N-myc* oncogene, deletions affecting chromosome 1 and gain of the long arm of chromosome 17(17q).

Pathology

Two-thirds of neuroblastomas are intra-abdominal tumours, of which 60 per cent occur in the adrenal and 40 per cent at other sites related to the sympathetic chain. The remaining one-third are divided between the chest, pelvis and head and neck region. In a small number of these tumours widespread metastatic disease may be present with no recognizable primary site.

Macroscopically, the tumour is usually encapsulated but soft and friable, containing areas of haemorrhage, necrosis, cystic degeneration and calcification.

Microscopically, there is a spectrum of appearances depending on the degree of differentiation. Typically, it is composed of densely packed, small round cells which may form rosettes. In the more differentiated forms neurofibrils and ganglionic elements and granule-containing chromaffin cells may be seen.

Natural history

Local infiltration of surrounding tissues is seen.

Regional lymph nodes may be involved but the predominant pattern of metastases is by early blood-borne dissemination, with around two-thirds of children having widespread disease at presentation, affecting, in particular, bone and liver. Lung metastases are relatively rare.

Spontaneous maturation and regression may occur. At post-mortem there is a much higher incidence of asymptomatic tumours in patients dying from unrelated conditions than in the general population.

Symptoms

These will depend on the site and age at presentation. Abdominal tumours which are the most common will present with abdominal discomfort and bowel or urinary obstruction. In the head and neck a painless mass may be the first manifestation. There also may be fever, anorexia, malaise and weight loss.

Metastatic disease may cause the first symptoms, particularly bone pain from bone metastases. Excessive catecholamine production from the tumour cells will cause flushing, palpitations, diarrhoea and headache.

Rarely, *in utero* it presents with pre-eclampsia in the mother.

Signs

These may include:

- a palpable mass;
- intrathoracic tumours, causing venous obstruction with dilated neck veins, plethora and oedema; and
- catecholamine secretion, causing hypertension.

There are rare neurological syndromes associated with neuroblastoma, in particular an acute cerebellar disturbance.

Differential diagnosis

A tumour presenting as a palpable mass must be distinguished from other types of tumour. In the abdomen this will include Wilms' tumour and in the neck a lymph node caused by lymphoma.

The differential diagnosis of a small round cell tumour in bone includes not only neuroblastoma but also Ewing's sarcoma and lymphoma.

Investigations

Routine blood tests may be unremarkable but extensive bone metastases may cause pancytopenia and there may be obstructive renal impairment.

Radiography

An X-ray of the tumour may demonstrate speckled calcification within it.

Computed tomography scan or magnetic resonance imaging

A CT scan or MRI is needed for more accurate definition of the tumour.

Bone marrow examination

This examination is important because of the high incidence of bone metastases.

Urine tests

Twenty-four hour urine collections will be made to measure catecholamines as vanillylmandelic acid (VMA) and homovanillylmandelic acid (HVA), the ratio of the two having prognostic importance. Other peptides such as vasoactive intestinal peptide (VIP) may also be raised.

Other tests

Because many of the tumours will contain cells synthesizing catecholamines from their precursors, a labelled precursor called meta-iodobenzyl guanidine (mIBG) may be used as a tracer in scanning when labelled with radioactive iodine. This also has therapeutic uses.

Staging

The Audrey Evans or COG (Children's Cancer Group) classification is used.

- Stage 1 – confined to the site of origin.
- Stage 2 – extending beyond site of origin but not crossing midline including lymph node involvement.
- Stage 3 – extending beyond site of origin across midline including lymph node involvement.
- Stage 4 – distant metastases.
- Stage 4S – infants (<2 years) with local tumour not crossing midline but with liver, skin or bone marrow involvement (without bone metastases).

Other classifications based on additional surgical findings are the POG (Paediatric Oncology Group) and INSS (International Neuroblastoma Staging System).

Treatment

STAGES 1 AND 2

Local treatment alone is given by radical surgical excision. Postoperative radiotherapy is given for older children (>1 year) or those with poor prognostic features on histology, in particular poorly differentiated tumours and those with aneuploidy or *N-myc* amplification. Neuroblastoma is very sensitive to irradiation and doses of only 20–30 Gy over 3–4 weeks are adequate.

STAGES 3 AND 4

Chemotherapy using a combination of cyclophosphamide and vincristine with the addition of Adriamycin, etoposide or cisplatin is given in those over 1 year of age. Resection of, or radiotherapy to the primary tumour may be considered before or after cytoreduction with chemotherapy.

Intensive chemotherapy using high doses of drugs such as melphalan with or without autologous bone marrow transplant may be of value, particularly in those with poor prognostic features.

Targeted radiation using iodine-131-labelled mIBG, which is actively concentrated in cells synthesizing catecholamines, is also used.

PALLIATIVE TREATMENT

Local radiotherapy for painful bone metastases or large tumour masses may be used.

STAGE 4S DISEASE

Spontaneous regression of tumour occurs with little or no treatment. Vincristine or low-dose irradiation may be indicated for pressure symptoms caused by a large liver or other tumour mass.

Tumour-related complications

Mediastinal, renal or intestinal obstruction may occur, depending on primary site. Excess catecholamine secretion may cause hypertension and tachycardia with arrhythmia. Diarrhoea may occur if VIP is produced.

Treatment-related complications

Irradiation of the abdomen of a child may cause bowel or renal damage. It is important to design symmetrical fields of irradiation to minimize deformity from growth retardation.

Prognosis

The prognosis for localized neuroblastoma is good, with virtually all patients with stage 1 disease and 80 per cent of those with stage 2 cured. Stage 4S also has a good outlook with cure rates approaching 80 per cent. In contrast, older patients with metastatic disease have a very poor prognosis with long-term survival between 10 per cent and 40 per cent. Important prognostic factors are hyperploidy conferring a good prognosis and diploidy or *N-myc* expression predicting a poor outcome.

Future developments

Evaluation of intensive high-dose chemotherapy regimes in those patients identified as having a poor prognosis on the basis of chromosomal changes. The use of 13-*cis*-retinoic acid has been shown to induce differentiation of neuroblastoma and is under evaluation as an adjuvant treatment following chemotherapy.

NEPHROBLASTOMA (WILMS' TUMOUR)

Epidemiology

Wilms' tumour is a tumour of young children with a peak incidence at 3 years and the majority occurring before the age of 5 years. The annual incidence is 1 in 20 000 children in the UK and there is equal distribution between boys and girls.

Aetiology

Wilms' tumour is familial in 1–2 per cent of cases. There is an association with certain rare congenital abnormalities, including Beckwith–Weidemann syndrome, hemi-hypertrophy, aniridia, Bloom syndrome and other abnormalities of the urogenital tract. Trisomy 18 is another associated disorder and a deletion on the short arm of chromosome 11 (11p13) is seen in around one-third of cases of Wilms' tumour, as well as certain other abnormalities of the genitourinary system such as hypospadias and cryptorchidism. The gene that causes aniridia is also located close to this position on chromosome 11. Other deletions are seen on chromosomes 16 and 1p.

Pathology

The tumour arises in the kidney and 5 per cent are bilateral. It may be lobular and is surrounded by a pseudocapsule as it compresses surrounding tissue. There may be areas of haemorrhage, necrosis and cyst formation.

Microscopically, there is often considerable variety within the tumour, with areas of primitive mesenchymal cells that may show differentiation into fat, muscle or cartilage within which are areas of recognizable embryonal glomerular and renal tubular elements.

Certain microscopic features are of prognostic importance. Anaplastic areas are associated with a worse prognosis, particularly if there are diffuse rather than focal areas of anaplastic change. Previously, subtypes labelled sarcomatous and clear cell are now thought to be distinct entities rather than variants of Wilms and also have a poor prognosis.

Natural history

Local invasion from the renal parenchyma into the renal pelvis and renal vein will occur. Lymph node involvement is relatively infrequent.

Blood-borne metastases are the usual means of spread beyond the kidney, the most common distant site being the lungs.

Symptoms

Abdominal pain is the most common presenting feature. Haematuria occurs in about 20 per cent and a similar proportion may have unexplained fevers. Other systemic symptoms are, however, unusual.

Pulmonary metastases may cause cough, haemoptysis or dyspnoea.

Signs

The majority have a palpable abdominal mass at presentation, which may be entirely asymptomatic. Hypertension may be present but is relatively unusual.

Differential diagnosis

Abdominal neuroblastoma may also present with a large abdominal mass but is usually associated with greater systemic upset and bone metastases rather than lung metastases.

Investigations

Blood tests

A full blood count may show anaemia and urea and electrolytes may be disturbed.

Urine tests

Urinalysis may show both blood and protein in the urine.

Radiography

Chest X-ray may demonstrate lung metastases.

Other tests

The primary tumour will be demonstrated on abdominal ultrasound and on intravenous urography (IVU). A CT and MR scan of the abdomen will give further information about its local extent, as shown in Fig. 18.3.

Staging

The largest group investigating Wilms' tumour is the National Wilms' Tumour Study Group in the USA and their staging system is commonly reported.

- Stage 1 – tumour completely excised and retained within capsule.
- Stage 2 – tumour completely excised but extending beyond capsule.
- Stage 3 – tumour incompletely excised but no blood-borne metastases.
- Stage 4 – blood-borne distant metastases.
- Stage 5 – bilateral tumours.

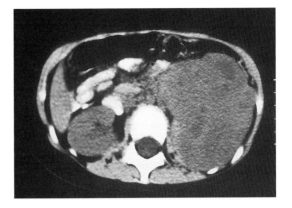

FIG 18.3 Computed tomography scan demonstrating large renal mass in nephroblastoma.

Around 5 per cent will present with bilateral tumours and a second tumour may develop in the contralateral tumour in up to 3 per cent.

Treatment

Surgery by laparotomy and radical resection of the tumour is performed, which will usually entail a nephro-ureterectomy and regional node dissection. An important feature of the operation should be mobilization and careful inspection of the contralateral kidney in view of the significant incidence of bilateral tumours.

Postoperative radiotherapy or chemotherapy are used as follows:

- stage 1 disease is given a short course of weekly vincristine injections;
- stages 2 and 3 disease are given radiotherapy to the renal bed delivering 20–30 Gy in 3–4 weeks together with chemotherapy using vincristine and actinomycin D; for tumours exhibiting anaplasia more intensive chemotherapy will be given as below;
- stage 4 disease is treated with intensive chemotherapy using vincristine, actinomycin D, Adriamycin, etoposide, and cyclophosphamide; in patients that respond satisfactorily, radiotherapy to the renal bed may also be considered.

Palliative treatment

This may take the form of chemotherapy or local radiotherapy for symptomatic disease. High-dose chemotherapy with bone marrow rescue has been used but may be no better than alternating chemotherapy regimens using ifosfamide, etoposide and carboplatin. Around 50 per cent of patients may be salvaged after recurrence. For chemotherapy-resistant lung disease low-dose whole-lung irradiation may be given, delivering 10–12 Gy in seven or eight small fractions.

Tumour-related complications

In bilateral tumours, preservation of as much renal tissue as possible will be attempted.

Treatment-related complications

Radiotherapy to the renal bed will include the lumbar vertebrae and there will therefore be growth retardation in this area. Because of this, it is extremely important that the radiotherapist includes the entire width of the vertebral body to avoid a scoliotic deformity resulting from differential growth across the vertebral body.

Immediate side-effects of chemotherapy may include nausea, vomiting and alopecia. In the longer term vincristine may be associated with a peripheral neuropathy, actinomycin D with liver dysfunction and Adriamycin with dose-related cardiomyopathy.

Prognosis

Wilms' tumour is both radio- and chemo-sensitive and the prognosis for localized disease is therefore very good with 80–90 per cent of patients with stage 1 or 2 disease being cured. Even those presenting with distant metastases (stage 4) have a cure rate of up to 40 per cent.

Rare tumours

The rhabdoid tumour of kidney is highly malignant metastasizing widely to lungs and CNS in particular. Clear cell sarcoma of the kidney also disseminates widely and both have a far worse prognosis than Wilms' tumour.

OTHER TUMOURS

Langerhans cell histiocytosis

This is a complex condition arising from a proliferation of histiocytes. Three distinct forms are recognized:

- Letterer–Siwe disease;
- Hand–Schuller–Christian disease;
- eosinophilic granuloma.

Letterer–Siwe disease affects infants and is usually rapidly fatal because of widespread infiltration of liver, spleen, skin and lymph nodes with proliferating histiocytes.

Hand–Schuller–Christian disease may occur at any age with a less fulminant course and is once again characterized by widespread infiltration by histiocytes which, in this case, is characterized by intracellular accumulation of lipid. Bones in particular are affected and patients survive for many years, although most ultimately succumb. It may be treated using drug combinations such as VAC.

Eosinophilic granuloma is the least aggressive form of the disease and is usually localized presenting as solitary lytic bone lesions. Deposits around the pituitary are a recognized cause of diabetes insipidus. They are characterized by accumulations of lipid-filled histiocytes, eosinophils and giant cells. They may regress spontaneously. If symptomatic they respond well to low doses of irradiation.

Retinoblastoma

This is a rare tumour present in around 1 in 20 000 live births in the UK. It may follow an autosomal dominant pattern of inheritance, although many have no preceding family history. A specific gene translocation has been identified in retinoblastoma with a deletion in the long arm of chromosome 13.

It usually presents in the first 2 years of life with reduced vision, white pupils or strabismus. As the tumour occludes fluid drainage within the eye secondary glaucoma may develop. The diagnosis is confirmed on examination of both eyes under anaesthetic. An example is shown in Fig. 18.4.

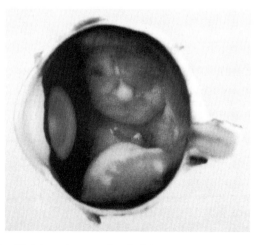

Fig 18.4 Lateral section of eyeball showing extensive primary retinoblastoma.

Small tumours may be treated by light coagulation using a xenon arc laser or cryotherapy. Larger tumours may be treated with radiotherapy, which may be delivered either by placing cobalt discs over the tumour or with external beam treatment, where most of the eye has to be included. Enucleation is avoided but may be necessary if the optic nerve is invaded.

Most tumours are cured using this approach, with preservation of vision.

Germ cell tumours

Teratomas may present in the first 5 years. The majority are benign but 20 per cent or so will be malignant. The common sites are the ovary and the sacrococcygeal region but they may also be found in the mediastinum, neck, nasopharynx, retroperitoneum or brain.

The management of these tumours is essentially the same as that of germ cell tumours in the adult. Initial treatment will be surgical removal, where possible, followed by appropriate adjuvant chemotherapy using combinations such as BEP (bleomycin, etoposide and cisplatin). Local radiotherapy may be considered where surgical excision is not feasible, as in the brain. Overall the prognosis, as in adult germ cell tumours, is good.

The skin is the largest organ in the body. Its large surface area and location make it particularly vulnerable to environmental carcinogens. Recent cultural, economic and environmental changes have resulted in many more people being exposed to high levels of ultraviolet radiation. As this is the main risk factor for developing skin cancer, many more cases can be expected in the decades to come.

SQUAMOUS AND BASAL CELL CARCINOMA

Epidemiology

There are 36 000 new cases and 400 deaths (nearly all from squamous cell carcinoma) registered in the UK per annum. Basal cell carcinoma (BCC) is twice as common as squamous cell carcinoma (SCC). The peak incidence is at 60–80 years and it is exceptional in the under 40s, in whom a strong aetiological factor can usually be identified (e.g. Gorlin's syndrome, arsenic exposure). There is a slight male predominance and they are more common in white people living in a sunny climate, particularly South Africa and Australia; the incidence increases as one moves closer to the equator. They are only rarely encountered in dark-skinned races.

Aetiology

Ultraviolet radiation is the most important cause accounting for the geographical and racial distribution of skin cancers. They are therefore most frequent on areas of the body exposed to the sun. Previous radiotherapy may lead to skin cancer at the entry or exit site of the radiation. Radiation-induced cancers were a particular problem to the pioneering

radiologists who used to calibrate their X-ray machines by exposing their hands to a dose sufficient to cause erythema of the skin.

Squamous cell carcinoma of the scrotum was described in nineteenth century chimney sweeps, where soot had become trapped in the rugose skin of the scrotum. Similarly, occupational exposure to tar and bitumen may lead to tumours on the exposed skin. Mineral oils were the cause of SCC described in yarn workers, where they were used to lubricate the spinning mules.

Arsenic is a potent cause of skin cancers and a history of exposure should be sought in patients with multiple BCCs and SCCs. It was once used as a 'tonic' and is found in some pesticides.

Squamous cell carcinoma has been described arising in chronic varicose (Marjolin's) ulcers, burn scars, cutaneous TB, sinuses from chronic osteomyelitis, and epidermolysis bullosa. Gorlin's syndrome is a very rare, dominantly inherited syndrome predisposing to multiple BCCs and should be considered in all cases arising under 40 years of age. Palmar pits are characteristic but other features include bifid ribs, a calcified falx cerebris, frontal bossing of the skull and mandibular cysts. Xeroderma pigmentosum is even rarer, recessively inherited, and patients inevitably develop multiple BCCs and SCCs at a very young age.

Chronic immunosuppression by agents such as azathioprine and cyclosporin in organ transplant recipients is associated with an increased incidence of BCC and SCC.

Pathology

The tumours usually arise on skin exposed to the sun, such as the scalp, nose, ears, periorbital tissues and dorsum of hand. Basal cell carcinoma is very rare in non-hair-bearing skin, such as the palms and soles. They are frequently multiple, with changes of solar damage in surrounding skin such as keratoses. An invasive SCC may arise in an area of *in situ* carcinoma such as Bowen's disease. Squamous cell carcinomas are usually well circumscribed, appearing as nodules, nodules with some central ulceration or ulcers with raised, everted, nodular edges (Fig. 19.1). A BCC may also appear predominantly nodular, ulcerating or mixed, and often have characteristic surface telangiectasia and a 'pearly' appearance (Fig. 19.2). They vary greatly in rate of growth, with some persisting unnoticed for many years and others growing rapidly over a period of several months. Large, neglected tumours (Figs 19.3 and 19.4) are accompanied by local tissue destruction and secondary infection. Both BCCs and SCCs may be found concurrently in the same patient.

Microscopically, these tumours are locally invasive, often for some distance beyond their macroscopic margins. The cell of origin of a BCC is uncertain, but is thought to be a basal cell of a hair follicle giving rise to small dark-staining cells. Squamous cell carcinomas arise from keratinocytes, are well differentiated, demonstrate intercellular bridges on electron microscopy and produce keratin. Sometimes the appearances are those of a mixed 'basisquamous' tumour.

Natural history

Both types of tumour are characterized by relentless local infiltration of the surrounding skin and normal tissues lying deep to, or adjacent to, the skin leading to their eventual destruction. About 5 per cent of SCCs and less than 0.1 per cent of BCCs spread to the regional lymph nodes (Fig. 19.5). Blood-borne spread is rare for SCCs and extremely rare for BCCs. Lung and bone are the most common sites of metastatic spread.

Symptoms

The patient may be asymptomatic, the lesion being noticed at a routine medical examination, or the patient may complain of a skin lesion which is causing concern or cosmetic defect. Ulcerating lesions may bleed spontaneously if traumatized and irritation is a common complaint, although pain is exceptional.

Signs

Careful inspection under a bright light with a magnifying glass is recommended as it is the most accurate way of defining the macroscopic extent of the tumour, which may be much greater than naked-eye inspection would suggest. Telangiectasia suggests a BCC. However, it may be difficult to distinguish an SCC from a BCC by appearance alone. The tumour may be tethered or fixed to

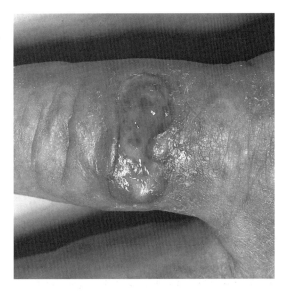

FIG 19.1 A typical ulcerating squamous carcinoma arising on the skin of a finger. Note the irregular, slightly everted edge.

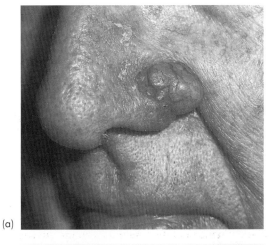

(a)

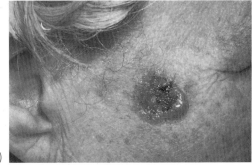

(b)

FIG 19.2 Basal cell carcinoma: (a) nodular variant; (b) ulcerating variant.

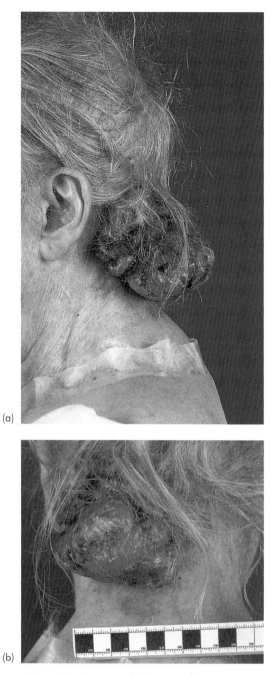

(a)

(b)

FIG 19.3 Basal cell carcinoma. This lesion had been neglected for 20 years and covered by a headscarf. Surgical excision was curative. (a) Side view; (b) rear view.

underlying tissues depending on the depth of invasion. There may be much destruction of the surrounding tissues and secondary infection of the tumour. Regional lymph nodes should be examined in all cases.

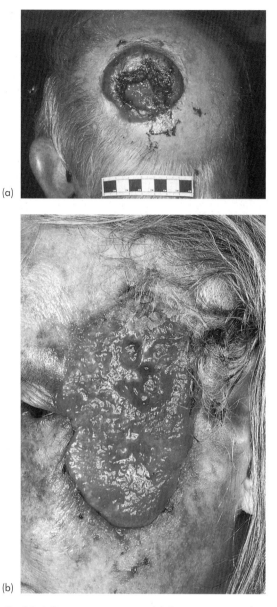

(a)

(b)

FIG 19.4 Squamous carcinoma. (a) Carcinoma arising from the skin overlying the vertex of the skull. Such tumours may penetrate into the skull and involve the underlying brain. (b) Large plaque of tumour arising from the temple.

Differential diagnosis

This includes:

- keratoacanthoma;
- solar keratosis;
- Bowen's disease.

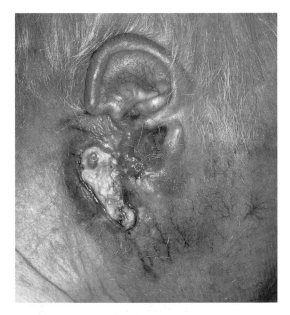

FIG 19.5 Nodal relapse of squamous carcinoma. This man has originally undergone surgery for a carcinoma arising from the pinna. There is now invasion and ulceration of skin overlying an enlarged lymph node.

Keratoacanthoma is a benign lesion. It is confused with an SCC and may grow very rapidly to form a large conical lesion with a characteristic central pit filled with keratin. It never spreads beyond the skin and usually resolves spontaneously within several weeks/months. Solar keratosis is a benign lesion seen in sun-damaged skin. It is usually a hyperkeratotic plaque with no evidence of nodularity, ulceration or invasion of the adjacent tissues.

Investigations

It is essential to obtain a tissue diagnosis in all cases prior to treatment.

Skin scraping cytology

This is the least traumatic means of obtaining a sample for analysis. A scalpel is used to scratch the surface of the tumour until the skin begins to bleed lightly, and the debris smeared onto a microscope slide. In conjunction with interpretation by a skilled cytopathologist, it is a sensitive test and can give a result within hours, but equivocal or obviously inconsistent results mean that a biopsy is necessary.

Incision biopsy

A wedge of tissue is removed, taking care to include representative tumour and surrounding normal skin. This is usually performed when the lesion is too extensive to be treated by surgery.

Excision biopsy

This is best for small lesions that can be easily excised as it provides an accurate histological diagnosis and may be curative if microscopically complete.

Fine-needle aspiration of any enlarged regional lymph nodes

Although unusual, enlarged lymph nodes should be sampled by fine-needle aspiration (FNA) to confirm malignancy.

Radiological investigations

Plain radiographs or a limited computed tomography (CT) scan are indicated for very large, deeply invasive tumours to delineate their margins when planning treatment.

Staging

There is no formal staging system in routine clinical use.

Treatment

Both surgery and radiotherapy achieve local control in about 95 per cent of cases. The choice is dependent on the anatomical site, size of lesion, convenience and previous treatment.

SURGERY

This is the treatment of choice for:

- very large tumours involving bone (radiotherapy would have a reduced local control and risk of osteonecrosis);
- scalp lesions (where radiotherapy would produce an area of permanent alopecia);
- tumours arising in regions that do not tolerate radiotherapy well (e.g. skin overlying lower third of tibia in the elderly);
- tumours of the upper eyelid where radiotherapy scarring could cause repeated trauma to the cornea;
- local recurrences after radiotherapy (Fig. 19.6) or tumours arising in previously irradiated skin.
- young patients in whom the late cutaneous effects of radiotherapy will have longer to manifest.

Excision is usually performed under local anaesthetic, although large lesions requiring a skin graft or flap reconstruction may be removed under general

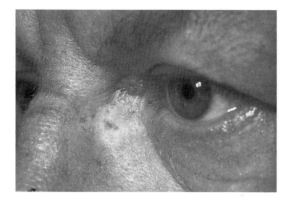

FIG 19.6 Recurrent basal cell carcinoma. This lesion has arisen at the edge of a previous radiation field. Such recurrences are best treated surgically.

anaesthetic. Facial lesions are best dealt with by a plastic surgeon to optimize the cosmetic result. Complete macroscopic and microscopic excision will be curative for SCC and BCC and so a margin of macroscopically normal skin of up to 10 mm (depending on size of tumour, cytological type and how well-circumscribed it is) should be taken away *en bloc*.

Surgery is the treatment of choice for cases with involved regional lymph nodes when a block dissection is indicated. Overall local control rates of 95 per cent or more are to be expected after excision alone. Patients with involved resection margins should be considered for re-excision or referred for radiotherapy as these patients will be at high risk of local recurrence.

RADIOTHERAPY

Radiotherapy is equivalent to surgery in terms of local control and is better for:

- tumours at sites where surgery would lead to an inferior cosmetic result (e.g. nasolabial fold);
- tumours at sites where surgery would lead to an inferior functional result (e.g. lower eyelid; Fig. 19.7).

Superficial X-rays or electrons are used to limit irradiation of subcutaneous tissues. Treatment can be given as a large single fraction or a course of daily treatment over 2–6 weeks. The former is preferred for patients with small tumours who would find travelling difficult owing to age or infirmity, but this approach gives an inferior cosmetic outcome. A custom-shaped lead cut-out is used to shape the beam to allow irradiation of a small annulus of apparently normal surrounding skin (Fig. 19.8).

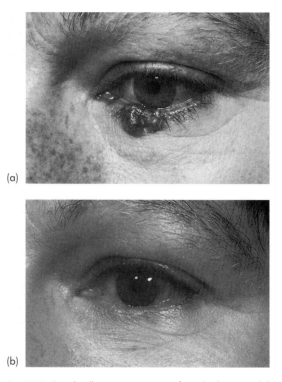

(a)

(b)

FIG 19.7 Basal cell carcinoma arising from the lower eyelid in a young woman: (a) before treatment; (b) after radiotherapy. Note the permanent loss of eyelashes along the lower eyelid.

CHEMOTHERAPY

Topical 5-fluorouracil (5-FU) can cause complete regression of Bowen's disease (squamous carcinoma *in situ*) and small, flat BCCs/SCCs, but has to be applied regularly, is inconvenient and requires careful follow-up. It is not routinely used.

CRYOTHERAPY

Thorough and sustained freezing with liquid nitrogen is very effective for small superficial tumours. It is usually administered by a dermatologist who will have the greatest expertise.

CURETTAGE

This is suitable for small (1 cm or less), well circumscribed and superficial tumours. However, there is a higher risk of local recurrence as the margins are more likely not to be free of tumour.

Tumour-related complications

Local tissue destruction will cause loss of function, disfigurement and predispose to secondary infection

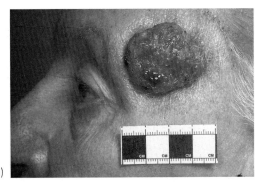

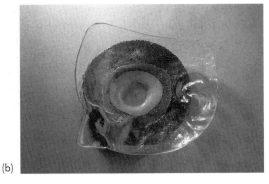

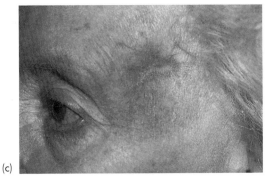

FIG 19.8 (a) A large squamous carcinoma. (b) Lead cut-out incorporated into a thermoplastic immobilization mask for the patient to wear during radiotherapy. (c) At 12 weeks after radiotherapy.

and bleeding. Secondary infection will lead to discharge and discomfort and may predispose to delayed healing after surgery or radiotherapy.

Treatment-related complications

After radiotherapy an acute skin reaction is inevitable, characterized by erythema, hyperpigmentation, itching, dry desquamation and, in some cases, moist desquamation. This begins after 10–14

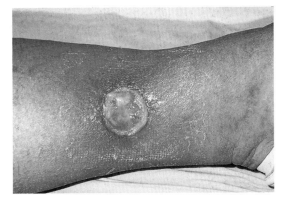

FIG 19.9 Necrosis after radiotherapy for a basal cell carcinoma arising from the skin of the lower calf region.

days of treatment and resolves within 2–4 weeks of completing radiotherapy. Occasionally, healing of a large area of skin may take many months. Chronic radionecrosis is a rare complication that may require skin grafting (Fig. 19.9).

Prognosis

It is exceptional for a patient to die from non-melanoma skin cancer. Local control should be expected in over 95 per cent, with most recurrences being successfully salvaged by further local treatment.

Screening/prevention

The risks of ultraviolet radiation need to be appreciated, particularly by children and young adults. Avoidance of the sun during the midday period and use of sun-block is recommended in sunny climates. Patients with a past history of skin cancer are at risk of subsequently developing others and benefit from surveillance and/or instructions regarding the early signs of a new tumour.

MELANOMA

This is a rarer but more serious form of skin cancer arising from the melanocytes of the skin. It is completely curable if detected and treated at an early stage.

Epidemiology

There are 34 000 new cases and 8500 deaths recorded in the European Union per annum and there has

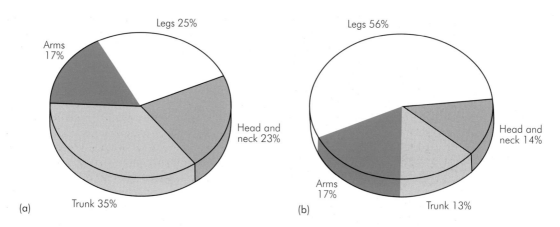

FIG 19.10 Site distribution of malignant melanoma: (a) males; (b) females.

been a 50 per cent increase in incidence over the last decade. It is one of the few cancers that has a significant impact on young adults, 22 per cent arising in the under-40s. It is very rare in children and is twice as common in women. The geographical and racial distribution is similar to that of non-melanomatous skin cancer. Malignant melanoma occasionally arises in dark-skinned people but is 10 times less common than in white people living a similar lifestyle. Severe sunburn (and therefore skin type) and childhood UV exposure are high-risk factors.

Aetiology

Ultraviolet radiation is the main causative factor, with sun exposure being very important in determining risk, particularly if exposed during childhood. Additional risk factors include blond or red hair colour, and intense episodic sun exposure, particularly in those that tan poorly and burn easily. The vast majority of naevi confer no additional risk of melanoma although individuals with large numbers (>100) are at increased risk. Dysplastic naevi may be congenital and are usually large lesions with irregular pigment and an irregular edge. Affected individuals should be monitored very closely.

Pathology

The site distribution in men and women differs and is shown in Fig. 19.10. Mucosal melanoma is rare and described in the upper aerodigestive tract, anus and vagina. Melanoma of the choroid of the eye is also described as the pigment cells are homologous with those of the skin. A melanoma is typically brown/black in colour owing to increased melanin

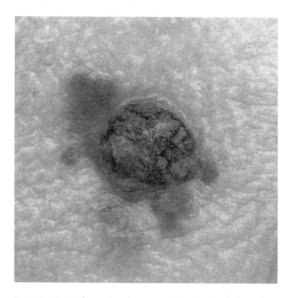

FIG 19.11 Malignant melanoma. Note the irregular edge, uneven pigmentation and nodular component.

production by the melanocytes, frequently with irregularity of pigment at its edge or centrally (Fig. 19.11). Amelanotic tumours are seen in about 5 per cent of cases. They may be nodular or flat and seen to be spreading along the superficial layers of the skin. Fifty per cent are superficial spreading melanomas and have a more favourable prognosis than nodular types, which have an early vertical growth phase. In advanced cases there may be associated ulceration or satellite lesions on the adjacent skin. Similar to hypernephroma of the kidney and neuroblastoma of the adrenal, spontaneous regression in both primary and metastatic tumours is recorded although this is seen in less than 5 per cent.

characteristically stain for S100, reflecting their origin from neural crest cells. A lymphocytic infiltrate is common, reflecting a host cellular immune response.

Natural history

Melanoma may remain at a superficial spreading phase for many months before it grows into the papillary dermis, reticular dermis and subcutaneous fat. Nodular melanomas tend to spread into the dermis at an early stage, which accounts for their poorer prognosis. Regional lymph nodes may be involved when the melanoma invades the deeper layers of the skin. Permeation of the dermal lymphatics may lead to satellite nodules adjacent to the main bulk of disease (Fig. 19.12). Melanoma is a tumour that disseminates to any tissue in the body. Lung, bone (Fig. 19.13), brain and skin metastases are the most common and it is one of the few extra-abdominal tumours to spread to the bowel and its mesentery. Primary melanoma of the choroid of the eye has a propensity to spread to the liver.

Symptoms

Presentation is usually with a pigmented skin lesion. Changes in a preceding naevus or appearance of a new pigmented lesion frequently go unnoticed, particularly if on the back. Itchiness or bleeding are sinister symptoms.

Signs

The lesion will usually be on a sun-exposed area. The degree and pattern of pigmentation is variable but is characteristically irregular, particularly at the edge of the lesion, and is ideally assessed with a magnifying glass. Ulceration is an ominous sign. Regional lymph nodes should be palpated for enlargement which may be caused by either tumour infiltration or reaction to the tumour/secondary infection. There may be signs of distant metastases such as hepatomegaly, pleural effusion/collapse/consolidation, or focal neurological signs. Patients with a heavy burden of metastases may have a slate grey complexion owing to increased circulating melanin released by the tumour cells. Skin metastases have a typical blue-black colour (Fig. 19.14).

Differential diagnosis

A number of benign pigmented skin lesions may be confused with melanoma, including benign naevi, seborrhoeic warts, dermatofibromata and pigmented BCC/SCC.

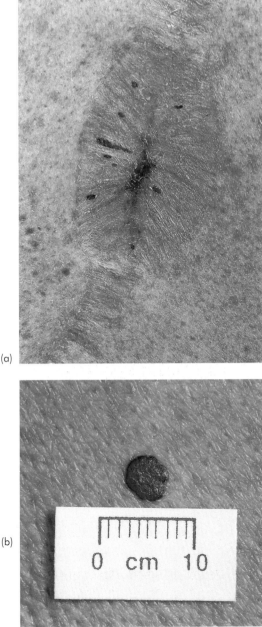

(a)

(b)

FIG 19.12 In-transit metastases from melanoma. (a) Spread radiating from site of original skin lesion. (b) Metastasis in skin some 20 cm away.

Microscopically, the tumour is composed of melanocytes which invade along the superficial layers of the skin and penetrate the basement membrane into the deeper layers of the dermis. The cells

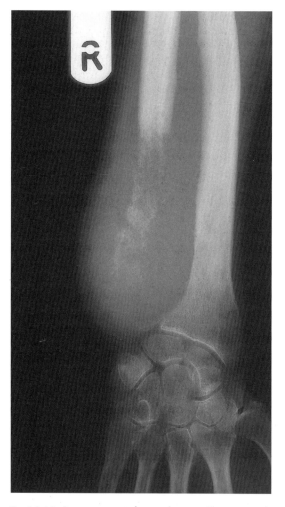

FIG 19.13 Bone metastasis from melanoma. There is significant bone destruction at a site that is less frequently affected by other solid tumours.

Lentigo maligna (Hutchinson's melanotic freckle) deserves special mention. It typically occurs in the elderly on the face as a large, slow-growing, superficial, pigmented and irregular lesion which represents a melanoma *in situ* and may become invasive.

Investigations

Excision biopsy

This is preferable to incision biopsy as it will provide a large specimen for detailed histological analysis and remove the lesion *in toto*. It is mandatory for any atypical pigmented lesion. Only a small macroscopic margin of normal skin is taken.

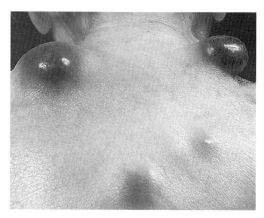

FIG 19.14 Multiple cutaneous metastases from malignant melanoma. Note the characteristic pigmentation of the lesions reflecting their origin.

Fine-needle aspiration (FNA) of any enlarged regional lymph nodes

This should differentiate between reactive and metastatic enlargement.

Exclusion of metastatic disease

A chest X-ray is performed in all cases to exclude lung metastases. A CT scan of chest, liver and regional lymph nodes is indicated in those at high risk of metastatic disease (e.g. 4 mm or deeper, lymph node-positive cases).

Staging

Clark's levels measure the depth in relation to histological landmarks.

- Level I – confined to the lamina propria.
- Level II – reaches the papillary dermis.
- Level III – reaches the papillary/reticular dermis.
- Level IV – reaches the reticular dermis.
- Level V – reaches subcutaneous fat.

The Breslow thickness measures absolute depth in millimetres and is the distance of the deepest malignant cell from the stratum granulosum. Thickness categories include:

- 0.75 mm or less;
- 0.76–1.50 mm;
- 1.51–4.0 mm;
- 4.0 mm or greater.

The TNM staging (see Chapter 2) incorporates both Clark's level and Breslow thickness.

Treatment

SURGERY

This is usually curative for localized lesions, a wide excision down to subcutaneous fat being necessary, including a margin of macroscopically normal skin the size of which is dependent on the depth (if known). A centimetre of clearance for every millimetre of depth (clinical estimate or from result of previous excision biopsy) up to a maximum of 2 cm is adequate and an immediate re-excision is necessary if the margins are not clear microscopically. A skin graft or vascularized skin flap may be needed to close the defect if too large to heal by itself. In the case of subungual melanoma, amputation of the digit is performed.

The role of elective regional lymph node dissection has always been controversial. To some extent, this debate has become less important with the development of sentinel lymph node mapping (see Chapters 4 and 8). This technique has proved valuable in the surgical management of melanoma. First, surgical clearance of all locoregional disease offers the only chance of cure; sentinel lymph node removal can be applied to all cases, ensuring that only selected patients undergo a full lymph node dissection, with its greater morbidity, while maximizing the opportunities for surgical cure. Second, for truncal melanomas, the regional lymph node region may not be obvious because of the highly variable pattern of lymph drainage; sentinel lymph node mapping overcomes this issue by guiding the surgeon to the appropriate zone. All patients relapsing in the regional nodes after successful local treatment and with no evidence of distant metastases should have a lymph node dissection.

Surgery also has a role in the management of distant metastatic relapses. If limited to one anatomical site, resection should be considered. This will occasionally result in successful salvage and long-term remission.

RADIOTHERAPY

Melanomas are considered relatively radioresistant tumours. The treatment technique is similar to that used for other skin tumours, and there is evidence that a few large doses are more effective than a prolonged course. In the rare case of melanoma of the choroid, very high doses of radiation administered using radioactive plaques sewn to the eye are curative in a high proportion. Otherwise, radiotherapy has little role as a curative treatment, being used when the patient refuses surgery or the tumour is inoperable (e.g. some mucosal melanomas). Low doses of radiation are valuable in palliating pain from skeletal metastases and focal, symptomatic metastases elsewhere.

CHEMOTHERAPY

Melanoma is not a chemosensitive tumour and is therefore incurable once distant metastasis has occurred. Adjuvant chemotherapy for high-risk patients does not have any proven benefit. The most active agents for metastatic disease are DTIC, BCNU/CCNU, cisplatin/carboplatin, vindesine and paclitaxel. Objective responses of 20 to 30 per cent are to be expected. In recent years, the oral drug temozolomide has been shown to yield objective response rates of 20–25 per cent.

BIOLOGICAL THERAPY

The recognition of spontaneous regression in melanoma and rich lymphocytic infiltrate seen in and around the lesions suggests that host immunity may play a role in the rate of growth of these tumours. Lymphokines are chemical messengers produced by T-lymphocytes which stimulate lymphocyte proliferation and in turn the body's capacity for immunosurveillance and lymphocyte cytotoxicity.

There is evidence from initial randomized trials that adjuvant α-interferon given for approximately 1 year after surgery for melanomas 1.5 mm or greater in depth may improve the 5-year recurrence-free survival from 40–50 per cent to 60–70 per cent. However, no significant survival prolongation has yet emerged from these studies. A similar improvement in disease-free survival has been shown for higher risk patients treated with high-dose α-interferon.

In metastatic disease, α-interferon, given subcutaneously at a dose of 3 MU three to five times weekly, produces objective responses of about 20 per cent. Similar response rates in metastatic disease have been observed to the lymphokine interleukin 2 (IL-2). Both drugs are expensive and have both physical and neuropsychiatric toxicity, which may prove worse than the symptoms they are being used to palliate (see below). Recipients of such treatment should therefore be selected carefully.

Other strategies under development and investigation include administration of gangliosides and the development of tumour-specific vaccines.

HORMONE THERAPY

There are reports of objective responses to the anti-oestrogen tamoxifen when given for metastatic disease. Tamoxifen also acts as a modifier of the chemotherapy agent DTIC and has therefore more often been used in combination with chemotherapy. In some trials, this did enhance the overall response rate. However, this is the subject of ongoing trials rather than routine practice.

Tumour-related complications

Secondary infection is an uncommon complication, predisposing to local discomfort, discharge and bleeding. Uncontrolled nodal disease may lead to lymphatic obstruction and lymphoedema of a limb.

Treatment-related complications

α-Interferon and IL-2 invariably have substantial systemic toxicity. The symptoms resemble influenza and include headache, malaise, fever, rigors, myalgia, lethargy, muscular weakness, depression, confusion, hypotension, renal failure and hypothyroidism.

Prognosis

Poor prognostic factors correlate with the risk of developing distant metastases and include:

- deep Clark's level;
- large Breslow thickness (5-year survivals for lesions <1.5 mm, 1.5–3.5 mm and >3.5 mm are approximately 90 per cent, 70 per cent and 40 per cent, respectively);
- ulceration;
- mucosal melanoma versus cutaneous (detected earlier);
- nodular melanoma versus superficial spreading (longer horizontal growth phase);
- male gender;
- age >50 years;

Overall 5-year survival is 50–60 per cent for men, and 70–80 per cent for women.

Screening/prevention

Four out of five melanomas are preventable. Health education is again vital to inform people to:

- avoid visible sunburn (e.g. avoiding midday sun by seeking shade, use of sunblocking creams and clothing to protect skin);
- take measures to protect skin of children;
- take care to avoid excessive UV exposure in northern Europe and not just when overseas;
- take extra care if involved in outdoor occupations and/or leisure pursuits.

People should be encouraged to visit their general practitioner or specialist dermatology clinic for an opinion if a pigmented lesion:

- increases in size;
- changes shape or colour, particularly if pigmentation becomes irregular;
- develops an inflammation at its edge;
- itches;
- bleeds or crusts.

Regular photographs of dysplastic naevi will aid early diagnosis of malignant change and screening of other family members should be undertaken if they have similar lesions.

METASTASES

The skin is frequently the site of distant metastases in patients with advanced cancer, particularly from breast and lung primaries (Fig. 19.15), usually presenting as one or more well-circumscribed subcutaneous nodules. They may be asymptomatic, cause irritation or fungate. If the diagnosis is in doubt, incision/excision biopsy or FNA provide the definitive diagnosis. Symptomatic lesions may be treated by any of the usual local/systemic cancer therapies to which the primary tumour is sensitive.

RARE TUMOURS

Hidradenocarcinoma

This is a carcinoma arising from the sweat glands.

Kaposi's sarcoma

This arises from vascular endothelial cells (see Chapter 20 for a detailed description).

Case history: melanoma

A 34-year-old woman with a fair complexion presents to her general practitioner with a mole on her right calf. This had been present for at least 10 years but over the last 6 months had enlarged in diameter, become more nodular, irregularly pigmented and itchy. She is referred to a fast-track dermatology clinic set up for such lesions.

Clinical examination reveals a pigmented lesion 1 cm in diameter suspicious for a melanoma. A detailed survey of the rest of the skin shows 20–30 benign naevi randomly distributed over the trunk and upper limbs. There is no popliteal, inguinal or femoral lymphadenopathy. There is no hepatomegaly. There are no other signs of disseminated malignancy.

Excision biopsy confirms a nodular melanoma, with strong S100 immunostaining, 12 mm in diameter with a Breslow thickness of 4 mm. The margins of excision are clear but by <1 mm at the superior and a lateral margin. She therefore undergoes a further wide excision and split skin graft to attain skin closure. Histology reveals a few residual nests of melanoma cells but the margins of excision are confirmed to be clear by 5 mm or more at all points. Baseline staging computed tomography (CT) scan of the thorax and abdomen shows no evidence of visceral disease.

In view of the depth of the melanoma, she receives 12 months of adjuvant α-interferon. Four years after diagnosis, she notices a lump in the right groin. Fine-needle aspiration confirms melanoma cells. Further CT scan shows no evidence of metastatic disease and no iliac lymphadenopathy. She therefore undergoes a radical groin lymph node dissection yielding three involved nodes.

Despite occasional swelling of the right lower leg, she remains well 8 years after diagnosis and hopefully cured of melanoma. She and her general practitioner keep the other naevi under regular surveillance and she always avoids excess sun exposure.

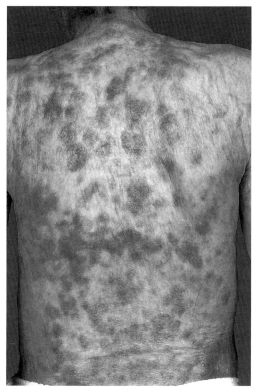

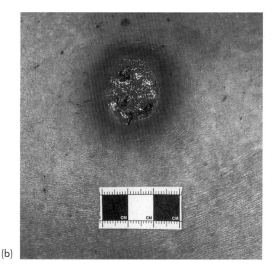

FIG 19.15 Cutaneous metastases from breast cancer. (a) Generalised rash; the skin infiltration was intensely irritating. (b) Solitary lesion: note the dark areas corresponding to diathermy used to treat bleeding.

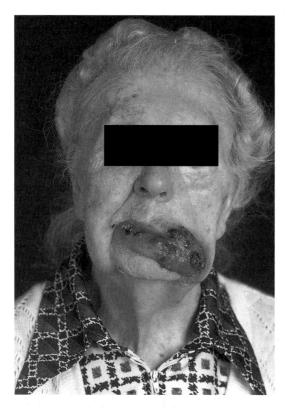

FIG 19.16 Cutaneous non-Hodgkin's lymphoma. There was no clinical or radiological evidence of disease elsewhere.

Merkel cell carcinoma

The mean age at diagnosis is 65–70 years and it presents as a solitary lesion, most frequent on the head and neck in sun-damaged skin. It arises from neuroendocrine cells and is locally aggressive, spreading to regional lymph nodes and to distant sites. Even with combined wide local excision and postoperative radiotherapy, over one-third will recur locally and about half will eventually die from their disease.

Mycosis fungoides

This is a cutaneous T-cell lymphoma with a peak incidence of 30–50 years. The eruption has a predilection for body creases, buttocks and face and is initially non-specific, resembling chronic eczema or psoriasis. This stage may last for several years before progression to plaques which are well-demarcated, erythematous, sometimes itchy lesions. The plaque stage progresses to the tumour stage, which consists of erythematous nodules arising in the plaques or in normal skin. Erythroderma is described when the whole skin is affected, and Sézary syndrome when abnormal lymphocytes are seen in the peripheral blood. Treatment options include phototherapy with UV light, steroids, radiotherapy either locally or to the whole skin, topical or systemic chemotherapy, retinoids and interferon. The clinical course is protracted and many will die of unrelated causes.

Non-Hodgkin's lymphoma

B-cell non-Hodgkin's lymphoma may also affect the skin (Fig. 19.16).

Sarcoma

These arise from the soft tissues of the skin and include leiomyosarcoma, liposarcoma, malignant fibrous histiocytoma, and angiosarcoma.

20 AIDS-RELATED CANCER

The acquired immune deficiency syndrome (AIDS) is a major health issue throughout the world, and its incidence continues to increase relentlessly. From the oncologist's perspective, it is an important disease since about 40 per cent of sufferers can be expected to develop some form of malignant disease, which has major implications for the planning of cancer services for the future. The types of tumours encountered are particularly rare in the rest of the population and present at a relatively advanced stage in patients who do not tolerate treatment well. Malignant disease may also be the first manifestation of infection with the human immunodeficiency virus (HIV), and should be considered in those presenting with Kaposi's sarcoma and primary cerebral lymphoma. In such patients, risk factors for AIDS should be sought:

- male homosexual sexual contact;
- sexual contact with an infected heterosexual partner;
- intravenous drug abuse;
- blood transfusion in an area where AIDS is endemic.

If appropriate, HIV positivity should be confirmed by a blood test after appropriate counselling.

MANAGEMENT PROBLEMS

COPING WITH THE DIAGNOSIS

The patient has already been diagnosed as having an incurable illness with a poor prognosis, which compounds any psychological difficulties in coping with the diagnosis of either condition alone.

POOR PROGNOSIS FROM THE TUMOUR AND AIDS

The prognosis from the underlying tumour will usually be very poor due to the tumour presenting at an advanced stage and growing rapidly in an environment of a suppressed cellular immune system. The combination of HIV infection and malignancy will make the risk of opportunistic infection extremely high and many may die from infection rather than their tumours. Much of the oncological management of such patients is therefore directed towards the prevention, early identification and treatment of opportunistic infections. However, the advent of high-activity anti-retroviral therapy (HAART) in recent years has improved life expectancy to an extent where the tumour poses a much more significant threat than AIDS itself.

POOR PERFORMANCE STATUS

Patients with AIDS may have a poor performance status which influences the treatment that they will tolerate, particularly as many present with advanced disease requiring aggressive chemotherapy.

RISK OF INFECTION TO HEALTHCARE PROFESSIONALS

All healthcare workers that could potentially come into contact with bodily secretions should be aware of the patient's illness. Surgeons should double-glove, consider wearing eyeshields during surgery, take care with any specimens obtained and notify the pathology laboratory of the risk of infection using appropriate biohazard labels. Radiographers should avoid routine use of skin tattoos, and take care with immobilization devices (e.g. bite blocks). Care should also be taken with needles and cannulae during and after administration of chemotherapy and when venepuncture is performed, and the laboratory should be notified of any blood specimens sent for analysis.

PREDISPOSITION TO MYELOSUPPRESSION

Some of the drugs used in the combination chemotherapy for HIV may cause bone marrow suppression and may therefore exacerbate the myelosuppressive effect of radiotherapy, chemotherapy and biological agents. This may in turn limit the intensity of anticancer treatment that may be given. Patients with CD4 counts of 200 or less are at particular risk in the context of their oncological management.

KAPOSI'S SARCOMA (KS)

This is the most common AIDS-related malignancy but also occurs sporadically in Eastern Europeans, Africans and renal transplant patients on long-term immunosuppressants. In recent years, with the emergence of combination antiviral therapy for AIDS, its prevalence in the HIV-positive population has declined. It has not been reported in HIV-positive patients that contracted the disease through intravenous drug abuse. Recent research has suggested that it is caused by infection with human herpes virus type 8. The tumour is derived from the vascular endothelial cells of the skin. There are usually multiple skin lesions, particularly on the lower limbs (Fig. 20.1). Extracutaneous disease is common, particularly in the oral cavity and gastrointestinal tract (Fig. 20.2). The lesions have a characteristic purplish hue, reflecting their vascular nature, appear as macules, plaques or nodules, and may ulcerate or bleed. Spread may occur to the regional lymph nodes or distant sites such as liver and lungs. Biopsy will confirm the diagnosis. Kaposi's sarcoma may lead directly to death when there is extensive gastrointestinal involvement leading to haemorrhage. Otherwise, most will die of other AIDS-related

complications. Indications for active management of KS lesions include:

- pain;
- ulceration;
- bleeding;
- oedema;
- disfigurement and stigma felt by patient;
- mass effects (e.g. upper airways obstruction).

Kaposi's sarcoma is a radiosensitive tumour and although it is difficult to assess response because of residual pigmentation, there is usually a visible regression in terms of flattening of the lesion and relief of symptoms, with 60–70 per cent attaining a complete response. A single fraction of radiotherapy is suitable for cutaneous sites. *Candida* superinfection of mucosal surfaces and enhanced radiation mucositis are problems when the oral cavity is irradiated.

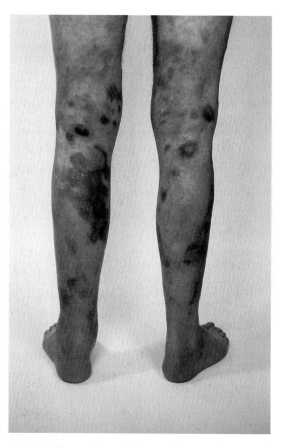

FIG 20.1 The multiple nodules and plaques of cutaneous Kaposi's sarcoma.

Immunotherapy has also been used as a therapeutic strategy in KS upon the following observations:

- regression of KS in renal transplant patients with a decrease in their immunosuppression;
- antitumour, antiviral effects of some biological modifiers; and
- recognized spontaneous regression of Kaposi's sarcoma (4 per cent) in the more immunocompetent patients.

Up to 40 per cent respond to high-dose interferon, with occasional complete responses. Objective responses have also been seen with chemotherapy. The drugs used are chosen to minimize the risk of myelosuppression and systemic toxicity. Bleomycin and vincristine are effective with response rates of 20–25 per cent, and are usually well-tolerated by patients. In recent years, liposomal doxorubicin has been shown to be active and well tolerated in HIV-positive patients with objective response rates of 50–60 per cent. Paclitaxel has activity comparable to liposomal doxorubicin.

PRIMARY CEREBRAL LYMPHOMA

This is an extremely rare primary extranodal site of lymphoma in the general population but relatively more common in HIV-positive patients, representing approximately 20 per cent of non-Hodgkin's lymphoma (NHL) in HIV-positive patients. It usually arises in the cerebral hemispheres and may be multifocal (Fig. 20.3). It presents with nonspecific symptoms such as headache, somnolence and epilepsy, which may mimic atypical CNS infections such as toxoplasmosis. Histologically, it is a high-grade B-cell NHL, which is associated with evidence of infection with the Epstein–Barr virus. It infiltrates the brain widely in the hemisphere of origin and may cross to the contralateral hemisphere. The CSF dissemination through the subarachnoid space will lead to nerve root deposits in the spine. It presents with focal or non-specific signs originating from the affected part of the brain. It must be distinguished from an opportunistic CNS infection

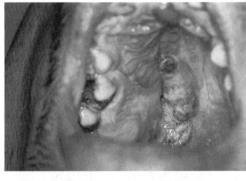

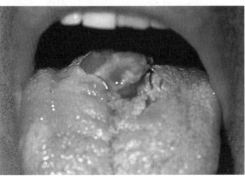

FIG 20.2 Kaposi's sarcoma. (a) Ulcerating plaques of tumour arising on the palate of a male homosexual. (b) Nodular tumour arising on posterior tongue.

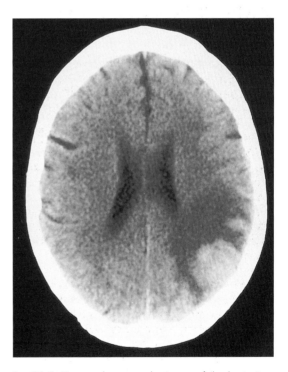

FIG 20.3 Computed tomography image of the brain in a patient with primary cerebral lymphoma. Note the two separate areas of contrast enhancement suggesting multifocality, and the surrounding cerebral oedema.

such as toxoplasmosis or tuberculosis to which HIV-positive patients are susceptible. The diagnosis is made by craniotomy and biopsy supplemented by whole-body CT scan and bone marrow trephine for staging as for lymphoma elsewhere. The tumour is not particularly sensitive to either radiotherapy or chemotherapy. The preferred treatment is whole-brain irradiation, with chemotherapy for those of good performance status. Intrathecal methotrexate and cytosine arabinoside may be used for proven spinal metastases. Primary cerebral lymphoma has an extremely poor prognosis in patients with AIDS.

NON-HODGKIN'S LYMPHOMA

Non-Hodgkin's lymphoma is relatively uncommon in the general population, but a significant proportion of HIV-positive patients will develop it within the natural history of their AIDS illness. Unlike KS, which has a higher prevalence among male homosexuals, NHL is seen in all HIV-positive subgroups. The human herpes virus type 8 implicated in the causation of KS may also cause a variant of NHL in these patients known as 'primary effusion lymphoma'. The diagnosis of NHL may be made before or at the time of discovery of positive HIV serology. These are usually high-grade B-cell lymphomas, frequently resembling Burkitt's lymphoma. Most patients present with extranodal stage 4 disease (Fig. 20.4). 'B' symptoms such as fever may mask or be confused with an opportunistic infection. Treatment is with combination chemotherapy such as CHOP, but tolerance of such treatment may be a problem owing to bone marrow suppression and poor performance status of some patients. Despite a good initial response to treatment, this is often short-lived and the prognosis remains very poor.

HODGKIN'S DISEASE

Hodgkin's disease (HD) is again uncommon in the general population but arises in HIV-positive patients at a rate of 2 per cent per annum. It is 10 times less frequent than NHL in this group. As with NHL in this patient group, it is more likely to present with extranodal disease. Mediastinal involvement is less frequent than with HD in HIV-negative cases and stage for stage the prognosis is worse for HIV-positive cases.

OTHER TUMOURS

Possible associations have been described for:

- carcinoma of the tongue;
- carcinoma of the anus;
- testicular tumours;
- hepatocellular carcinoma.

Many of these tumours are thought to have a viral aetiology (e.g. human papilloma virus and carcinoma of the anus) which may account for their prevalence in this immunosuppressed population.

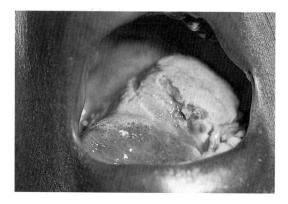

FIG 20.4 Non-Hodgkin's lymphoma of the tongue in a 27-year-old Ugandan woman.

21 CARCINOMA OF UNKNOWN PRIMARY

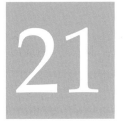

Some patients are diagnosed as having disseminated cancer but with no evidence of the site of origin; many present with their disease as an incidental finding such as, for example, enlarged cervical lymph node(s), bone metastases or pulmonary metastases on chest X-ray. Their management is a problem, with the oncologist having to determine whether the patient has a curable tumour such as a teratoma or lymphoma, one that can benefit from systemic therapy (e.g. a hormone-responsive cancer such as from the breast or prostate) or one where treatment would not be justified.

A detailed history should be taken. Questions should be aimed at eliciting symptoms of the underlying primary neoplasm, judging its time course and rate of progression, as well as gauging the performance status of the patient. The presence of 'B' symptoms may suggest an underlying lymphoma. The possibility (albeit rare) of choriocarcinoma should be considered in a young woman with a recent history of pregnancy. The development of breast tenderness in a young male may suggest an underlying trophoblastic germ cell tumour.

A detailed physical examination should include the skin, oral cavity, thyroid, breasts, peripheral lymph node groups (cervical chains, Waldeyer's ring, supraclavicular fossae, axillae and groins), spleen, rectum, including prostate and testes in males, and pelvic examination in females. If the patient has presented with lymphadenopathy, the region that drains to those nodes should be examined particularly thoroughly. For example, inguinal lymphadenopathy should prompt a thorough survey of both lower limbs, perianal region and anal canal, penis and scrotum in males, vulva and vagina in females.

Differential diagnosis

The most likely primary sites vary with histology (Table 21.1). The common solid tumours (lung,

TABLE 21.1 Most likely sites of primary carcinomas according to histology

Histological type	Most likely sites of primary
Adenocarcinoma	Lung
	GI tract (stomach, colon, pancreas)
	Breast
	Prostate
	Ovary
	Kidney
Squamous carcinoma	Lung
	Head and neck
Small cell carcinoma	Lung (always consider lymphoma)

breast, colorectal, prostate and pancreas) should be considered. Anaplastic tumours are mainly poorly differentiated carcinomas, the rest being undifferentiated teratomas, lymphoma, melanoma (particularly amelanotic variant), sarcomas and neuroendocrine tumours.

Investigations

Patients with distant metastases should not undergo exhaustive investigation in the relentless search for a primary that is ultimately likely to be incurable and where local treatment of the primary will not be justified. For those with distant metastases, localization of the primary tumour site is unlikely to affect materially the diagnosis or immediate management. However, histological typing of the tumour will influence assessment of prognosis and the type of systemic therapy chosen.

Biopsy

A balance has to be struck between the need to confirm the histological diagnosis, how it will affect ultimate management, and what is reasonable for the patient to undergo. The general principle is to obtain a sizeable piece of tissue from a representative part of the tumour that is not necrotic. This should ensure adequate tissue for immunocytochemistry so that an accurate histological analysis is possible. If several sites of bulk disease are accessible, the safest and least traumatic route of access should be followed. The simplest option is fine-needle aspiration of a palpable lump with immediate cytological examination. However, this does not always yield adequate material for an accurate pathological diagnosis, particularly for conditions such as lymphoma. A needle biopsy, open biopsy or excision biopsy is therefore preferred in most circumstances. The lesion for biopsy may need to be localized using computed tomography (CT) (Fig. 21.1) or ultrasound depending on its anatomical location and accessibility.

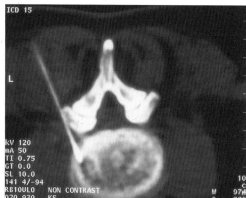

(a)

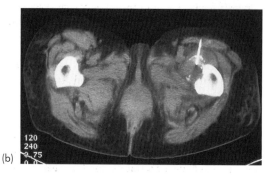

(b)

FIG 21.1 Computed tomography-guided percutaneous biopsy for a tissue diagnosis (a) vertebra; (b) pelvic lymph node.

Immunocytochemistry

Some tissues have staining characteristics depending on their embryological origin and constituent cells:

- α-fetoprotein (AFP) – teratomas, hepatomas;
- β-human chorionic gonadotrophin (HCG) – teratomas, choriocarcinomas;
- prostate-specific antigen (PSA) – carcinoma of the prostate;
- carcinoembryonic antigen (CEA) – gastrointestinal cancers;
- CA125 – carcinoma of the ovary;
- oestrogen receptors and/or CA15-3 – carcinoma of the breast;
- CA19-9 – carcinoma of the pancreas;
- leucocyte common antigen – lymphomas;
- pancytokeratin/epithelial membrane antigen – squamous carcinomas;
- desmin – leiomyosarcomas, rhabdomyosarcomas;
- myoglobin – rhabdomyosarcomas;
- vimentin – sarcomas;
- neurone-specific enolase – neuroblastomas, primitive neuroectodermal tumours (PNETs);
- calcitonin – medullary carcinoma of the thyroid;
- thyroglobulin – follicular carcinoma of the thyroid;
- α₁-antitrypsin – hepatomas;
- S100 – melanomas, small cell lung cancers;
- chromogranin – carcinoids;
- CD117 (c-kit) – gastrointestinal stromal tumours (GISTs).

Cytogenetic studies

These are of value in tumours arising in children and adolescents because many tumours have characteristic chromosomal abnormalities, for example translocations in Ewing's sarcoma (t11;22), rhabdomyosarcoma (t2;13), non-Hodgkin's lymphoma (t8;14). Extragonadal germ cell tumours may have abnormalities of chromosome 12. These are of less value in adult solid tumours.

Radiological investigations

A CT scan of the thorax, abdomen and pelvis not only allows a detailed radiological survey of a number of possible sites of origin of the metastases which are clinically impalpable (e.g. pancreas or ovaries), but also allows full staging, which is of prognostic value and of use in planning treatment. An isotope bone scan is useful to assess the skeleton for staging purposes. Bilateral mammography should be considered in women with adenocarcinoma of unknown primary to exclude an occult breast primary, which would be amenable to aggressive locoregional therapy or hormone manipulation. A transrectal ultrasound should be considered if the prostate feels suspicious or the PSA is elevated, and if clinically indicated, will facilitate a needle core biopsy of the prostate under direct vision.

Blood tests

Serum tumour marker assays can be useful for providing a clue as to the likely origin of the metastases and therefore allow a more focused approach to investigations. A normal PSA makes carcinoma of the prostate unlikely. A very high CEA may suggest a gastrointestinal primary. CA15-3 and CA125 should be measured in women presenting with adenocarcinoma of unknown primary to exclude carcinoma of the breast and ovary respectively. Young adults presenting with undifferentiated cancers should have blood taken for AFP and HCG to exclude a germ cell tumour. In an urgent situation, a urinary pregnancy test is a crude way of checking for excess HCG levels in a male.

Other investigations

Patients presenting with squamous carcinoma in lymph nodes draining the head and neck region must be referred to an ear, nose and throat (ENT) surgeon for an endoscopy of the upper aerodigestive tract (especially nasopharynx, tonsils, posterior third of tongue, supraglottic larynx and pyriform fossa) as the patient may still have a curable occult primary cancer.

Management

The problem is usually one of systemic disease at the outset and so it is logical to consider some form of systemic therapy. The patient should be managed according to their age, general condition, site and stage of disease, and symptomatology. In cases of widespread distant metastases in a patient with a very poor performance status, local treatment directed towards symptom relief is likely to be most appropriate as the patient will be incurable and unlikely to profit from chemotherapy. Conversely, the patient should be treated with curative intent if there are distant metastases and the tumour is particularly chemosensitive (e.g. teratoma or lymphoma) or if there are regional lymph node metastases from a tumour that may be cured by aggressive

locoregional therapy (e.g. in the head and neck or breast). For this reason, women presenting with isolated axillary lymphadenopathy containing adenocarcinoma and no other primary site should be assumed to have an occult carcinoma of the breast and treated accordingly. A young person presenting with a rapidly enlarging mediastinal mass or retroperitoneal mass and a biopsy showing poorly differentiated tumour cells and negative lymphocyte markers should be suspected as having a nongonadal germ cell tumour, and treated accordingly with a cisplatin chemotherapy regime, even if serum AFP and HCG levels are not elevated.

Most patients fall between these two extreme ends of the spectrum, in which case systemic therapy may be employed to maximize the symptom-free interval, with the expectation that this may in turn lead to a prolongation of survival. Hormonal therapy should be initiated in selected tumours, such as prostate cancer and breast cancer. Chemotherapy is frequently used in good performance status patients. For those where the primary tumour origin is found or suspected from biopsy, the regimes specific for that disease are most appropriate. For those where it is impractical to obtain a histological diagnosis, it is rational to select several drugs that cover the most common solid tumours (e.g. an anthracycline, an alkylating agent, 5-FU and/or platinum derivative). Examples therefore include combinations such as:

- ECisF – epirubicin, cisplatin, protracted infusion of 5-FU;
- CAP – cyclophosphamide, Adriamycin, cisplatin.

Prognosis

The prognosis is poor, with a median survival of approximately 3–4 months in most studies with less than 25 per cent and 10 per cent of patients alive at 1 and 5 years, respectively. Male sex, increasing number of involved organ sites, adenocarcinoma histology and hepatic involvement are all unfavourable prognostic factors. Only the few with lymphoma or a germ cell tumour have a greater chance of cure.

Unfortunately, the site of the primary tumour may never be found during life. A post-mortem examination may be very instructive for the clinicians and relieve uncertainty for the next of kin, although even then the primary origin may prove elusive.

Case history: carcinoma of unknown primary

A previously fit 51-year-old woman is well until she joins a gym. Following a quadriceps toning exercise, she develops persistent discomfort in the right thigh. This persists for 2 weeks despite the use of a topical anti-inflammatory gel. She is climbing a flight of stairs when she hears a loud 'crack', and collapses with severe acute pain in the thigh. She is taken to the Accident and Emergency Department where a plain radiograph confirms a transverse fracture of the femoral mid-shaft. There is some lysis of the cortex either side of the fracture, suggesting a pre-existing condition that had led to bone absorption. The diagnosis of a pathological fracture is made, the radiologist confirming that there is almost certainly a metastasis at this site. She is referred to an orthopaedic surgeon and undergoes an emergency open reduction and internal fixation. A specimen is sent for histology but this shows normal connective tissue and bone.

Postoperatively, she is referred to an oncologist. A full history fails to reveal any symptoms of an underlying malignant process and therefore does not give any clue as to the likely underlying cause. She has had a recent cervical smear which was normal and her first screening mammogram was unremarkable. A detailed physical examination reveals a hard, solitary 1.5 cm lymph node in the left supraclavicular fossa. There is no abnormality within the breasts or axillae and all other lymph node groups are normal. The thyroid is unremarkable and there is no mucosal abnormality within the oral cavity and oropharynx. The chest is clear and there is no hepatomegaly. Digital examination of the rectum and vagina examinations are normal. There are a few benign naevi but no obvious cutaneous manifestation of primary or secondary malignancy.

Full blood count is normal. Liver function tests show a moderate elevation of both gamma-glutamyl-transferase and alkaline phosphatase at 125 U/l and 340 U/l respectively. The serum calcium corrected for the serum albumin is 3.2 mmol/l (normal range 2.1–2.6 mmol/l). Fine-needle aspiration of the supraclavicular lymph node reveals adenocarcinoma cells which are both carcinoembryonic antigen (CEA)-negative and oestrogen receptor-negative. Bilateral mammography is normal. Chest X-ray is clear while computed tomography (CT) scan shows low-volume bilateral lung metastases and multiple liver metastases. Isotope bone scan confirms increased isotope uptake at the site of recent bone surgery and in the dorsal spine, lumbar spine and contralateral humerus. Plain radiographs are obtained of the last which confirm that this area is not at risk of imminent fracture and therefore does not require prophylactic internal fixation. The CA15-3, CA125, thyroglobulin and CEA tumour markers are all within the normal range. Taking account of the extent of metastatic disease, it is not felt appropriate to investigate the gastrointestinal tract for an occult primary.

In view of the presentation and asymptomatic hypercalcaemia, she is encouraged to maintain a high fluid intake and commenced on infusions of 90 mg disodium pamidronate 4-weekly. A short course of radiotherapy is delivered to the fracture site to consolidate the surgical fixation. Bearing in mind her good performance status and extent of disease, and having discussed the option of best supportive care with chemotherapy kept in reserve for symptomatic progression, an indwelling venous catheter is inserted and she starts chemotherapy with continuously infused 5-fluorouracil (5-FU) and 3-weekly boluses of epirubicin and cisplatin. Restaging after three cycles shows stable disease but after six cycles there is evidence of progression within the thorax and liver. Repeat physical examination at this point reveals an ill-defined 2 cm lump within the left breast. Core biopsy confirms adenocarcinoma cells with similar staining characteristics to those obtained from the original lymph node. The tumour is HER2-negative. The chemotherapy is changed to docetaxel and she attains a good partial response which is sustained for 4 months. At second relapse, she fails to respond to further chemotherapy and dies of her disease. The certified cause of death is metastatic breast cancer.

22 ONCOLOGICAL EMERGENCIES

There are few conditions in the management of malignant disease which are true emergencies. However, it is important to identify those patients in whom urgent treatment is required. The following conditions can be associated with rapid deterioration and even death, and should be considered emergency situations:

- hypercalcaemia;
- spinal cord or cauda equina compression;
- superior vena cava obstruction;
- neutropenic sepsis;
- tumour lysis syndrome.

HYPERCALCAEMIA

Malignant hypercalcaemia is the most common cause of a raised serum calcium in practice. It is associated, in particular, with lung cancer, breast cancer, prostatic cancer and myeloma. It is generally found in patients with disseminated metastatic disease, although this is not always the case.

Aetiology

There is increasing evidence that hypercalcaemia associated with malignancy is due principally to the effects of chemical agents released by the tumour, which disturb the normal mechanisms of calcium balance. A number of chemicals have been identified. The effect of these substances is to have actions similar to parathyroid hormone and they include parathyroid hormone-like peptides, prostaglandins, interleukins and transforming growth factor β (TGFβ). The result is osteoclast activation and mobilization of calcium from bones.

Symptoms

These include anorexia, nausea, vomiting, constipation, confusion, polyuria, thirst, polydipsia and bone pains.

Signs

There are usually no specific physical signs. The patient may appear drowsy and have signs of confusion. They may have signs of dehydration.

Differential diagnosis

Other causes of a similar constellation of symptoms may include diabetes mellitus, causing polyuria, polydipsia and confusion, cerebral metastases, hepatic or renal failure or neutropenic sepsis.

Investigations

The diagnosis is made on the basis of a raised serum calcium. It is important to correct the total level for the serum albumin, which is often low in patients with advanced malignant disease. The simple correction is to add to the serum calcium level 0.02 mmol/l for every g/dl of albumin below 40, which is the conventional standardization level. For example, a reading of calcium at 2.3 mmol/l with an albumin of 30 gives a corrected serum albumin of 2.5 mmol/l. The usual range after correction is between 2.1 mmol/l and 2.6 mmol/l.

Treatment

There are two components to the treatment of malignant hypercalcaemia:

- correction of dehydration and establishing good urine flow;
- specific therapy to reduce calcium levels.

To correct dehydration and establish good urine flow, an intravenous infusion of normal saline giving 1 litre every 6 h should be established. Careful attention to fluid balance is essential, particularly in the elderly, who may easily become fluid overloaded. Frusemide may be added which, in addition to acting as a diuretic, also promotes urinary excretion of calcium. Thiazides should be avoided as they increase calcium reabsorption.

The management of hypercalcaemia in these patients has been revolutionized in recent years by the introduction of the bisphosphonates, which are a class of drugs acting primarily through stabilization of osteoclast activity. They are given by short intravenous infusion once good urine flow has been established. The drugs currently available are pamidronate, clodronate, zolendranate and ibandranate.

With the advent of bisphosphonates the use of other drugs in this condition such as calcitonin, mithramycin or steroids has become of historical interest only.

Unfortunately, although rapid correction of serum calcium is often possible with the above approach, rebound hypercalcaemia is also very common and regular bisphosphonate infusions may be required.

The ultimate prognosis for malignant hypercalcaemia is poor, with most patients that present with this surviving for only a few months, succumbing to either refractory hypercalcaemia or the effects of widespread malignancy.

SPINAL CORD AND CAUDA EQUINA COMPRESSION

This condition arises most commonly as a result of extradural tumour, typically secondary to carcinoma of the lung, breast or prostate. It should be treated as an emergency because the outcome in terms of final neurological disability is determined by the speed of diagnosis and treatment.

Aetiology

Extradural metastases are usually a result of blood-borne dissemination. Less often, paravertebral tumour or tumour within the vertebral body may infiltrate directly into the spinal canal.

Symptoms

Spinal cord compression presents with neurological symptoms of weakness and reduced or altered sensation below the site of cord damage. This is accompanied by constipation and hesitancy in micturition leading to urinary retention.

Cauda equina compression similarly presents with weakness and sphincter disturbance. The sensory disturbance may be of reduced or altered sensation but also nerve root pain affecting the lumbosacral segments.

Signs

Spinal cord compression causes a spastic paraparesis or, if affecting the cervical spine, quadriparesis, with a cut-off of sensory changes corresponding to the anatomical level of the compression – a sensory level. In contrast, cauda equina compression will result in a flaccid paraparesis with loss of sensation in a dermatome pattern affecting the lumbosacral segments (the lower limbs and buttocks). Reflexes are increased with cord compression and plantars extensor while with cauda equina compression reflexes are reduced or lost with flexor plantar responses.

Sphincter function may be disturbed and with cauda equina compression a distended bladder may be palpable and anal tone will be lax.

Differential diagnosis

This will include intrinsic spinal cord tumours and paraneoplastic neuropathies. Transverse myelitis will give a similar clinical picture to cord compression and in cancer patients may be due to viral infection and rarely as a side-effect of chemotherapy or radiotherapy. Other unrelated causes include prolapsed intervertebral disc, subacute combined degeneration of the cord and a parasagittal intracranial tumour.

Investigations

Urgent investigations are required to confirm the diagnosis. Plain X-rays of the spine may demonstrate associated vertebral disease. Magnetic resonance

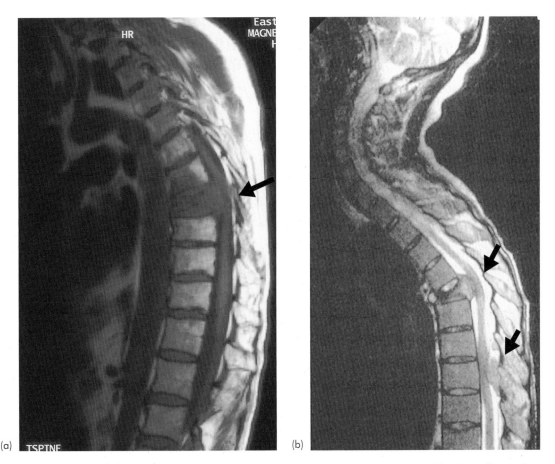

FIG 22.1 Magnetic resonance imaging scans demonstrating metastatic spinal canal compression caused by direct infiltration from a bone metastasis (a), vertebral collapse (upper, b) and an extradural metastasis (lower, b).

imaging (MRI) of the spine is now the definitive investigation, as shown in Fig. 22.1. In the rare patient where MRI is contraindicated, for example those with a pacemaker or metal fragments, then a myelogram combined with computed tomography (CT) scanning at the level of obstruction may be performed.

Treatment

In the presence of a known histologically confirmed malignancy, treatment should proceed immediately with the following:

- all patients should start on high-dose steroids using dexamethasone 4 mg q.d.s. with, if necessary, prophylactic omeprazole or misoprostol and monitoring of urine for diabetes in those with borderline glucose tolerance;
- definitive treatment will usually be local radiotherapy starting on the same day as the diagnosis

is made – a course of 20–30 Gy over 1–2 weeks will usually be prescribed;

- certain patients should be referred for surgery (these are those where there is instability of the spinal column with extensive vertebral collapse or spondilolisthesis);
- certain patients may be more appropriately treated with chemotherapy, in particular those with lymphoma, small cell lung cancer and germ cell tumours who have not been previously treated.

In addition, appropriate general measures should continue. Patients with sphincter disturbance may require catheterization and analgesia should be given as necessary. Active physiotherapy and rehabilitation is a further important component of the management to optimize the chances of neurological recovery.

When cord or cauda equina compression is the presenting feature of a malignant condition it is important to establish a histological diagnosis. This can usually be achieved by a needle biopsy of the affected region performed under CT control.

Prognosis

Survival following cord compression is defined by the underlying condition and the performance status of the patient. It is often a reflection of disseminated disease and average survivals are usually measured in only a few months from diagnosis.

The prognosis for neurological recovery is dependent almost entirely on the speed of diagnosis and instigation of treatment. In patients that are mobile at the start of treatment the majority (85 per cent) will walk after treatment. In contrast, less than 15 per cent of paraplegic patients will regain useful neurological function despite intensive treatment. For this reason, there should be a high index of suspicion for this condition, particularly in patients known to have metastatic disease, with urgent referral to a specialist centre for treatment.

SUPERIOR VENA CAVA OBSTRUCTION

This refers to the clinical picture arising from a large mediastinal tumour mass causing obstruction to venous return to the right side of the heart and is often associated with other symptoms of mediastinal compression including dysphagia and stridor.

Aetiology

Any tumour involving the mediastinum may be the cause. The most common cause is carcinoma of the bronchus. In young patients in particular it is important to consider malignant lymphomas and germ cell tumours. Rarely, a thymic tumour or retrosternal thyroid tumour may be the cause.

Post-mortem studies suggest that in most patients although mechanical obstruction to venous flow may be the first event, thrombosis within the large veins inevitably follows, although emboli are almost unknown.

Symptoms

Dyspnoea, stridor or dysphagia may be presenting symptoms. Intracranial venous congestion may cause headache or confusion. There may be swelling of the face, neck and arms.

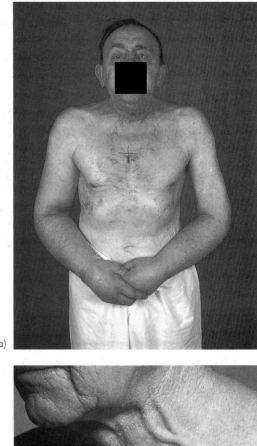
(a)

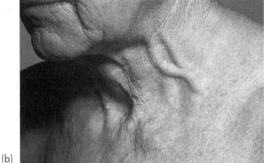
(b)

FIG 22.2 Superior vena cava obstruction characterized by arm and facial oedema, distended veins, plethora and conjunctival suffusion (a) and distended, raised neck veins which do not empty on lying flat ('fixed veins') (b).

Signs

Oedema of the face, neck and arms may be apparent, with fixed engorged jugular veins and dilatation of superficial skin veins over the chest, neck, face and upper limbs. Typical appearances are shown in Fig. 22.2. There may be obvious respiratory distress or stridor. A tumour mass may be palpable, arising out of the mediastinum in the supraclavicular fossae. Papilloedema may be present on fundoscopy.

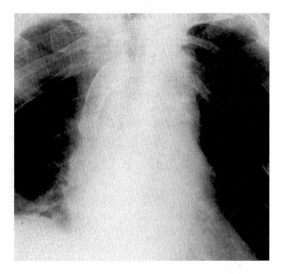

FIG 22.3 X-ray showing superior vena cava stent in situ.

Investigations

A chest X-ray will usually demonstrate a mediastinal mass which will be better defined on CT scanning. Unless a diagnosis of malignancy has already been made it is important to obtain a tissue diagnosis if at all possible. Other readily accessible disease sites should be sought such as a peripheral lymph node. If the mediastinum is the only site of disease then a needle biopsy under CT control will usually be possible. More invasive approaches are usually avoided because of the theoretical risk of excessive haemorrhage from the area of raised venous pressure.

Treatment

Immediate treatment should take the form of high-dose steroids using dexamethasone 4 mg q.d.s. Initial management should include consideration of vascular stenting, which is the most effective means of overcoming the venous obstruction in the early stages of superior vena cava obstruction (SVCO) and will result in immediate restoration of blood flow. An example is shown in Fig. 22.3.

Definitive treatment will be either radiotherapy or chemotherapy. Where a diagnosis of lymphoma or germ cell tumour is made, further staging investigations should be completed as soon as possible, followed by immediate chemotherapy. In small cell lung cancer chemotherapy may also be the treatment of choice unless there has been previous exposure to chemotherapy or the patient is elderly or frail. All other patients should receive a course of radiotherapy to the mediastinum.

Prognosis

The prognosis of superior vena cava obstruction depends on the underlying condition and in itself this is not a poor prognostic factor. For this reason, it is important to identify those patients with lymphoma and germ cell tumour so that correct radical treatment can be given despite the acute nature of their presentation.

Most patients will benefit symptomatically from local treatment, although recurrence of symptoms may occur at a later date.

NEUTROPENIC SEPSIS

Neutropenic sepsis is a major hazard and the principal cause of treatment-related death associated with the use of cancer chemotherapy. However, if promptly identified and aggressively treated most episodes can be successfully controlled.

Aetiology

Neutropenia will occur after most chemotherapy treatment and may also be a problem with irradiation of large areas of the spine. Bone marrow infiltration by tumour is a further cause. Life-threatening infection is most likely to occur when the total neutrophil count falls below $1.0 \times 10^9/l$. The major cause of infection is from host organisms in the bowel or skin. The presence of a central venous line is a further risk factor. The common pathogens are Gram-negative bacteria such as *Escherichia coli*, *Klebsiella* and *Pseudomonas* and Gram-positive organisms including *Staphylococcus aureus*, *Staphylococcus epidermidis* and *Streptococcus faecalis*. Less often, the organism may be an anaerobe, *Pneumocystis carinii*, *cytomegalovirus* or a fungal infection.

Symptoms

The patient may be initially asymptomatic or have non-specific symptoms such as malaise and anorexia. Specific symptoms related to a site of infection may include dysuria, cough or sore throat.

Signs

Any fever over 38.5°C in a patient with less than $1.0 \times 10^9/l$ neutrophils should be considered as caused by systemic infection even in the absence of any other positive findings. There may be specific signs of infection in the oropharynx or chest.

Sites of intravenous catheters should be carefully inspected for erythema or discharge. In more severe cases there may be obvious septicaemic shock with hypotension and tachycardia.

Investigations

Any patient that is at risk of neutropenia and found to be febrile requires an urgent blood count. If a low white count is confirmed, blood cultures, a midstream urine, throat swab and chest X-ray are required, together with swabs from other clinically relevant sites, such as a catheter or cannula site, and collection of sputum if produced.

Treatment

Intravenous antibiotics should be instigated as a matter of urgency. The results of cultures should not be awaited as life-threatening septicaemia may develop if there is any delay. The precise antibiotic combination to be used will be guided by individual hospital antibiotic policies but will take the form of broad-spectrum cover against both Gram-negative and Gram-positive organisms. Typical combinations are an aminoglycoside with an extended spectrum penicillin (e.g. gentamicin or amikacin and carbenicillin, ticarcillin or piperacillin). Alternatively a single-agent cephalosporin may be used, such as ceftazidime or cetotaxime. If the fever does not settle after 48 h and there have been no positive results from culture then it may be necessary to add metronidazole for anaerobic organisms or amphotericin for fungi. If there is clinical evidence for *Pneumocystis* then treatment with high-dose co-trimoxazole will be required.

Once the results of cultures become available then antibiotics can be adjusted appropriately. They should be continued for at least 5 days or for 48 h after the fever has settled, whichever is the longer period.

Persistent fever in patients with a central intravenous line suggests colonization of the line and will require removal of that line to eradicate the source of infection.

Antibiotic prophylaxis is recommended in patients at high risk of infection. This includes those with leukaemia and lymphoma undergoing intensive chemotherapy. Daily co-trimoxazole is as good as more complex regimes together with oral antifungal agents such as nystatin or amphotericin.

TUMOUR LYSIS SYNDROME

This is a syndrome arising as a result of rapid breakdown of large numbers of cells, usually at instigation of chemotherapy for a highly sensitive tumour such as lymphoma or leukaemia, which results in extensive metabolic disturbance characterized by hyperkalaemia, hyperuricaemia, hyperphosphataemia and hypocalcaemia.

If clinically significant, the syndrome may present as acute renal failure or acute cardiac arrhythmias with the risk of sudden death.

Treatment

Tumour lysis should be anticipated in any patient with a bulky lymphoma or leukaemia about to undergo chemotherapy. Preventative measures should be instigated prior to chemotherapy with 24 h of prehydration, ensuring good renal output and urine flow, and oral allopurinol should be started to prevent hyperuricaemia.

In patients that develop metabolic disturbances after chemotherapy then intravenous hydration should be continued. Rasburicase will achieve a rapid fall in uric acid levels in high-risk patients and established tumour lysis. Alkalinization of urine with sodium bicarbonate may increase tubular excretion of potassium and phosphate. Specific measures to reduce very high levels of potassium may be required using insulin and glucose in order to prevent cardiac arrhythmias. In the most severe cases, particularly where renal function deteriorates, then dialysis may be required.

Prognosis

In most cases, the metabolic sequelae of tumour lysis should be predictable and preventable. Where metabolic disturbance does occur, prompt treatment is usually successful and the effects are usually self-limiting with resolution within 5–7 days of chemotherapy.

# PALLIATIVE CARE

Medical care of a cancer patient does not stop when there is no curative treatment to offer and indeed over 50 per cent of 'cancer treatments' are palliative. In this area lie many of the greatest challenges of patient care: controlling pain, dyspnoea, vomiting, haemorrhage and other tumour-related symptoms.

PAIN CONTROL

Cancer pain is a chronic pain distinct from that associated with acute events such as trauma, postoperative pain or a toothache. An important feature for its management is that it will often be associated with a significant affective component alongside the physical cause of pain. Most cancer patients have associated anxiety, fear, depression and anger, which will modulate their perception of pain and attention to these features will be of equal importance to the use of analgesic drugs. Three components to the pain of advanced cancer have been described:

- physical;
- emotional;
- spiritual.

Careful evaluation of pain is important in this group of patients in order that treatment can be directed to the principle underlying cause. Measurement of pain on an objective scale is of value, particularly in monitoring response to treatment. The use of a 10-point scale is common, sometimes in the form of a visual analogue scale (VAS), that is a 10 cm line on which the patient is asked to place a mark representing the severity of their pain. An example is shown in Fig. 23.1.

Another important principle in the management of pain in this setting is that few patients will have

a single cause of pain, the average will have three or four individual pains identified and, in some circumstances, several more. Such pains may be interrelated, but around one-quarter may not be directly caused by the cancer but reflect pre-existing pathology (e.g. osteoarthritis) or be associated pains from the effects of treatment interventions. The overall picture for an individual patient may therefore be quite complex. Assessment and monitoring may be aided by the use of a 'pain diagram' alongside the use of pain scores as shown in Fig. 23.1.

The incidence of pain in patients with advanced cancer is between 70 per cent and 80 per cent. This can be effectively controlled in almost all cases by the application of simple rules governing the use of analgesics and related drugs.

1. Make a precise diagnosis of the cause of pain (e.g. whether a bone metastasis or nerve root pain).
2. Remember that many patients will have more than one pain and that pre-existing causes of pain such as arthritis will still be important.
3. Prescribe analgesics regularly, not as required, to prevent pain rather than wait for pain to return before the next dose.
4. Use and be familiar with a small number of drugs based on the analgesic ladder shown in Fig. 23.2.
5. Consider specific cancer treatments (e.g. radiotherapy for bone pain) whenever appropriate.
6. Establish realistic aims and expectations; not all patients will experience complete pain relief within a full range of activity and this should be made clear. Three levels of pain relief are described: pain-free at night, pain-free sitting at rest and pain free on movement. While the first two should be expected by most patients, pain control for movement-related pain is often much more difficult to achieve without limitation to movement.

PAIN CHART

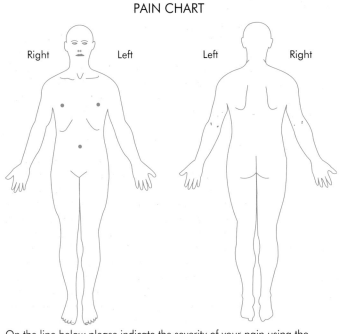

On the line below please indicate the severity of your pain using the scale from 0 to 10

0   10
No pain   Worst imaginable
                                                             pain

FIG 23.1 Pain assessment chart showing pain diagram on which the patient is asked to mark sites of pain and 10-cm visual analogue scale (VAS) on which the patient is asked to mark severity of pain (0 = no pain, 10 = worst imaginable pain).

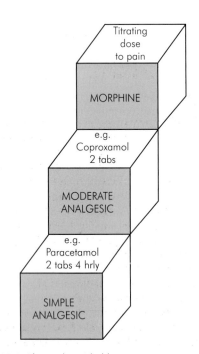

FIG 23.2 The analgesic ladder.

7. Continually reassess the response to treatment and be prepared to modify regimes as the patient's condition evolves. The use of analgesics in this situation should be based on a simple three-step analgesic ladder progressively escalating the potency of drug used. Alongside this it is important to consider more specific causes of pain, which may respond to additional treatment (e.g. radiotherapy for bone metastases).

Level I analgesics

Although these drugs may be considered inadequate for 'cancer pain', in patients that have not experienced regular analgesics around 20 per cent will achieve good pain control simply by starting regular level I analgesics. Paracetamol or ibuprofen are the drugs of choice and are available 'over the counter' in many countries. They are, nonetheless, highly effective drugs when given on a regular basis. Paracetamol has the advantage of a very low incidence of side-effects while ibuprofen or a similar non-steroidal anti-inflammatory drug (NSAID) may be better where an anti-inflammatory action is required, although it is associated with gastrointestinal side-effects, particularly in the elderly.

Level II analgesics

When level I analgesics are no longer effective the next step is to use regular level II analgesics. These drugs are weak opioids, that is, they act by binding to the same opioid receptors as morphine but are less potent. Because of this, however, they tend to have a similar side-effect profile, in particular being associated with nausea and constipation. The drugs that are available in this group are:

- codeine, given as codeine phosphate 4- to 6-hourly;
- dihydrocodeine, a derivative of codeine;
- combination formulations of the above with paracetamol (co-codamol or co-dydramol);
- dextropropoxyphene, a synthetic weak opioid, used in combination with paracetamol (co-proxamol);
- tramadol, a newer synthetic opioid.

There is no evidence to suggest that any one of the above is superior in the treatment of cancer pain; choice will be based upon availability, patient tolerance and physician preference.

Level III analgesics

MORPHINE

Morphine should be used when the pain is no longer responsive to a level II analgesic. The following principles apply to the use of morphine in this setting.

1. Start treatment with regular 4-hourly morphine solution or tablets. These are much more flexible for dose titration than controlled-release tablets.
2. Start a regular laxative such as co-danthramer with morphine.
3. Start or be prepared to introduce a regular antiemetic such as haloperidol.
4. Slowly increase the dose from an initial 10 mg 4-hourly until pain control is achieved. Initially, the dose may be doubled every 24–48 hours; beyond 60 mg 4-hourly increments of 50 per cent may be better tolerated.
5. Warn the patient that during the introduction and dose titration they may feel drowsy and that this will improve once on a stable dose.
6. Reassure the patient that addiction does not occur in this setting.

Parenteral opioids

Injection of opioid drugs such as morphine does not make them more potent when equivalent doses are given and should only be considered when oral or rectal administration is not possible. Remember, however, that because of its greater bioavailability, when injected the oral dose should be approximately halved to give an equivalent analgesic action.

Controlled-release morphine

Morphine tablets giving a 12- or 24-hourly release of morphine are generally preferred by patients once their dose requirements have been defined. Conversion from one morphine preparation to the other is simple as they are equivalent and a 12-hourly dose may therefore be given as a single controlled-release tablet or divided into three doses of immediate-release morphine at 4-hourly intervals.

If pain recurs then the cause should be investigated. Immediate-release morphine may be given in addition to controlled-release tablets to redefine morphine requirements or the patient changed back to 4-hourly morphine.

Spinal opioids

Epidural or intrathecal administration, usually using diamorphine, may have a place in patients with very high morphine requirements or who are resistant to oral medication.

ALTERNATIVES TO MORPHINE

There are very few drugs which have advantages over morphine in this setting.

Fentanyl

This is a highly potent opioid drug with a short half-life. It is available in the form of skin patches, allowing continuous transdermal absorption. This may have advantages over morphine in patients experiencing limiting side-effects or in those where oral administration is difficult. A single patch will provide analgesia for 72 hours at a time and a dose of $25\,\mu g$/hour gives equivalent analgesia to a 24-hour morphine dose of approximately 100 mg. There is, however, less flexibility with patches available in $5\,\mu g$/hour increments, up to $75\,\mu g$ strength in a single patch. If necessary, breakthrough morphine doses can be combined with the use of fentanyl patches, but because of the delay in immediate absorption, the previous full dose of morphine should be continued for the first 24 hours starting fentanyl patches to avoid withdrawal symptoms.

Hydromorphone

This is a synthetic strong opioid, similar to morphine but in some patients better tolerated. It is therefore a useful alternative to morphine when side-effects intrude. It is available in the same oral formulations as morphine, but because it is more potent a dose reduction is needed, with 1.5 mg hydromorphone giving equivalent analgesia to 10 mg morphine.

Oxycodone

This is another alternative strong opioid. It has for many years been available as a suppository, but is now also produced as an oral drug in both immediate-release and controlled-release formulations. With hydromorphone it represents a suitable alternative to morphine for patients that cannot tolerate morphine because of limiting side-effects, although since it is also a strong opioid a similar spectrum of unwanted effects are to be expected with both these drugs, in particular nausea and constipation. The use of these drugs should therefore follow similar guidelines to those for morphine, with the accompanying use of regular prophylactic laxatives and antiemetics.

Phenazocine

This is also sometimes tolerated better in patients that are having specific side-effects with morphine. It is a less flexible preparation, being available in only 5 mg tablets, each of which is equivalent to around 25 mg of morphine when given in a regular schedule.

Diamorphine (diacetylmorphine)

This is preferred for injections because of its greater solubility. Otherwise, it has no advantages and is converted to morphine rapidly on passing through the liver.

MORPHINE-RESISTANT PAIN

While the above approach will work well for most patients, there is undoubtedly a group of patients whose pain is not sensitive to morphine or other opioid drugs. It is important to recognize these patients and not submit them to ever-increasing doses of morphine for no benefit. In particular, musculoskeletal pains and neurogenic pains may fall into this category. A further group of patients have been identified whose pain has been described as 'morphine irrelevant pain'. This refers to those where the over-riding aetiology of their pain is due to an affective or spiritual component.

Therefore, in patients who after dose titration to 40 or 60 mg morphine 4-hourly are reporting no pain reduction with medication it is important to reconsider the further use of morphine and explore alternative approaches with coanalgesics, non-drug treatments or specific treatment such as local radiotherapy. A small group of patients can be identified that have true 'morphine resistance'. This has been attributed to an adaptive central response resulting in 'wind up', with altered perception of painful and non-painful stimuli (hyperalgesia and allodynia). This is thought to be mediated by a specific neurotransmitter, N-methyl-D-aspartate (NMDA). Specific NMDA inhibitor drugs are available, of which ketamine is sometimes used in these situations. However, its use can be associated with troublesome psychotomimetic side-effects and such measures should only be considered under careful supervision in a specialist pain unit.

ADJUVANT ANALGESICS

This includes all drugs that do not have intrinsic analgesic activity but in specific situations will help in pain relief.

Non-steroidal anti-inflammatory drugs

These are useful in bone pain and soft tissue infiltration by tumour. They include drugs such as aspirin, ibuprofen or naproxen and may be adequate used alone as step 1 analgesics in some patients. Their main disadvantage is their association with gastritis and gastrointestinal haemorrhage. The risk is least with ibuprofen and greatest with ketorolac. Where there is a previous history of dyspepsia or proven peptic ulceration then particular care is required and concomitant use of a protective drug such as omeprazole, lansoprazole or misoprostol is recommended.

Steroids

These are of value in nerve root pain, raised intracranial pressure, hepatomegaly and soft tissue infiltration. Dexamethasone may be more convenient than prednisolone but both are effective in moderate doses (e.g. dexamethasone 4 mg twice daily or prednisolone 20–40 mg daily). There may be the added advantage of increased well-being experienced by many patients on taking steroids but care should be taken not to induce steroid-related side-effects, in particular fluid retention, restlessness and insomnia. The last may be avoided by taking single early-morning doses.

Bisphosphonates

Both pamidronate and clodronate may be effective in metastatic bone pain even in the absence of hyper-calcaemia. Oral absorption is poor and variable and therefore intermittent infusions are usually required, but as new more potent drugs in this class become available such as olendronate and ibandronate, oral use will be more widespread. Hypocalcaemia and transient fevers during administration may occur and serum calcium requires occasional monitoring.

Anxiolytic drugs

Small doses of drugs such as diazepam may be required where anxiety is either a major component of pain or a debilitating condition in its own right. In patients in the final days of life who become rest-less and agitated then midazolam given by sub-cutaneous infusion is effective.

Antidepressants

These may be required for some patients that are sig-nificantly depressed and may also be of value for neuropathic pain in particular. Their efficacy in this setting may arise from both an effect on peripheral nerve transmission and by raising the mood of the patient. At present, evidence for a role in neuropathic pain is greatest for drugs such as amitriptyline, while where a true antidepressant effect is sought, newer drugs with selective serotonin uptake inhibitor activ-ity such as fluoxetine, paroxetine and sertraline may be preferable.

Muscle relaxants

Baclofen may be of value where muscle spasm is a significant component of pain, for example in para-plegia or associated with underlying bone or soft tissue metastases.

Anticonvulsants

Pain caused peripheral nerve damage either from tumour infiltration or other associated conditions, for example herpes zoster, can be particularly diffi-cult to control and is often not very responsive to pure analgesics. It is typically a burning or stabbing pain within the affected dermatome. Alongside amitriptyline, drugs with anticonvulsant activity such as carbamazepine, sodium valproate or clon-azepam are helpful for this neuropathic pain. They each appear equally effective and are usually chosen on the basis of tolerance: carbamazepine and clonazepam are associated with drowsiness and valproate with gastrointestinal symptoms.

Specific cancer treatments for pain control

For local pain from a growing and infiltrating tumour, specific therapy aimed at a reduction in tumour bulk and growth arrest is often the most effective approach.

RADIOTHERAPY

This is highly effective for metastatic bone pain and is also of value in relieving headache caused by raised intracranial pressure from primary or metastatic intracranial tumours. In this setting it is, however, important to select those patients with good performance status whose symptoms cannot otherwise be controlled with medication, or those in whom medication such as morphine and steroids causes troublesome side-effects.

In other situations, where tumour is invading nerve roots or plexuses, as with an apical lung tumour invading the brachial plexus or presacral rectal tumour invading the lumbosacral plexus, radiotherapy is indicated for pain control.

CHEMOTHERAPY

In sensitive tumours such as small cell lung cancer, breast cancer and myeloma, chemotherapy may be of value for both bone and soft tissue pain where tumour infiltration is the main cause of pain. Again, careful patient selection is required to optimize benefits and avoid unnecessary treatment in the face of inexorable progression of disease.

Other pain treatments

Pain may have many components to it and, in par-ticular, the pain associated with malignant disease is recognized to have a major affective (emotional) component. Such pain has been termed 'morphine irrelevant' pain. Alternative non-drug treatments may be very successful in selected patients that do not respond well to the above approach:

- transcutaneous electrical nerve stimulation (TENS) may be particularly valuable for neuro-pathic pains;
- specific nerve blocks can be dramatically suc-cessful in selected cases;
- neurosurgical procedures such as cordotomy, rhizotomy or thalotomy may occasionally be indicated;
- massage, including the use of heat and cold to painful and tender areas, is often helpful;

- acupuncture may be particularly successful for difficult neurogenic pains;
- relaxation and techniques such as aromatherapy may also have a place in alleviating distress related to advanced malignancy.

OTHER SYMPTOMS

Because of the systemic nature of metastatic cancer, many other symptoms may affect the patient with advanced cancer. These include anorexia, nausea and vomiting, constipation, sore mouth, confusion, cough and dyspnoea. The basic principle of making a diagnosis of the precise cause for each symptom should be adhered to in order to choose the most effective treatment.

Anorexia

This may be due to anxiety, nausea, pain, liver metastases, sore mouth or uraemia, each of which may require specific treatment. In addition, appetite may be stimulated by the use of low doses of steroids such as dexamethasone 4 mg daily or prednisolone 10–20 mg daily, or alternatively progestogens such as medroxyprogesterone or megestrol, which have the advantage of fewer steroid side-effects. However, it is important to have clear goals and realistic expectations. Patients with advanced cancer do not typically regain weight lost prior to diagnosis and there is no evidence that specific dietary approaches will prolong life at this stage. Often considerable anxiety and tension develop between patients and those caring

for them who, with the best possible motives, wish to see them eating heartily. Small, perhaps more frequent, meals with the emphasis on patient enjoyment and avoiding dehydration rather than high-calorie intake is a preferable approach.

Nausea and vomiting

This may be a side effect of many drugs used in this situation, in particular morphine. Other potential causes include mechanical bowel obstruction, hepatic metastases, uraemia or hypercalcaemia. A simple biochemical profile is therefore of value in all these patients.

In addition to correction, where possible, of biochemical disturbance, antiemetic drugs will be required. It is important to consider a rational choice of the many drugs available based on their site of action, as shown in Table 23.1.

Where there is no apparent cause, or it can be attributed to any one of a number of drugs, then treatment should be started with metoclopramide 10 mg 4- to 6-hourly, haloperidol 1.5–3 mg nocte or cyclizine 50 mg 8-hourly. A similar principle of regular medication to prevent symptoms rather than 'as required' medication equally applies to the use of antiemetics and analgesics. Often, patients end up on a cocktail of three or four drugs and it is important to evaluate carefully the response to each and discontinue them if there is no clear benefit.

Patients with nausea and particularly those that are already vomiting may have difficulty taking oral medication which may, if anything, simply provide an additional stimulus to emesis. In this situation, rectal administration using domperidone or

TABLE 23.1 Antiemetic drugs in advanced cancer

Site of action	Drugs	Indication
Vomiting centre	Cyclizine	May be useful in all causes as this is the final common pathway for vomiting reflex
Chemoreceptor trigger	Prochlorperazine Chlorpromazine	Drug-induced Metabolic (e.g. hypercalcaemia, uraemia, hepatic) metastases
	Haloperidol Metoclopramide Domperidone Ondansetron	
Peripheral	Metoclopramide Domperidone Ondansetron	Gastric stasis

prochlorperazine suppositories may be helpful. Where the patient already has a subcutaneous infusion running for analgesic administration, antiemetics can be added, with benefit, to this; metoclopramide, cyclizine and haloperidol are all compatible in this setting.

Constipation

This may be a side-effect of drugs, in particular morphine, or related to dehydration, hypercalcaemia or mechanical restriction of the bowel from an intra-abdominal or pelvic tumour. Good hydration and, where appropriate, a diet containing fruit and other fibre should be encouraged. Fruit juices are often welcome when solid food is no longer taken.

Laxatives should be given regularly to all patients receiving opioid medication. Co-danthramer, which has a combination of a bowel stimulant and faecal softener, is useful for opioid-related constipation and the dose can be titrated to the patient's requirements. Alternatives such as Senna formulations, bisacodyl, docusate, osmotic salts, and lubricants such as liquid paraffin are also effective. While oral agents are generally preferable in stubborn constipation, glycerine suppositories or phosphate enemas may be necessary to break a difficult cycle, particularly when preventive measures have not been used.

Sore mouth

This may be caused by dryness of the oral cavity as a side-effect of drugs, including morphine and phenothiazine antiemetics, radiotherapy to the mouth, or mucositis related to chemotherapy or candidiasis.

Oropharyngeal candidiasis can cause severe symptoms in these patients and should be treated actively with topical nystatin or amphotericin and using systemic ketoconazole for resistant cases. Regular mouthwashes, sucking ice cubes, carbonated drinks or ascorbic acid are also recommended.

Confusion

This can be one of the most difficult symptoms to deal with. There is usually an identifiable precipitating cause including drugs, in particular morphine, hepatic or renal dysfunction, hypercalcaemia, hypoxia, infection or cerebral metastases. In addition to specific attention to the above, mild sedation with low doses of a benzodiazepine may be of value. In severe cases with hallucinations, haloperidol may be required in the acute phase. However, drugs should not take the place of sympathetic psychological

support and reassurance counteracting the cycle of misinterpretation and over-reaction which builds up.

Cough and dyspnoea

This will usually arise as a result of intrathoracic tumour causing bronchial irritation or obstruction, lung collapse, lung metastases or pleural effusion. Chest infections are also common in this group of patients.

Treatment may include aspiration of effusion and antibiotics. Specific cough sedatives based on codeine linctus may be tried but are often unsuccessful, as are bronchodilators unless there is preceding obstructive airways disease. Small doses of morphine (10–20 mg 4-hourly) are often the most useful and steroids may be of value in diffuse lung infiltration of lymphangitis carcinomatosa.

Common patterns are seen to emerge when considering the above symptoms. In particular, many symptoms may be attributable to biochemical disturbance and simple investigations including blood urea and electrolytes, liver function tests and serum calcium are often rewarding in providing a cause for specific problems. It is always important to take a full and detailed drug history, since many of the problems encountered will reflect some degree of drug side-effect. Renal and hepatic dysfunction will also influence drug handling and a change in these may suddenly destabilize a previously satisfactory drug schedule. In particular, remember that active metabolites of morphine are excreted through the kidney and in impaired renal function morphine toxicity can quickly develop due to their accumulation if appropriate dose adjustments are not made.

THE DYING PATIENT

Inevitably there will come a time when death is imminent. This may require changes in medication to minimize the physical distress for both the patient and their relatives. The following points should be considered.

Place of death

Only a small minority of patients die in a specialist palliative care setting such as a hospice. The majority die in a general hospital ward or at home. When it is clear that the terminal course of the disease is approaching it is helpful to broach with the patient and their relatives the issue of their mode of death and the place they would choose to die. The extent to which this is possible will depend upon the individual patient, their wish to discuss freely such issues and to take part in such decisions. It is often a greater burden for the family of the patient, who may worry about their ability to care for them at home while having misgivings about the care available in local institutions. This is a particular concern where the patient expresses a strong wish to die at home but may live with only one elderly spouse whose physical capacity to provide the care required is limited. It is therefore important to identify the level of support that may be required for each individual, to have realistic plans for their care and to enable them, as far as they wish, to die in the surroundings in which they and their family are most comfortable.

Medication for the dying patient

Diminishing levels of consciousness will require a switch from oral medication. It is rarely necessary to give drugs intravenously or intramuscularly and the subcutaneous route should be chosen. If the patient is expected to succumb within a day or so, intermittent injections may be acceptable but it is often easier and less traumatic to set up a continuous infusion pump. Diamorphine or morphine can be given by this route (remembering to reduce the oral dose by 50 per cent) and if antiemetics are required, haloperidol or metoclopramide can be added to the infusion. Alternatively these may be given in suppository form.

Agitation and restlessness

There may be terminal agitation and restlessness. This is best treated by rectal diazepam or using haloperidol or midazolam in the subcutaneous infusion.

Respiration

Pooling of secretions may make respiration unpleasantly noisy and uncomfortable. This is best controlled with subcutaneous hyoscine in doses of 0.2–0.4 mg. Methotrimeprazine is also a useful drug in this setting, compatible with subcutaneous infusions and, as a phenothiazine, it also has antiemetic actions if required.

Reassessment of medication

Many patients continue to be left on large numbers of oral medications, most of which are irrelevant in these final hours. It is important, therefore, to review carefully all medication and, in general, most routine oral medical treatments such as anti-hypertensives, anti-inflammatory drugs, laxatives and H_2 antagonists can be discontinued without causing distress to the patient or hastening death.

Acute haemorrhage

Acute deaths are unusual in oncology but rarely a tumour may erode a large enough blood vessel to cause acute haemorrhage. The typical sites for this are the carotid artery in the neck, femoral artery in the groin or an intrapulmonary vessel. These are inevitably terminal events and can cause considerable distress. Sedation with parenteral diamorphine and local pressure to control blood loss should be administered. A dark-coloured blanket is also of great value in masking the dramatic loss of blood.

Resuscitation

It is always distressing following a chronic illness and inevitable death for the final moments to be submitted to inappropriate resuscitation procedures. It is important, therefore, that clear policies regarding resuscitation are given to those caring for the patient, arrived at only after full discussion with the patient and their family.

APPENDIX 1

Cancer: the scale of the problem in Europe (adapted from WHO database, 2001)

Country	Number of new cases per year	Number of deaths per year
Austria	33 018	18 737
Belgium	46 339	27 293
Denmark	23 474	15 037
Finland	20 154	10 036
France	244 622	143 316
Germany	367 641	212 453
Greece	34 145	22 218
Ireland	11 891	7367
Italy	250 508	147 455
Luxembourg	1692	977
The Netherlands	64 116	37 150
Portugal	35 021	20 213
Spain	136 629	86 380
Sweden	39 681	20 707
United Kingdom	241 875	155 807
European Union	1 550 806	925 146

APPENDIX 2

Data for 12 commonest malignancies in order for more-developed countries according to site (adapted from WHO database, 2001)

Site	Number of new cases per year	Number of deaths per year
Males		
Lung	470 836	430 043
Prostate	415 568	128 185
Colon/rectum	318 694	152 178
Stomach	208 282	138 699
Bladder	163 648	48 891
Non-Hodgkin's lymphoma	80 181	38 575
Kidney, etc.	79 090	35 700
Liver	73 270	68 992
Pancreas	66 186	65 773
Larynx	62 196	31 108
Leukaemia	58 416	43 928
Oral cavity	59 959	22 392
All sites except skin	2 503 772	1 488 212
Females		
Breast	579 285	189 203
Colon/rectum	291 897	149 470
Lung	175 392	151 159
Stomach	125 029	91 240
Corpus uteri	113 618	25 529
Cervix uteri	91 451	39 350
Ovary, etc.	91 307	59 113
Non-Hodgkin's lymphoma	66 148	32 742
Pancreas	61 230	62 957
Melanoma of skin	53 511	11 048
Bladder	48 129	18 308
Kidney, etc.	47 936	22 182
All sites except skin	2 175 974	1 157 634

APPENDIX 3

Data for 12 commonest malignancies in order for less-developed countries according to site (adapted from WHO database, 2001)

Site	Number of new cases per year	Number of deaths per year
Males		
Lung	430 919	380 389
Stomach	350 176	266 514
Liver	325 108	314 611
Oesophagus	224 071	177 465
Colon/rectum	180 059	102 640
Prostate	127 419	76 127
Oral cavity	109 553	58 454
Bladder	96 118	50 162
Non-Hodgkin's lymphoma	86 436	54 738
Leukaemia	85 912	65 372
Larynx	79 972	47 460
Other Pharynx	63 934	44 148
All sites except skin	2 814 132	2 034 163
Females		
Breast	471 063	183 768
Cervix uteri	379 153	194 025
Stomach	192 850	150 100
Lung	161 719	141 538
Colon/rectum	154 064	88 121
Liver	132 298	128 305
Oesophagus	117 092	96 095
Ovary, etc.	101 060	55 121
Corpus uteri	75 336	19 177
Oral cavity	72 687	39 490
Leukaemia	65 366	49 429
Non-Hodgkin's lymphoma	54 659	35 076
All sites except skin	2 561 666	1 528 670

APPENDIX 4

Data for 12 commonest malignancies in order for the UK according to site (adapted from WHO database, 2001)

Site	Number of new cases per year	Number of deaths per year
Males		
Lung	23708	24433
Prostate	21302	10062
Colon/rectum	17249	9341
Bladder	9593	3670
Stomach	6178	5101
Non-Hodgkin's lymphoma	4402	2414
Oesophagus	4264	4214
Leukaemia	3585	2180
Kidney, etc.	3356	1891
Pancreas	2978	3240
Melanoma of skin	2398	769
Brain, nervous system	2380	1802
All sites except skin	123791	84722
Females		
Breast	34815	14415
Lung	13423	13231
Colon/rectum	15924	9047
Ovary, etc.	6138	4560
Corpus uteri	5000	1112
Bladder	3837	1795
Non-Hodgkin's lymphoma	3760	2131
Stomach	3579	3199
Cervix uteri	3537	1906
Melanoma of skin	3375	795
Pancreas	3144	3475
Leukaemia	2932	1808
All sites except skin	123876	76923

INDEX